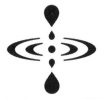

LEARNING ACCEPTANCE AND COMMITMENT THERAPY

The Essential Guide to the
Process and Practice of
Mindful Psychiatry

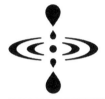

LEARNING ACCEPTANCE AND COMMITMENT THERAPY

The Essential Guide to the Process and Practice of Mindful Psychiatry

Debrin P. Goubert, M.D.

Niklas Törneke, M.D.

Robert Purssey, M.D., FRANZCP

Josephine Loftus, M.D., MRCPsych

Laura Weiss Roberts, M.D., M.A., DLFAPA, FACLP

Kirk D. Strosahl, Ph.D.

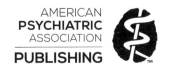

AMERICAN
PSYCHIATRIC
ASSOCIATION
PUBLISHING

American Psychiatric Association Publishing
800 Maine Avenue SW, Suite 900
Washington, DC 20024-2812
www.appi.org

Library of Congress Cataloging-in-Publication Data
Names: Goubert, Debrin P., author. | American Psychiatric Association, issuing body.
Title: Learning acceptance and commitment therapy : the essential guide to the process and practice of mindful psychiatry / Debrin P. Goubert, M.D., Niklas Törneke, M.D., Robert Purssey, M.D., FRANZCP, Josephine Loftus, M.D., MRCPsych, Laura Weiss Roberts, M.D., M.A., DLFAPA, Kirk D. Strosahl, Ph.D.
Description: First edition. | Washington, DC : American Psychiatric Association Publishing, [2020] | Includes bibliographical references and index.
Identifiers: LCCN 2020016602 (print) | LCCN 2020016603 (ebook) | ISBN 9781615371730 (paperback ; alk. paper) | ISBN 9781615373550 (ebook)
Subjects: MESH: Acceptance and Commitment Therapy—methods | Case Reports
Classification: LCC RC489.C63 (print) | LCC RC489.C63 (ebook) | NLM WM 425.5.C6 | DDC 616.89/1425--dc23
LC record available at https://lccn.loc.gov/2020016602
LC ebook record available at https://lccn.loc.gov/2020016603

British Library Cataloguing in Publication Data
A CIP record is available from the British Library.

To my children, Eva, Isaac, Lucia, and Linn, who have taught me about acceptance. And, most of all, to my husband Will, with whom I've learned to appreciate commitment. —D. P. G.

To Birgitta, for walking side by side with me through all these years. —N. T.

To my children, George, Dexter, Nish, and Talita, for their infinite joy and love; my wife, Su, for her kind, continual support; my mother, Daphne, for her endless nurturance; and my father, Brian, recently retired at 92 years from his life in medicine—as a surgeon, medical administrator, and old-fashioned doctor—whose lifelong learning and willingness to move with the evidence has been a huge inspiration. —R. P.

I would like to thank my parents for the sacrifices they made for me; my patients for their generosity; and my daughters, Gina and Chiara, for their patience and understanding. —J. L.

For Eric, my love, take care. —L. R.

To all the patients I've worked with over the years, who have shown the courage to endure suffering and the wisdom to transcend it. To Patti, my spouse, soulmate, and fellow traveler on my life journey, love for 1,000 lifetimes. —K. S.

Contents

PART I
What Is ACT?

1 The Benefits of ACT in Psychiatric Practice

2 An Overview of ACT

From Basic Behavioral Science Foundations

PART II
How to Do ACT

3 The Practice of Functional Psychiatry

4 Learning to Treat Your Patient With CARE

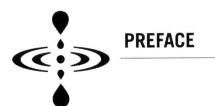 **PREFACE**

A journey is a person in itself; no two are alike. And all plans, safeguards, policing, and coercion are fruitless. We find that after years of struggle, that we do not take a trip; a trip takes us.

—*John Steinbeck*

The six authors who took a life journey together for more than a year to craft this book come from highly divergent personal and professional backgrounds. Not only do they reside in four different countries but they also practice in contexts ranging from a private, multidisciplinary psychiatry clinic, to a "solo" psychiatric outpatient practice, to a consultation-liaison psychiatry service situated within a large commercial health care system, to an inpatient affective disorders unit, and to a university-based psychiatry department and associated psychiatric residency program. Despite their divergent professional experiences, what brought this group of authors together was both a belief in the value of the practice of psychiatry and a shared conviction that systematically integrating an evidence-based psychotherapeutic approach within the current practice of psychiatry can increase patient well-being and promote better clinical outcomes. Most importantly, we believe that when you see the positive benefits of this new approach unfold, even with your "difficult" patients, it will make the practice of psychiatry more professionally and personally rewarding.

The evidence-based clinical approach described in this text is called *acceptance and commitment therapy* (pronounced as the word "ACT"). ACT is an innovative cognitive-behavioral therapy that combines principles of acceptance and change to create a new type of clinical conversation with our patients (Hayes et al. 2011). Our clinical experience, as well as an already substantial and growing body of clinical research, suggests that applying ACT to the common (and uncommon) psychiatric problems we treat will expand the breadth, depth, and longevity of clinical benefits. ACT has many unique and somewhat counterintuitive features, the most salient being the proposition that it is the patient's attempts to get rid of distressing, unwanted thoughts, feelings, memories, urges, or sensations—rather than the direct experience of these private events, per se—that lead to mental and emotional dysfunction. A corollary belief is that "psychological health" is not defined by the absence of distressing mental experiences. Rather, the patient's ability to "make room" for these natural human experiences and not let them function as barriers to effective action in the patient's external world is what defines healthy functioning.

Cultivating the ability to accept what is present inside, while organizing subsequent behavior in the world to be consistent with closely held personal values, is the hallmark of the ACT approach. Going back to the acceptance and change motif: we cannot directly control or eliminate what naturally arises inside of us in any particular life moment, but we can control our behaviors in the moment. We can also choose how we are going to "relate to" what is going on inside the skin. In so doing, we choose how we wish to respond to the immediate demands of the social environment.

Although the dynamics of acceptance and change seem rather simple and straightforward at first glance, they require us as psychiatrists to rethink some of our most basic assumptions about the goals of psychiatric care. What if the natural resting state of humans is not to be symptom free, "happy," and free from emotional concerns but instead involves having ongoing contact with our harsh, self-critical thoughts; painful emotions; invasive and distressing memories; powerful, unpleasant urges; or uncomfortable bodily sensations? If symptom control and elimination do not automatically lead to psychological health and well-being, then what goes into living a full and satisfying life? What additional activities should the psychiatrist engage in to produce more broad-ranging health and clinical outcomes? How should the symptom-focused approach be modified in situations in which patients are likely to endure chronic, treatment-refractory symptom distress for months or years to come? Indeed, is it possible that at least some distressing private experiences (symptoms) have an adaptive role to enact? Is it possible that symptoms play an important function in the patient's ongoing attempts to adapt to the demands of the external environment? Could symptoms of distress be signals that the patient's life context is out of balance in some important way? Are there situations in which the goal might be to leave the patient's symptom distress unabated so that the distress can motivate the patient to make needed behavior changes? In this text, the first of its kind to translate ACT into a clinically focused psychiatric framework, we grapple with these important questions and many other clinically relevant considerations that arise along the way.

How to Use This Book

We have organized this text into three parts. Part I ("What Is ACT?") delves into the clinical benefits of using ACT in an everyday psychiatric practice and provides an in-depth analysis of the ACT model, from its basic science origins in the study of the functions of human language to a fully elaborated model for clinical assessment and intervention. Part II ("How to Do ACT") describes the practice of functional psychiatry, including not only how to organize assessment and intervention activities within a functional framework but also how to optimize the flow of each clinical session. You will also have the opportunity to learn both basic and advanced ACT clinical concepts and intervention methods. In addition, we examine the intricacies of blending medication treatment and management with ACT interventions. Part III ("ACT in Practice") provides chapter-length examples of how to deliver ACT in an ambulatory psychiatric setting, in a hospital consultation-liaison service, and in an inpatient psychiatric context. We finish this part with a chapter examining the all-important issue of teaching ACT to psychiatric residents as well as affiliated health professionals working in medical or psychiatric treatment team contexts.

Some psychiatrists learn best by reading, others learn best by watching, and still others learn best by doing. To address these different learning styles, we have developed various learning strategies that you, the reader, can take advantage of. If you learn best by reading, you will want to pay close attention to the numerous real-life clinical dialogues included in nearly every chapter. These dialogues illustrate how the ACT-informed psychiatrist performs core assessment and intervention activities. We do not merely "talk" about what to do; we demonstrate how to do it by offering commentaries about how to analyze information and formulate a response to the patient as the clinical dialogue unfolds sequentially.

Similarly, if you learn best by watching, we have assembled an instructional video library available at https://www.appi.org/Goubert. When you see this icon 🎥 it means you can access and watch a video demonstration of the clinical assessment or intervention activities being discussed in that particular section of the chapter.

Now, if you learn best by doing, we have assembled a nice portfolio of ACT-consistent self-report measures, case analysis and treatment planning forms, practice tips, and guidelines as well as patient engagement and intervention tools for you to use as you begin doing ACT in your practice. When you see this icon 📝 it means one of these clinical tools is available at https://www.appi.org/Goubert in a downloadable, reproducible format for use in your practice.

Finally, just as Rome was not built in a day, your ACT clinical skills will not suddenly appear in their finest form as a result of reading this book. Refining your clinical skills takes practice and persistence. To this end, additional ACT training and supervision are available in many ways. You can access our website (www.ACTinpsychiatry.com) for information about local ACT trainings, as well as local options for online, real-time case supervision and consultation. The website also contains periodic postings about new developments that psychiatrists using the ACT approach will want to incorporate into their clinical practices.

A Final Word

Although ACT has a multifaceted theoretical flavor, we tried to keep the theory limited to clinically relevant aspects of the overall model. Indeed, the ACT model is so theoretically rich and diverse in its implications that each member of this authorship team might have very different interpretations about how to apply it to specific patient care situations. Thus, in every chapter we give the reader additional reading resources to pursue, should a particular theoretical or applied clinical concept create a desire to learn more. We can say without reservation that this book has been a labor of love for all of us. It is our gift to the profession of psychiatry. It reflects our desire to give practicing psychiatrists around the world a new, optimistic perspective on the problem of human suffering and what to do about it. If you, the reader, are interested in learning more about this innovative and clinically powerful approach, then let's get started!

Acknowledgments

Jennifer Gilbreath was responsible for oversight of book copy editing, proofing, and production. Justin Kerr, Webology 501, was responsible for the design of the book cover and all book graphics. Rick Prather was responsible for the book layout and design.

Reference

Hayes S, Strosahl K, Wilson K: Acceptance and Commitment Therapy: The Process and Practice of Mindful Change. New York, Guilford, 2011

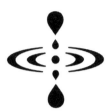

INSTRUCTIONAL VIDEO GUIDE

Callouts in the text identify the instructional videos by name, as shown in the following example:

🎥 Video #: Video Title

The instructional videos are streamed via the internet and can be viewed online by navigating to https://www.appi.org/Goubert and using the embedded video player. The videos are optimized for most current operating systems, including mobile operating systems.

Instructional Videos Discussed by Chapter

CHAPTER 4

Video 1: Brief Contextual Assessment (8:41)
Video 2: "A-B-C" Analysis of an Emotionally Charged Situation (5:08)
Video 3: The Bullseye Values Exercise (6:28)
Video 4: Analyzing Avoidance (4:54)
Video 5: Linking Emotional Pain to What Matters (2:49)
Video 6: Eliciting Simple Awareness of Experience (5:29)
Video 7: Promoting a Sense of Self as Separate From Inner Experiences (3:37)
Video 8: Promoting Observational Distance From Distressing Inner Experience (4:40)
Video 9: Analyzing Barriers to Valued Living (2:21)
Video 10: Passengers on the Bus Metaphor (3:18)
Video 11: Life Path Goal Setting Exercise (4:51)
Video 12: Introducing the ACT Matrix Model (4:30)

CHAPTER 6

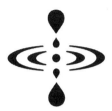

CLINICAL TOOLS GUIDE

Many of the measures and screens discussed in the text are available online. These are identified by name, as shown in the following example:

 Clinical Tool #: Tool Title

These tools can be viewed and downloaded for use in your ACT approach by navigating to https://www.appi.org/Goubert.

Clinical Tools Discussed by Chapter

CHAPTER 3

CHAPTER 4

CHAPTER 5

CHAPTER 10

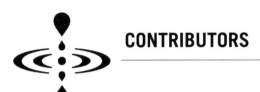

CONTRIBUTORS

Debrin P. Goubert, M.D.
Psychiatrist, Hospital Psychiatry, Northwest Kaiser Permanente, Clackamas, Oregon

Josephine Loftus, M.D., MRCPsych
Head of Mood Disorder Unit and Expert Bipolar Centre, Department of Psychiatry, Centre Hospitalier Princesse Grace, Monaco

Robert Purssey, M.D., FRANCZP
Director, Brisbane ACT Centre; Clinical Senior Lecturer, University of Queensland, Brisbane, Australia

Laura Weiss Roberts, M.D., M.A., DLFAPA, FACLP
Chairman, Katharine Dexter McCormick and Stanley McCormick Memorial Professor, Department of Psychiatry and Behavioral Sciences, Stanford University School of Medicine, Stanford, California

Kirk D. Strosahl, Ph.D.
President, HeartMatters Consulting LLC, Wheeler, Oregon

Niklas Törneke, M.D., Ph.D.
Private practice, Kopingsvik, Sweden

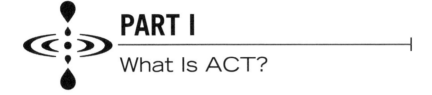

PART I

What Is ACT?

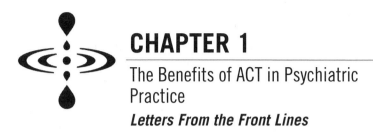

CHAPTER 1

The Benefits of ACT in Psychiatric Practice

Letters From the Front Lines

Life is never made unbearable by circumstances, but only by lack of meaning and purpose.

—Victor Frankl

Psychiatrists are asked to deal with a vast array of mental health, substance-related, and social issues, often within the same clinical encounter. Addressing the full set of biopsychosocial concerns can be a daunting task, particularly if the primary—or only—tool in our toolbox is limited to prescribing medications. Although medications and other somatic treatments can be very effective for the syndromes we treat, the sad truth is that many patients respond only partially, or not at all, to medication treatment. Some initial responders experience medication "burnout" and find themselves receiving increasing medication regimens, with increasing side effects, in an attempt to get symptoms under control again. Other patients have difficulty taking their medications as prescribed. Aside from issues with medications, some patients live in such dire social circumstances that the prescriptions we write are little more than bandages on the source of their pain. Significant issues with drugs and alcohol and other addictive behaviors can create chaos and lead to more psychiatric symptoms. Even with more straightforward patients, many do not comply with our suggestions to use sleep hygiene, exercise, socialize, or engage in other behaviors that will improve their health.

As psychiatrists, part of our meaning and purpose is to help our patients "get better," but what does "better" mean? Does it mean helping them achieve freedom from symptom distress? What if we have become so preoccupied with controlling and eliminating the symptoms of mental disorders that we are actually teaching our patients the wrong lesson about life? What if distressing symptoms are not the enemy within but rather are important signals about needed life changes that our patients should be listening to?

Take chronic pain as an analogy for the chronic symptom distress that many of our patients endure. In the treatment of persistent pain, the limitations of current medication treatments designed to eradicate pain have led to a change in treatment focus. The goal has changed from getting rid of pain to helping the patient live a full and vital life despite the pain that remains after we have done all we can to reduce it. Similarly, current somatic treatments for painful thoughts and emotional states also have limitations. Frequently, persistent emotional pain cannot be vanquished without drastically dulling our ability to engage meaningfully with the world. This approach of "numbing the pain" begs the question: Can we help our patients live richer, more satisfying lives despite the presence of uncomfortable emotions? In the treatment of these complex mental health and substance abuse issues, is there an additional approach we can take to complement medication management? Even more fundamentally, is there an approach we can use to help increase our patients' personal strengths and natural resilience so that they can bear their pain and move into the future with hope and health?

Acceptance and commitment therapy (ACT), the subject of this book, suggests that the path forward is to support patients in becoming more psychologically flexible so that they become better able to manage distressing, unwanted symptoms while choosing behaviors that lead them in the direction of vital, rich, and meaningful lives. Indeed, ACT holds that many of the patient's distressing symptoms may be the direct result of *not* living according to one's values, in a futile attempt to avoid experiencing distressing and unwanted emotional reactions to failure, setback, or disappointment. This complementary, alternative perspective on symptoms encourages the psychiatrist to be far more curious about the patient's values and current life context, leading to a new type of clinical conversation.

ACT affirms our view of our patients as human beings with important life values and aspirations that are being achieved, or not achieved, in a specific life context. This approach allows us to help patients navigate through the inevitable ups and downs in life and to help them understand that their attempts to avoid pain paradoxically keep them stuck in a self-perpetuating spiral of unworkable coping behaviors. We can share in our patients' life journey, helping them engage in behaviors that help them move in a more values-consistent life direction and to persist in positive behaviors even when they encounter the emotional pain of disappointment, setback, or failure. This sense of striving for a valued life both justifies and dignifies the ups and downs of living.

A Little About ACT

In essence, ACT involves teaching patients to be *psychologically flexible*. Psychological flexibility involves being able to make direct contact with distressing, unwanted inner experiences without struggling to control or eliminate them and to act according to one's personal beliefs and values in the presence of these distressing experiences. ACT helps patients develop the ability to contact the present moment fully and without defense and make contact with and accept the presence of distressing, unwanted mental experiences while connecting with their personal values and choosing behaviors that push them in the direction of those values. ACT can be useful in various treatment settings with a wide range of clients. It can be applied in a brief initial evaluation, a 15-minute medication check, a 50-minute therapy session, a group therapy session in the psychiatric ward, a one-time consultation in the emergency department, or a case discussion with a treatment team.

ACT helps us as psychiatrists reframe our definition of the "problem to be solved" away from eliminating or reducing symptoms and toward thinking about the patient as a whole person situated within a dynamic life context. The goal is to help our patients achieve their best interests within that context. In this way, no two patients are ever alike, even though their symptoms of distress may be similar. ACT helps patients identify ways that they can engage in life-enhancing behaviors despite the reality of physical or emotional pain, reframe emotional discomfort as a potentially useful signal of a discrepancy between the life they want to live and the life they are actually living, and identify and engage in values-consistent behaviors that create a sense of vitality, purpose, and meaning.

To summarize, ACT teaches patients to recognize painful thoughts, feelings, and memories not as unquestioned reality but rather as a product of their minds. Being in mental pain is not a sign of being broken; it is a sign of being human. As patients get over the need to control, eliminate, or avoid distressing, unwanted mental experiences, they improve their ability to behave in ways that provide balance, insight, and joy in their lives. ACT helps both psychiatrists and patients adopt new perspectives on the meaning of personal pain and what to do about it. We have found that incorporating ACT principles within a wide range of difficult clinical situations leads to more thoughtful prescribing of medications, increased patient motivation, better adherence to treatment plans, and improved patient outcomes.

A Brief Review of the Evidence for ACT

An exhaustive review of the research literature on ACT is beyond the scope of this chapter. Suffice to say, in excess of 300 studies have been published in peer-reviewed journals that demonstrate the benefits of ACT-consistent interventions for a wide range of mental health, substance use, and health-related problems. ACT has been applied not only to "garden variety" mental health problems (e.g., depression, anxiety, panic, OCD) but also to severe mental health concerns such as psychosis and chronic PTSD. Maybe the most remarkable thing about the ACT approach is how quickly it has spread to the treatment of various chronic and acute medical problems (i.e., cancer, diabetes, chronic pain syndromes, migraine, multiple sclerosis, epilepsy), as well as to the treatment of health risk behaviors (i.e., smoking cessation, weight control, exercise). In general, published meta-analyses have consistently demonstrated that ACT produces clinical benefits that are at least comparable with, if not superior to, those achieved with other empirically supported cognitive-behavioral therapies (A-Tjak et al. 2015). Furthermore, ACT treatment benefits appear to be sustained over time. Anecdotally, some clinical studies have shown that ACT treatment benefits continue to "grow" over time, such that the largest effect sizes are noted during follow-up assessments. Patients seem to get better and better at balancing the roles of acceptance and change in their lives as a function of practicing these important life principles. Finally, the basic tenets of the ACT approach suggest that it will also be effective across cultural, ethnic, and sexual minorities, and this broad applicability is already evident in the empirical literature (Woidneck et al. 2012). Clinical studies of ACT have already been conducted in such diverse cultures as India, Iran, South Africa, and Turkey.

The Benefits of ACT in Psychiatric Practice: Case Examples

Although the ACT model has many nuances, the basic tools are pretty straightforward to learn and use in daily practice. As the saying goes, "this isn't rocket science." In the remainder of this chapter, we describe case examples that demonstrate some of the clinical benefits of integrating the ACT model along with our more traditional psychiatric treatment approaches.

ACT HELPS PATIENTS ACCEPT WHAT CANNOT BE CHANGED

Bea is a 69-year-old married woman who is mourning the loss of her physical functioning in the context of progressive Parkinson's disease. She was originally referred by her primary care physician for treatment of refractory depression and has just completed a third antidepressant trial with mild but inadequate response. She has failed a trial of lithium augmentation, and she is not a candidate for antipsychotic augmentation because of the Parkinson's disease. Recently, she has expressed feelings of hopelessness, and her family is concerned that she has lost weight and seems disengaged from her daughters, who have been the centerpiece of her life. The next step might be a trial of electroconvulsive therapy (ECT), but the patient is refusing ECT. Her physician offered to refer Bea to see a therapist, but she does not want to go.

Rather than sending Bea away with a sense that she is broken and that nothing will work to help her, we can normalize her grief. We can validate, in a humane, empathic way, the anxiety she experiences about what is yet to come. We can then help her clarify what steps she can take to continue to live according to her values, even in the midst of her declining physical and cognitive health. Rather than focusing on treating her depression, which is a completely understandable emotional reaction to the stress of her illness and encroaching disability, we can help her focus on creating meaning and purpose in the context of her growing physical limitations.

> Psychiatrist: Bea, it makes sense that you feel sad. I'm hearing that the life you were counting on is lost. You had plans to travel, and now it's difficult for you to get around. You're worried about what this illness means to your independence in the long run. Do I have this right?
> Bea: Yes. I've always been able to stand on my own two feet. I used to want to travel. That's impossible now. I don't know if I'll even be able to take care of myself, and I don't think my husband will be much help.

The psychiatrist will try to shift the conversation to the things that matter in Bea's life, to begin a conversation about her values and the ability to continue to make choices in her life.

> Psychiatrist: You've told me that you've always valued being strong, reliable, and independent. What about now? What do you want to model for your daughters about how to manage adversity?
> Bea: I haven't thought about it like that. [She starts to tear up.] I want to show them that I'm still strong.
> Psychiatrist: This looks hard. What's coming up for you?
> Bea: I feel ungrateful. I've always tried to teach the girls to be grateful for the blessings we have. I've been focusing on what I don't have. But I can't stop it; I'm so depressed. My daughters keep offering to help me out. Trisha even offered that I could move in with her if I need to. God has given me all of these blessings, and I'm so ungrateful.

Bea is judging herself for having the normal thoughts that come up in these situations. These judgments are adding to her suffering and making it more difficult for her to choose behaviors that support her values. The psychiatrist will try to normalize these thoughts and other products of the mind.

> Psychiatrist: You are blessed. And it's normal for you to both have the thought that you are blessed and to feel sad, in this situation. It's normal to feel pain about what you were hoping for and what you now have to cope with. Many people notice thoughts coming up such as, "This isn't fair," or "What did I do to deserve this?" I don't know if that happens with you?
>
> Bea: Yes. I keep thinking that it's not fair and wondering what I did to deserve this. I just don't want to be a burden to my girls.
>
> Psychiatrist: Let me see if I have this right. It sounds like you're having the thought of not wanting to be a burden and the thought that it's not fair that you have Parkinson's disease. And you're having a hard time being kind to yourself during this difficult time. You're calling yourself "ungrateful." Do I have this right?
>
> Bea: Yes, that's what I do.
>
> Psychiatrist: Do you think that you could just start noticing all of these thoughts? Could you try not judging them and not beating yourself up for having them? It's hard to imagine anyone not being pretty sad about their health failing. Most of us kind of know that eventually something is going to come along that causes our health to decline, but we keep that knowledge locked away because it's a bit scary.
>
> Bea: But it feels so heavy.
>
> Psychiatrist [again validating the feeling]: You're grieving a big loss. This isn't easy.
>
> Bea: It's foolish. I feel so worried. If I let myself grieve, I'll just get back into bed and never get up.
>
> Psychiatrist: It's not all or nothing. We're talking about learning to notice the pain you're feeling without being drowned by it. What would you tell a friend to do, if she were diagnosed with Parkinson's disease? Should she try to ignore feeling sad? Should she spend all day isolating herself so no one else can see how sad she is? Is there a middle ground?
>
> Bea [pausing to think]: Maybe allow some time every morning to let yourself feel sad, but then get up and wash your face and do what you can do. I don't want to be a burden to my daughters. I want to be strong for those girls.
>
> Psychiatrist: Do you want to model being so strong that you are not allowed to have feelings?
>
> Bea: No. I also want to work on being kind to myself, to model it to my daughters, especially Trisha. I really liked that self-compassion group last week.

In this brief exchange, the psychiatrist has helped shift the conversation away from "getting rid of" depression and toward living according to personal values. The psychiatrist has also built on skills that the client has learned in psychoeducational groups she has attended.

ACT HELPS INCREASE MOTIVATIONAL READINESS

Talking with chronically distressed patients about what matters to them in life and how they are moving toward or away from those things can be a powerful motivational intervention. As the following case example demonstrates, even listless, unmotivated patients respond positively to being treated with respect, curiosity, and authenticity.

> Owen is a 27-year-old single white man with a history of anxiety and depression since his early twenties. He has attempted suicide by overdose three times, twice in the past year. Owen lives with his parents in his childhood home. He does not have a job. He sometimes walks to the local library during the day, but he typically stays in bed until late afternoon. He used to read a lot, but less so recently. Most evenings he will sit with his parents and watch television. His parents no longer leave the house during the evenings so that he will have company and so that they can "make sure he is okay."
>
> Each night Owen relates his fear that the police are coming to get him because he ran a stoplight. He says he knows it is irrational, but he worries that the police will take him to Guantanamo Bay, where they will torture him. Night after night, his parents listen to his fears and the details of how he will be tortured. No matter what they say, they are unable to reassure him. "He just can't let the worries go," says his mother. Nine months ago, Owen overdosed on his medications. He was hospitalized and his antipsychotic was changed to clozapine. His mother did not notice any improvement. Three months ago, he overdosed again. During that hospitalization, his antipsychotic was changed again, to perphenazine. His mother says she has still seen no improvement. She thinks her son is sinking further and further into "a hole." "He has no energy," she says, and "feels so afraid of everything." Owen no longer does chores around the house. He no longer bathes or brushes his teeth with any regularity. He has barely left his bedroom in the past month. This morning he told his case manager that he was thinking about overdosing again and was referred to the hospital for readmission.

As Owen's psychiatrist, looking at the daunting list of anxiolytics, antipsychotics, and antidepressants Owen has been tried on might make you anxious about your ability to help. What are the options, other than to try yet another medication? *Incorporating ACT interviewing strategies into the psychiatric evaluation process* might stimulate Owen to try some new strategies around his home that might lift his mood, energy, and motivation. You also wonder whether the perphenazine is helping with symptoms or adding to lethargy and poor functioning.

Psychiatrist: Owen, your mother told me you were very social and out-going when you were younger and that this shifted by the time you went to high school. I'm wondering, if a miracle happened and you woke up tomorrow cured of your symptoms, what would you be doing with your life?

Owen: A miracle?

Psychiatrist: Yes, a miracle. You wake up and you have no symptoms. What would you be doing in your life if your symptoms just vanished?

Owen: Well, I wouldn't be scared. I'm always worried about getting arrested.

Psychiatrist: What if you weren't scared? What if someone were making a movie about your life now that you're no longer scared? What would you be doing differently? What would I see you doing if I were watching this movie about your life after this miracle happened?

Owen: I wouldn't be in bed all day.

Psychiatrist: Would you be different with people? With your parents or old friends?

Owen: I'd like to stop scaring my mom. I sit with them every night. We watch TV, and it's nice for a minute, but I always end up talking about how I'm going to get arrested and tortured. Then my mom cries, and I feel worse, and then I usually go to my room. I hate feeling so scared, and it always seems like it will help if I tell them.

Psychiatrist: Does it help you to tell them?

Owen: Yes. Well, no. I just feel like I need to tell them. Then I feel bad about making my mom upset. But it always feels like it's going to help when I start.

Clarifying the unworkability of current strategies while validating the uncomfortable feelings that lead to them opens the door for Owen to begin to make behavioral changes.

Psychiatrist: Let me see if I have this right. You have this urge to tell them because it seems as though it might make these painful thoughts less intense. It helps for a minute but not in the long run, and you feel bad because it also makes your mother upset.

Owen: Yeah. Yeah, that's just what happens. And I'm not sure it even helps for a minute. It just always seems like it *should* help.

Psychiatrist: Have you thought about different ways of behaving when these thoughts come up?

Owen: Not really.

Being patient, giving him some time to think, and asking what he would suggest to a friend can be helpful here. You can also introduce some strategies by prefacing your statement with the phrase, "Can I share something with you that might be worth considering?"

Psychiatrist: Can I share with you what some other people with problems with these kinds of thoughts have tried? Would you be willing to consider some of those ideas?

Owen: Other people have had these kinds of thoughts?

The psychiatrist now has the opportunity to relabel and reattribute
Owen's painful obsessional thoughts. This is an important part of ACT
for conditions in which obsessional thoughts and fears recur and are
frightening, such as OCD, PTSD, and many forms of psychosis and depression—and of ACT in general.

Psychiatrist: Do you remember that questionnaire I had you fill out
about thoughts you have that come back again and again and don't
seem to go away, even when you try to make them? Although most
of our minds generate some uncomfortable thoughts, some people's minds seem to get stuck with particular painful thoughts, almost like a hiccup. It's usually helpful to call these thoughts that are
bothering you again and again your "mental hiccups." Your mind
has this urge to give you this thought, and it comes out just like that,
bang, just like a hiccup.
Owen: You mean the thought that the police are going to arrest me and
send me to Guantanamo and torture me? I know it's irrational,
but I can't stop thinking about this stuff.

It's important here both to validate the discomfort of the thought or
feeling and also to begin helping the patient relabel it.

Psychiatrist: Exactly. What an uncomfortable thought! That could make
anyone feel anxious. Will you write that down here? Are there
other hiccups that come up a lot? Does "hiccup" work for you as
a name to call those thoughts?
Owen: It's pretty much the one thought. And that name works, or maybe
"The Evil Hiccups."
Psychiatrist: Great. It sounds like the enemy in a video game. If you can
bear with me stretching a metaphor, if you were playing a video
game and the evil hiccups were trying to destroy you, what goal
would you be trying to reach? I'm guessing in video games it's gold
or power points or something, but with people, your parents for example, if you could stand up to the evil hiccups, what would your
strategy be? What would I be able to see you doing differently
when you spend time with your parents?

Owen reports that he would feel as though he is moving toward being
the son he wants to be, if he could sit with his parents for the entire evening without talking about his fears of being arrested and tortured. Having come up with that goal, Owen and the psychiatrist discuss different
ways to notice but not be so pushed around by the thoughts—mindful-

ness exercises, observing self, writing down the thoughts, and keeping count of how often they occur while he is sitting there. They discuss how rebalancing his medications will probably help make the thoughts less "sticky" but may not take them away completely, so it will be important for him to practice his skills. Owen agrees to let his parents know if he is having any thoughts about harming himself or others. Owen states that he would rather let his parents know about his goal of sitting with them but would prefer to keep his "evil hiccups" to himself. Owen and his psychiatrist rehearse out loud what he will say to his parents about this goal and what he will request from them in the way of support and encouragement. Most importantly, Owen and his psychiatrist address Owen's reluctance to seek support from his parents should he become fearful during one of his "sitting quietly" experiments.

Owen: I hate making my mother cry—and it doesn't make me feel any better. But I don't want to hang out in my room all of the time. I really think this is a good idea.

Psychiatrist: On a scale of 1–10, 10 being the most likely, how likely are you to be able to sit with your parents all evening without talking about those fearful thoughts and images we've talked about?

Owen: 4 or 5?

Psychiatrist: What makes it a 4 or 5 and not a 0?

Owen: I hate making my mom cry, and my parents worry more than they have to. Asking them for reassurance doesn't help me, so this is something I want to do.

Psychiatrist: And what makes it a 4 or 5 and not a 10?

Owen: Well, they watch TV for an hour, or maybe two. That feels like a long time.

Psychiatrist: Would it be better to start shorter, with the goal of increasing the time later?

Owen: Yeah. Can I start with 30 minutes? Also, I'm not sure how I'm going to remember to wait.

Psychiatrist: Is there anything that might help you remember?

Owen: Well, I could ask my dad to remind me. Oh, I have an idea! I'm going to write it on my arm in pen. I always look at this tattoo on my arm. I can write underneath, "Wait." When I tell my parents about the plan, I'll ask my dad to remind me if I start talking before the time is up. And I could use the timer on my phone.

Psychiatrist: That sounds like a good idea. With that plan, where are you on the 1–10 scale?

Owen [looking more excited and energized than he has since admission]: Oh, I'm a 9, maybe even a 10.

Psychiatrist: That's great. Is there anything else important that you could take some steps toward when you get home? Do you want to think about getting out of the house and seeing people? You said that was important to you. Or maybe beginning to get healthier, walking to the library, getting

going with exercise again—you had said that was helpful
in the past.

Owen: I've been eating better here and walking laps. Last year
I lost a lot of this extra weight and felt better; I know how
to do it. I think one of my pills was making me really tired,
and I was depressed.

The psychiatrist could use this as an opportunity to help Owen
make this into a measurable goal or refer Owen to a class given by the
health system or a local Y.

Psychiatrist: What about work? You're on disability now. Your mom
said you used to want to be a translator. If you were magically better, do you have any sense of what you'd want to do with your
time?

Owen: I don't think I should get off of disability. But I've thought about
becoming a volunteer at the library, and maybe a peer counselor
for the NAMI[1] groups that they have at the library on Wednesday
nights.

This style of change-oriented interviewing helps you, the psychiatrist, summon up more compassion and creates a sense of hope. It is easier to see beyond Owen's morbid obesity and limited hygiene and to
ask about the content of the paranoia and about his behaviors, leading
to a more accurate diagnosis. Having this picture of Owen allows you
to support him in considering what he might want his life to be about if
these symptoms were no longer pushing him around. It is easier to discuss medications as "training wheels," to teach mindfulness and rela-
beling strategies, and to use his values to give direction to his efforts.

ACT HELPS IMPROVE TREATMENT ADHERENCE

How can we best intervene with patients who are having difficulty adhering to their treatment? As the following case example demonstrates,
ACT focuses not on the patient's resistance but on his values related to
living a vital, purposeful life.

George is a 74-year-old widower who lost his wife of 50 years to a heart
attack about 2 years ago. Other than coming back on a monthly basis to
get his lorazepam refilled, George does not seem to be benefiting from
treatment. Despite various medication trials, he remains depressed and
anxious and looks forward to dying and joining his wife, although he denies active suicidality. George reports that he used to be very happy. He
loved his wife, attended a weekly coffee group of retired men at church,

[1]NAMI=National Alliance on Mental Illness.

spent time with their daughter and her two children, and put in an annual vegetable garden that not only fed the family but also helped stock the church's food pantry. He always verbalizes plans to restart the garden, go to the Tuesday coffee group, or spend time with his grandchildren, but he never follows through. The psychiatrist has tried to get him to be more specific about the timing of these plans, their value, and their benefit. Each visit George promises he is going to do "it" this time. Yet, without fail, at the next visit George lets the psychiatrist know, with a hang-dog expression, that he has failed again.

Should the psychiatrist give up on behavioral goals? Conclude that George is a hopeless case? Maybe, but she could also help George clarify his values about living life without his partner and identify the mental processes that are functioning as barriers to him following through on his commitments.

Psychiatrist: George, how are these visits working for you?

George: I don't know. I'm useless without Carol. I'll never get over her.

Psychiatrist [validating the emotion]: That's true. Your life will never be the same. You don't want to forget her, and you'll never stop missing her. You may have another 10 or 20 years on this planet without Carol. I'm wondering, when it's your turn to pass, what do you want to be remembered for during those years you lived without her? [Pausing] What did you and Carol stand for? What would Carol want for you?

George: Well, family…and church. [He looks down and picks invisible lint off of his pants, with a heartfelt sigh.]

Psychiatrist: I'm wondering what you're thinking right now. Could you let me in on it?

George: I'm not proud of myself. I think I'm going to do the things we talk about and then I don't. I'm sitting on the couch watching baseball, trying not to feel sad and thinking about how disappointed Carol probably is for me. I don't know if she can see me from heaven, but if she can, I'm sure she's disappointed.

Psychiatrist [finds this interesting]: I would imagine that she would feel love for you, and compassion for your struggle to adjust, and certainly concern that you're having a hard time moving on. But why disappointment?

George: I just can't. I'm stuck. I leave here meaning to do things differently, but I just can't.

Psychiatrist: Would it be okay to look at what's making it hard for you to do the things you feel are important? For instance, you had said you were going to start going to dinner with your daughter's family. What stops you?

George: I don't know. I want to. I know she worries about me.

Psychiatrist: Can you take me back to the last time she invited you?

George: Well, she invites me to dinner on Tuesday night every week.

Psychiatrist: And you tell her no?

George: No, I usually tell her "I'll see."

Psychiatrist: Does that mean "no"?

George: No. I guess it means....It means that I'm going to try.

Psychiatrist: Hmm. Today's Wednesday, and I'm guessing she invited you to last night's dinner. Could you walk me through this? I'm curious as to how the "I'll see" turns into a "no." What happened last night? [The psychiatrist's goal here is to get George to really drill down to see what happens.]

George: When I woke up yesterday morning, I was thinking I would go. I was feeling a little anxious, but then I started to get more anxious—it gets really bad in the afternoon, when I think about how Carol and I used to have dinner together every night, and I miss her even more—and I called my daughter, feeling all panicky, and I told her "no."

Psychiatrist: What were you anxious about? What was going through your head?

George: I don't even know. But my heart starts racing, and it feels like I can't breathe, and I get tingly and shaky inside. I was thinking of asking you if I could take more lorazepam so I could try to go.

Psychiatrist: That's one approach we could take. But before we go there, could we talk a little more about this? You're feeling anxious, and it feels like you can't go because you are anxious. What's your mind telling you might happen if you go? What picture is your mind drawing for you?

George: It's ridiculous.

Psychiatrist: Would you be willing to let me in on the picture?

George: Well, I guess you're my doctor. [He looks down and tears up. The psychiatrist passes him tissues.] I'm afraid I'll start crying when we're eating dinner. [Collecting himself, he wipes away tears. He looks down at his knees and brushes off more invisible fuzz.] Carol loved those kids, and she should be here with them. I don't deserve to be the one that's left. [He begins crying.]

Psychiatrist [after giving George some time]: Those sound like very painful thoughts. I can see why it would make sense for you to not go. That would be one way to keep your fear of breaking down at bay. But I'm wondering how trying to avoid these thoughts—that Carol should be here with the grandkids, that you don't deserve to be the one that's left—how will avoiding your fears about grieving in front of your children help you to be the person you want to be? You've told me how much you love your family. If Carol could talk to you right now, what would she think of you not going over?

George: She'd be mad as a hornet.

Psychiatrist: Maybe there is a better way for you to relate to your fearful thoughts and images, like the thought that Carol should be here, or the image of you breaking down and sobbing at the dinner table. You don't have to give in to those thoughts and images [holding his hands up to his face], and you don't have to eliminate them either [pushes one hand away with the other].

George: But I don't think I can go over to my daughter's for dinner. I miss Carol, and Carol should be there, not me. I don't think I can go—at least not while I'm feeling this way.

Psychiatrist: Sometimes we do things we feel are important even when we feel anxious and our minds are giving us these uncomfortable thoughts and images. You're a veteran, aren't you?

George: Yes.

Psychiatrist: Weren't you ever scared, but you did your job as a soldier anyway?

George [starts to chuckle]: I guess so! But it wasn't my idea.

Psychiatrist: Did you ever think "I'm going to get killed" or feel afraid of something bad happening to you during your service?

George: Oh, yes, many times.

Psychiatrist: You told me you practically rebuilt your house on weekends and after work on weekdays. Didn't your mind ever tell you that it was too hard, and you should just go out fishing instead of working on the bathroom?

George: All the time.

Psychiatrist: So how did you get yourself to do things when your mind was telling you not to?

George: Well, when I heard that voice in my head saying, "I don't want to work on the bathroom," I'd tell myself right back, "But you've got to because your family is depending on you."

Psychiatrist: So it sounds as though, if the situation is right, you're able to overrule your mind's advice. I'm wondering, how can you do what you need to do in this case? Right now, it seems like you're letting your mind run the show.

George: I guess I hadn't thought about it like that.

Psychiatrist: Now, what did you tell me your mind says to you when you think about going for Tuesday dinner?

George: I guess that I don't deserve it, that I don't deserve to be happy now that Carol is gone. And I'm afraid I'll cry in front of them; I only started crying after Carol died, but now it feels like it's always about to happen.

Psychiatrist: You might cry in front of them the first night. In the long run, in terms of you having the life you want, is it more important to you that they never see you cry or that you get to see your family and be part of your daughter's and the grandkids' lives?

George: It doesn't feel good to always be making excuses to my daughter for not showing up.

Psychiatrist: Yeah. To have what you want in life might mean just accepting that you're going to have these thoughts and feelings, but you don't have to let them run the show. Would you be willing to experiment with that? Just allowing yourself to notice whatever uncomfortable thoughts, images, or feelings come up? Not fighting with them, but just doing what's important for you and letting those thoughts and feelings come along for the ride?

ACT moves the clinical conversation toward "both/and" choices patients can make. They can choose behaviors that reflect deeply held values while at the same choosing to accept the presence of distressing and unwanted emotions, memories, thoughts, urges, images, or physical sensations that arise in the context of values-based behaviors. All of this is done in a very respectful and nonjudgmental way. When patients are allowed to approach important life commitments in this way, they can move forward more easily in their lives in ways that are meaningful to them.

ACT PROMOTES EMOTIONAL RESILIENCE

A basic tenet of ACT is that it is not distressing, unwanted mental experiences per se that create dysfunction; rather, the attempt to avoid making contact with unwanted experiences is what leads to trouble. As the next case example demonstrates, ACT fosters emotional *approach* rather than emotional *avoidance*, thus supporting the health-producing integration of difficult emotional experiences in life.

> Anna is a 48-year-old happily married middle-school music teacher and mother of a 10-year-old son. She has always been high energy and mildly anxious but has developed overwhelming anxiety over the past year. She finds the anxiety intolerable and ruminates about what is causing her anxiety and her "dark thoughts." She worries the anxiety will never go away. She reports being very sensitive to medications and had stopped Lexapro at 10 mg/day because she thought it was making her more anxious and suicidal. She was recently admitted for psychiatric inpatient care due to lack of sleep and appetite and started on low-dose clonazepam and fluoxetine. She was discharged after showing indications she was experiencing less anxiety and fewer depressive symptoms. She returned to the hospital the next evening complaining of intolerable "dark thoughts," increased anxiety, and hopelessness. She had written a suicide note and was thinking through where she could best run her car into a tree when she decided to call her husband for help.

What are the treatment options? The psychiatrist could increase her fluoxetine, and maybe her clonazepam, and possibly add an antipsychotic. However, medication treatment alone is unlikely to rid someone permanently of painful thoughts or anxiety. Alternatively, the psychiatrist could explore the content of Anna's "dark thoughts" and show her how to use acceptance and mindfulness skills to defang them.

> Psychiatrist: Can we talk about your dark thoughts? Would that be okay with you?
> Anna [frowning and looking down]: Hmm, okay.
> Psychiatrist: Can you be more specific about them? Like yesterday, when you were thinking about killing yourself, or writing the note, what was showing up inside of you?

Anna: I was thinking about how I'm a failure as a mother. Justin [her son] had some homework he needed checked, and he asked his father to help; he just walked right past me and ignored me. I know that's not a big deal, but then I just—I felt angry at him. What kind of mother feels angry at her son because he asks his father for homework help? There's something wrong with me. I never used to be like this. I don't know what happened. Something is wrong with me. I'm falling into a pit, and there's no way to fix it.

Psychiatrist: Okay, so part of these dark thoughts is feeling that you're broken, that it's never going to get better, and that you're a monster for feeling hurt when your son bypassed you to ask his father for help with homework. Is that it?

Anna: Yes, that I'm not a good mom. And I worry that my husband is getting tired of me. I didn't used to be like this, but I don't know how to stop these dark thoughts.

Psychiatrist: It's normal to sometimes feel possessive of our children's attention and to experience jealousy when we don't get as much "love" as we want. Those feelings just show up on their own, and we can't do much to stop them, no matter how uncomfortable they are. When we add in self-judgment and the need to control or get rid of those feelings, they somehow seem to get even stronger. You told me you used to meditate. Did you go to yesterday's class on mindfulness?

Anna: It was a good class, but it's not working for this anxiety. I have a hard time sitting still, and even when I do, the anxiety and darkness just stay.

Psychiatrist: The goal of mindfulness, at least in this context, is not to get rid of uncomfortable thoughts and feelings but just to set an anchor so we can notice them. We're not pushing them away, but we're also not getting pushed around by them.

Anna: Oh. I thought it was supposed to help me feel better.

Psychiatrist: Well, the eventual goal is for you to stop getting pushed around by these uncomfortable dark thoughts so you can make peace with them, so to speak. You don't have to like their tone or the feelings they bring up inside, but you must learn to make room for them if you want to live in a vital way. Sometimes, these painful thoughts, images, memories, or feelings actually tell us about what we want in life. You know, if you didn't love your son, you wouldn't care who he asked for help with his homework. You wouldn't be hurt or jealous at all, and you wouldn't have put yourself through these harsh self-judgments. The goal is just to notice the thoughts, images, and feelings without engaging in a struggle with them. You can respect their role in helping you be the person you are, rather than allow them to keep you from living your life.

Anna: I can be anxious and have dark thoughts without having to get rid of them somehow? I don't know if I can manage that. It's so different from how I used to be.

Psychiatrist: The key is to recognize that trying to control or get rid of these thoughts makes them seem bigger and more threatening.

The harder you try to have "light thoughts" instead of "dark thoughts," the more dark thoughts you will have.

Anna: That's so weird, but it is exactly what's been happening to me!

Psychiatrist: It's hard to resist the temptation to stamp out painful feelings, memories, or images. The trick is to create a place you can go where you can just accept what is happening without judging it or judging yourself. How about I talk you through a brief exercise that will help you practice being aware and nonjudgmental at the same time? You could practice the technique when you're feeling fine, but you can definitely use it when it feels like those "dark thoughts" are pushing you off course.

In this brief exchange, the psychiatrist normalized Anna's uncomfortable thoughts and feelings, clarified the purpose of mindfulness practice, and introduced a basic mindfulness skill. The psychiatrist can now try to shift Anna's response to her uncomfortable thoughts.

Psychiatrist: Being here in the hospital, and in the outpatient group you were in, you were learning a lot of distress tolerance tools. Have you been practicing them?

Anna: Yes. I'm feeling much better being here, in the hospital. I'm hardly anxious.

Psychiatrist: It's sort of a problem, isn't it? I wonder if we could almost encourage you to be anxious, so you can practice not having the thoughts push you around?

Anna: Should I stop taking the clonazepam?

Psychiatrist: That's an interesting idea. How about we lower your dose tomorrow so you can practice working with the thoughts and the anxiety while you're here in this safe place? You'll want to invite the dark thoughts and anxiety in so you can practice unhooking from them. You may want to start by writing down some of the thoughts or feelings that come up and practicing the noticing exercise we just ran through.

By shifting the focus of the conversation from controlling and eliminating distressing mental events to being willing to make direct contact with them, the psychiatrist helps Anna create a new definition of the task at hand. This shift of focus from "feeling better" to "feeling it better" is a powerful ACT message. It can be used to manage the challenge of patients who feel better in a structured inpatient or outpatient setting but then feel overwhelmed when the painful thoughts and feelings re-emerge after discharge.

ACT HELPS SIMPLIFY THE TREATMENT OF COMPLEX CASES

Another singular feature of ACT is its emphasis on the *function* of symptoms and unworkable coping behaviors, rather than their *form*. In traditional psychiatry, we have long been focused on the form symptoms take. Our diagnostic system is largely based on the form, or pattern, of presenting symptoms. In ACT, seemingly different clinical problems are often seen as birds of a feather. The dysfunctional behaviors look different on the surface, but underneath they enact the same psychological functions for the patient. When we take this approach with complex, refractory cases, we are able to group seemingly different forms of behavioral dysfunction into the same functional class. As the following case example demonstrates, this allows the psychiatrist to use the same basic intervention principles to tackle an array of seemingly different clinical problems.

> Miguel is a 41-year-old machinist who has been treated for depression in the past. He has a history of alcohol use disorder and had 2 years of sobriety until experiencing a brief relapse last month. He is now "back on the wagon." His partner of the past 2 years, the woman for whom he "got clean," told him not to call because she needs some time to think about things. The psychiatrist has met with Miguel in the past but has not seen him over the past year because Miguel had been doing well and had been transferred back to his primary care physician for medication maintenance. Miguel returns, reporting sharply increased depression as well as anhedonia, helplessness, hopelessness, and passive suicidal ideation. He talks about his new girlfriend and how upset he is that she is cutting off their relationship. "I'm nothing without her," he says. His depression is mostly focused on the loss of the relationship. He reports that he has been attending Alcoholics Anonymous (AA) and that work has been going well. He notes that he and his partner had been enjoying going for walks and cooking together. Because he has been eating healthier and not drinking, he has been able to lose 30 lb and get his diabetes under control.

The psychiatrist will certainly address the medication issue. Is Miguel still taking the naltrexone and sertraline that he had benefited from previously? However, the psychiatrist also wants to inquire about relationships, work, leisure, and health so she and Miguel can focus not only on recent setbacks but also on what Miguel wants in life and the progress he has been making toward those life ends. The psychiatrist also hopes to help Miguel explore his recent relapse, guessing that he relapsed as a way to avoid unwanted thoughts, feelings, or memories.

> Psychiatrist: Miguel, I haven't seen you in some time. It sounds like you were doing better for a while, but things have been more challenging lately. What have you been up to?
>
> Miguel: I've been working my program, doc. I'm exercising more regularly tand watching my eating. My sugar diabetes is getting better; I've lost almost 30 pounds. I'm up for a promotion at my job; it will mean a pretty nice pay raise if I get it. The biggest thing was

meeting Vivienne, and we hit it off instantly. She keeps me in line. Really, I don't think I'd be doing well without her. Now she's closing the door on me.

Psychiatrist: Can you tell me about the relapse?

Miguel: I just had a slip.

Psychiatrist: It sounds like you're trying to create a life you want, a life in touch with your values. You're exploring being in a committed relationship with Vivienne, and you're actively working your program in AA. You've been getting to work regularly, without being hungover, and are in line for a promotion. That's great! It sounds like you're also taking much better care of your body. You've had this recent relapse, but overall it sounds like you've been working hard to stay sober, get regular exercise, and eat better. Do I have that right?

Miguel: Well, it's important for me to be reliable. I want people to be able to trust me. I want to be a man of my word. I want to be the guy Vivienne wants to spend her life with. [He stops talking and looks down at the floor.]

Psychiatrist: What's going on now? If I could hear your mind, what would it be saying?

Miguel: What's the use? I'll always mess up. Without Vivienne—I just don't want to do it. I'll fall apart without her. I can't believe how stupid I am, what a jerk I am.

Psychiatrist: What else does your mind say to you, when you get in this dark space?

Miguel: That I'm a loser, and I'll never amount to anything. That I will end up alone with no one to love me.

Psychiatrist: I'm guessing that drinking helped drown out that noise?

Miguel: Yeah, it was the only way I could get away from the thoughts. My dad messed me up really bad before he walked out on us.

Psychiatrist: You had a hard childhood, and frequently that makes it harder to be kind to ourselves, even as adults. Did any of this mind chatter come up before this recent relapse?

Miguel: Yes. Vivienne and I had this fight. She told me I'm smothering her. I couldn't stand it. [He looks down at the floor, pausing.]

Psychiatrist: You couldn't stand it. You couldn't stand what came up when she said that?

Miguel: Yes, it just feels terrible.

Psychiatrist: Do you have any strategies to use when those kinds of bad feelings show up?

Miguel: I learned some in rehab. I stopped using them because when I tried them, they didn't work for me anyway.

Psychiatrist: They didn't work for you?

Miguel: Yeah. I try to relax and let go. I'm still doing it, the slow breathing, but I still feel upset.

Psychiatrist: It sounds like you're using those strategies to try to get rid of those feelings, as a way to control them.

Miguel: Well, I guess it could be that I'm hoping those feelings will just go away if I relax and breathe deep.

Psychiatrist [holds her left hand in front of her face]: Yes, when our uncomfortable thoughts and feelings and memories are drowning us, it makes it hard for us to live our lives.

Miguel [smiling]: Definitely.

Psychiatrist [pushes her left hand away with her right hand]: But pushing this stuff away all the time gets tiring, doesn't it?

Miguel: Yes.

Psychiatrist [brings her left hand back to her face]: Then what happens?

Miguel: I'm back where I started.

Psychiatrist: I'm wondering if we can find a third option here, maybe an approach that is really different from what you've tried before. That is, to just be aware that this uncomfortable stuff is around, to not let yourself drown in it [raises a hand to her face], but to not push it away either [pushes her hand away]. To just let it be there [rests her hand upturned in lap]. Not to say "yes" to it, but not to say "no" either. If you could get rid of that stuff, you would have, right? Have you been able to get rid of this stuff?

Miguel: No. I think I see what you're saying. I used to use drinking as a way to avoid dealing with my memories.

Psychiatrist: Did drinking to numb out the memories work?

Miguel: No. Well, maybe a little at the beginning. But it made everything worse. I don't want to go back there.

Psychiatrist: If I'm hearing you right, your life experience has been that you can't get rid of those thoughts and feelings from your childhood, but you can learn how to not let them run the show. You can learn how to have those thoughts and feelings and still do the things that make your life work.

Miguel: She's just trying to make our relationship work by setting these limits with me. She says she's not sure how she feels about the relationship now that I've relapsed, and I reacted by being upset and ashamed of myself, all of those old feelings from my childhood—about being wrong somehow, about always saying the wrong thing, about not being okay. I've been thinking that I can't stay sober without her. She's like my new Jack Daniels.

Psychiatrist: She can't help you get rid of those old thoughts and feelings any better than alcohol could. Would you be willing to practice just being aware of those old thoughts and feelings when they show up? You could almost wave at them and say, "Hi, I know you." When they try to push you in the wrong direction, you can remember to breathe in and set an intention to live according to your values and to do the things that are in line with where you want your life to go. Maintaining sobriety, staying in touch with your brother, giving Vivienne space, doing your job, exercising, eating well, taking good care of your diabetes, and spending time outdoors.

Miguel: Yes. This makes it a lot clearer to me. I've already called my AA sponsor. Being with Vivienne has been a good thing, no matter how it turns out; having a partner is a move toward what I want in life. I want to be with her, but I want to be okay without her as well. I think that's the only way it's going to work.

In this conversation, the psychiatrist helped Miguel see how his use of alcohol and his "addiction" to Vivienne both function in the service of emotional avoidance. This allows Miguel to use the same approach to support his sobriety and create a healthier balance in his current relationship—and weather the storm if the relationship does not last. He later stated that he knew he could go on with his life even without the relationship and that it was ultimately up to Vivienne if she wanted to continue to date him. The functional approach of ACT helped meld his two seemingly different problems into one, which in turn allowed him to exercise better control over his behaviors going forward.

Summary

In this chapter we reviewed some of the global benefits of using ACT in daily psychiatric practice. ACT, when used alone or in conjunction with medication, gives us several new avenues for effective intervention. Including ACT in their repertoire of treatment approaches allows psychiatrists to feel less "stuck" when medications are not working as well as hoped for or are contraindicated for some reason. In these instances, the psychiatrist can simply shift gears and refocus the conversation onto the patient's values and willingness to pursue those values in daily life. Furthermore, ACT allows psychiatrists to undermine unhealthy forms of emotional avoidance and to teach patients various acceptance and mindfulness strategies that they can use for a lifetime. In the next few chapters, we delve more deeply into the particulars of the ACT approach, from the theory aspects of the model to the applied clinical steps needed to promote powerful, lasting change. If you are interested in or intrigued by ACT at this point, we encourage you to read on!

The Essentials

ACT helps patients

- Question culturally transmitted rules that portray painful private experiences as toxic to personal health and something to be avoided, controlled, or eliminated at all costs.
- Use mindfulness strategies to recognize and accept—without becoming enmeshed with—distressing, unwanted thoughts, emotions, urges, memories, and sensations.
- Learn to live in the here and now rather than residing largely in the past or future.

- Gain perspective on harsh self-narratives so as to increase the capacity to adopt novel, flexible coping strategies.
- Clarify deeply held values and link meaningful life actions to those values in the pursuit of a vital, purposeful life.

ACT helps psychiatrists

- Disconnect from the prevailing paradigm—that our job essentially consists of finding the right medications to help clients get rid of their painful thoughts and feelings.
- Respond to patients' distressing, unwanted private experiences in a new, more compassionate and accepting way.
- Help patients gain skills to increase their psychological flexibility and personal vitality despite emotional hardship.
- Change the conversation with patients from a singular focus on symptom relief to a broader discussion of how symptoms fit into the context of their lives.
- Realize we usually do not have the power to cure the unavoidable pain that comes from being human.

Suggested Readings

Hayes S, Strosahl K, Wilson K: Acceptance and Commitment Therapy: The Process and Practice of Mindful Change. New York, Guilford, 2011

Strosahl K, Robinson P, Gustavsson T: Brief Interventions for Radical Change: Principles and Practice of Focused Acceptance and Commitment Therapy. Oakland, CA, New Harbinger, 2012

References

A-Tjak JG, Davis ML, Morina N, et al: A meta-analysis of the efficacy of acceptance and commitment therapy for clinically relevant mental and physical health problems. Psychother Psychosom 84(1):30–36, 2015 25547522

Woidneck M, Pratt K, Gundy J, et al: Exploring cultural competence in acceptance and commitment therapy outcomes. Prof Psychol Res Pr 43(3):227–233, 2012

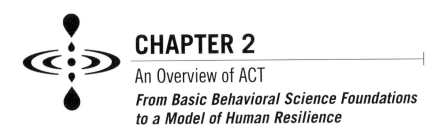

CHAPTER 2

An Overview of ACT

From Basic Behavioral Science Foundations to a Model of Human Resilience

I used to think that the brain was the most wonderful organ in my body. Then I realized who was telling me this.

—*Emo Phillips*

In this chapter we examine the underlying theories that collectively contribute to the ACT approach. This is a difficult task, because the ACT model has an amazing amount of depth and breadth as it evolves. ACT draws key concepts from wide and diverse scientific traditions such as evolution science, behavior analysis (both experimental and applied), experimental psychopathology, developmental psychology, basic language research, and affective neuroscience. The foundations of ACT also include a heavy dose of clinical theory related to motivational enhancement, health behavior change, human growth and development, habit formation, and self-directed behavior change. To top it off, many of the clinical principles that arise from this collage of scientific traditions bear a striking resemblance to the spiritual principles of Eastern religious traditions. We cannot do justice to such a complex theoretical, clinical, and spiritual framework in a single book chapter, but we introduce you to the most important features of the ACT approach, starting with its roots in the basic behavioral sciences and ending with a fully elaborated clinical model of psychopathology and psychotherapeutic intervention. Should you, the reader, become interested in a particular feature of the model and want to learn more, we provide you with a list of recommended source readings at the end of the chapter.

In essence, the founders of ACT started out trying to answer a question that most practicing psychiatrists have probably asked themselves on more than one occasion: How is it that bright, well-intentioned, motivated patients employ the same unworkable behaviors over and over again, often just moments after admitting in session that these behaviors do not work? Why does the saying "insanity is doing the same thing over and over again and expecting different results" [1] ring such a bell for us? How can we get patients who are stuck in a rut to try something different rather than leave our office and do exactly what they have done before, sometimes minutes after telling us that their coping strategies do not work?

Before we explore answers to this question, one important "note to self" should be made: We *all* do this! This phenomenon is not confined to patients with mental health problems; it is part of what we as humans do. The more important questions to answer are why this happens and what can be done about it through psychiatric assessment and intervention. The short answer—before we go into the long answer—is that human language functions as a sophisticated form of behavioral control so ubiquitous that these control functions generally operate automatically, unless we bring them under voluntary control and regulate their influence in a systematic way. Because language and thought are everywhere, all the time, we seldom interfere with this habitual process, even though it may not be serving our best interests in a particular setting or circumstance. Instead, we tend to let the system of language and thought do its thing because most of the time it is extraordinarily effective. However, when the powerful regulatory functions of language are extended into areas where they do not belong, we can and do end up trapped in unworkable, rigid patterns of behavior. When people present for help with mental health concerns, their presenting complaints and underlying issues are often directly connected to following these habitual—and for the most part invisible—mental rules.

The solution, therefore, is to teach people how to become more aware and skeptical of the dictates of mind by seeing rules as products of mind rather than as mandates that must be followed at any cost. We want people to *have* a mind without *becoming* their mind. All of the core techniques of ACT, in one way or another, play a role in creating this distinction between the thought and the thinker, the emotion and the feeler, the memory and the one remembering. Only by driving a wedge between the human being and the mind can we short-circuit the mind's most destructive and unworkable regulatory functions. Once the hegemony of mind is reversed, we are in a position to offer patients an alternative form of regulatory control: consciously chosen behaviors that

---

[1]Attributed to Albert Einstein.

reflect their personal values and associated aspirations in life. To get to this point, however, the contributors to the ACT model spent many decades conducting the basic and applied research needed to both inform and substantiate their approach. In the following sections, we work our way from the ground up to show how the ACT model evolved into what it is today.

The Basic Behavioral Science Origins of ACT

ACT is somewhat unique in the field of psychotherapy because its origins are rooted in a philosophy of science called *functional contextualism* and a behavioral analytic account of human language known as *relational frame theory* (RFT; Hayes et al. 2001). *Functional contextualism* has long been the basic model used in applied behavior analysis, a discipline that has attained widespread recognition for its success in treating individuals with developmental disabilities and autism spectrum disorders. We examine functional contextualism and its relevance for psychiatric practice in more detail in Chapter 3. For now, we want to touch upon a few major tenets of this scientific and epistemological theory.

The first principle of the functional contextual approach is that it is impossible to separate the behavior of humans from the surrounding contexts in which their behavior is embedded. The contextual approach holds that all behavior is controlled by specific antecedents (triggering events) or consequences (rewards or punishments following a behavior). Throughout this book, in various ways, we use this method for analyzing behavior, often called the A-B-C approach. The "A" stands for determining which factors are functioning as *antecedents,* or factors that trigger a specific response; "B" stands for the *behavior* triggered by the antecedent; and "C" stands for the results, or *consequences,* of the behavior in question. This is not a single, linear process but rather is iterative in nature. This means that behavior interacts with and modifies its controlling factors. Thus, all behavior is in a dynamic, ever-changing relationship with its surroundings, and pragmatically speaking, we cannot influence and control behavior unless we can influence and control its surroundings. In the functional contextual view, all behavior is organized and purposeful, even if it falls outside of social norms and even if the human being is not completely aware of what the function of a behavior might be.

The second key principle is that human behavior is triggered not only by influences in the external world but also by events in the mental context of human language. The context of human language is a rich playground mentally constructed antecedents and consequences. Often, the external and internal worlds work iteratively, in a repetitive series of feelings, thoughts, and actions. For example, a parent may criticize a child for something the child did not actually do; the child believes he or she is being treated unfairly and throws a temper tantrum, which in turn elicits another aversive consequence from the parent. If the parent brought the child in for treatment of temper tantrums, the psychiatrist could only make sense of this problem by working backward up the chain of behaviors on both sides of the problematic interaction. A behavior analytic approach grounded in functional contextualism would automatically involve looking closely (and sometimes even directly) at the back and forth going on between the child and the parent. Any intervention would have to somehow change how this chain of action/reaction unfolds (Ramnerö and Torneke 2011).

Relational Frame Theory

Although many behavior analytic theorists have become well known over the decades, no doubt the "poster child" for this approach is B.F. Skinner. Skinner's contributions to the field of behavioral psychology continue to exert a strong influence on behavioral analytic theories and applied practices to this day. Skinner was not a big fan of what is called "mentalism" in behavior analysis. *Mentalism* involves using unobservable and unmeasurable features of human experience to explain observable behaviors. In Skinner's view, then, thoughts, emotions, memories, and urges could theoretically be studied but also presented a host of potential problems for accurate scientific inquiry and analysis. He argued that we can predict and control human behavior without attempting to use such unobservable mental experiences as causes of behavior. He was, of course, assailed for this perspective by his critics in the humanistic, psychoanalytic, and cognitive-behavioral wings of clinical science.

At the same time, Skinner acknowledged that human language and thought were "real" but simply could not be studied because they had no observable end products, no behavioral reference points upon which everyone could agree. Skinner speculated near the end of his life that if language ever were studied within a behavior analytic framework, the laws governing the acquisition, maintenance, and functions of language would mirror those explaining the acquisition, maintenance, and functions of other forms of observable human behavior. In other words, language would be nothing special.

In the early 1980s, almost 20 years before the first book on ACT was published, behavior analytic researchers who disagreed with Skinner's skepticism about the utility of including private events within a behavioral analytic framework began conducting basic research into the *functions* of human language and how those functions emerge in a developmental sequence for humans. The groundbreaking results of this research led to a behavior analytic account of human language (RFT) and eventually to ACT as a clinical model. These researchers discovered core features of human language that can result not only in powerful forms of human problem solving but also in powerful and enduring forms of human dysfunction and suffering. They demonstrated that language is both the source of human flexibility and resiliency and the source of behavioral rigidity and psychopathology (Törneke 2010).

The Evolution of Language as a Behavioral Control System

The first thing to understand about language is that it likely evolved to promote social organization, conformity, procreation, and survival. Having an organized social group that behaves in largely predictable ways provides a huge evolutionary advantage both in terms of protecting the group from predators and in promoting procreation and sustained social order.

To function as a member of a tightly organized social group requires that infants learn to follow rules that support the interests of the group. Humans learn these rules in two basic ways: contingency-based learning and symbolically derived relations. *Contingency-based learning* refers to learning directly from the consequences of one's own behavior. Certain actions have certain consequences, and these consequences affect the way we act in a new but perhaps similar situation in the future. Another type of contingency-based learning is to associate events in time and space, such as when Pavlov's dog learned to salivate upon hearing the sound of a bell after several trials of first hearing a bell and then having a bowl of food arrive. Some things occur together in time or in close physical proximity, and that affects how we respond to new situations that might share similar properties. If a certain smell was present during an episode of sexual abuse, then contacting that smell again is likely to elicit many of the thoughts, feelings, memories, or sensations that were present during the original episode of abuse. Both humans and animals rely on contingency-based learning, and this allows them to engage in fairly complex patterns of behavior.

Considering the evolutionary importance of promoting widespread social organization and control, contingency-based learning suffers from one great flaw: the human or animal must directly experience the consequence in order to learn the rule that must be followed. To create and sustain complex social systems and cultural practices requires a far more potent system: symbolically derived relationships that can be readily transmitted through verbal signals rather than learned by direct experience. The evolutionary advantage of human language is directly tied to the fact that it is a far, far more potent way to create complex social systems and cultural practices without being burdened down by the need to transmit this information through contingency-based learning. Human language achieves this feat through a system of *arbitrary, symboli-*

cally derived relations. These arbitrarily derived rules in turn exert direct regulatory influence (control) over the behavior specified in the rule. This means someone else can give us a rule about something we have not directly experienced, and we can use that rule to guide our behavior without directly testing it. For example, when a parent says, "Don't ever touch the burner when it's red or you'll get a nasty burn that will hurt for a long time," the child is not compelled to go up and touch a red-hot burner to learn not to touch the burner. The specification of the behavior (do not touch the burner) and the symbolically derived consequence (you will get a burn that will hurt for a long time) are sufficient to get the job done. Once the ability to both influence and control behavior in this manner was established in human language, it quickly became the dominant way cultural practices and social norms were transferred from one generation to the next. The vast majority of how we behave is controlled, quite simply, by this type of explicit (or implicit) verbal instruction.

Language as a Relational System

In RFT, the building blocks of language are known as *relational frames.* Surprisingly, a limited number of basic relational frames are needed to produce the entire system of symbolic activity we call human language and thought. For example, if you have a relational frame that establishes "now" as different from "then," you are able to relate backward to forward in time. If you also have the ability to create "if/then" relationships, you are able to predict upcoming events based upon selected features of the current context. Another important relational frame, called the *deictic* frame, creates a distinction between *I* and *you*, thus establishing a basic distinction between the originating source and the target of a communication. Once the perspective of *I* is established, it is possible to distinguish between *your* experiences and *my* experiences. This allows us to express our needs, justify and explain our actions, and receive precise verbal instructions from others.

Relational framing allows us to symbolically interact with the world without having to make direct contact with the world. Language helps us do this by allowing us to relate one symbol to another. A sentence such as "I am going to the store" actually contains at least three different symbolic relations. *I* (not *you*) is the subject of this relation. I am moving from where I am to some other place. That place is the store. As this example shows, even simple examples of human language have a lot of moving parts. Notice that this entire communication refers to an action that has not yet happened. This allows the recipient of the communication (*you*) to understand where *I* will be in the immediate future. The listener can infer that if *you* need me to be "here" at a specific time when *I* will be "there," *I* will not be able to help *you* out.

Once we are able to derive symbolic relations, we can relate one thing to another not only on the basis of the physical characteristics of the perceptual target but also by associating perceptual targets together in space and time. We can also relate one thing to another on the basis of signals given by other humans, not only using a unique combination of sounds that we call "words" but also through gestures. We learn, for example, to interact with a ball as "larger" not necessarily because of its physical properties but because of a specific social signal—the word *larger*. Imagine that we gave you two balls that are identical in size, one blue and the other red, and we tell you that the red ball is larger. If we then ask you which ball is the smallest, you would answer "the blue one."

Another example: here are two symbols: φ and Δ. Now, Δ is worth $10,000, and φ *is worth twice as much as* Δ. Which of the two would you rather have? You would likely choose φ. When completing these tasks, you are not responding to the two balls or written symbols in terms of their physical properties but rather based upon their symbolic properties as established by words alone. Language is a shared game that seamlessly transforms the stimulus properties of objects and events. This transformation occurs when we learn to relate objects on the basis of specific verbal signals or cues, such as "smaller," "larger," and "twice as much." This way of relating is called *relational framing*. This behavioral repertoire allows us to put virtually anything in a relational frame. Humans can, in principle, relate anything to anything else, in any possible way.

Rule-Governed Behavior

The ability to relate multiple things to each other in complex ways bestows tremendous evolutionary leverage on humans. One of our most important skills is that we can do something that has painful immediate consequences and keep doing that same behavior because of another symbolic relation that overrides what we would do if we relied only on the immediate consequences. Subject any animal to an action with painful consequences, and the animal will stop engaging in that behavior and likely will avoid being put back in the same basic setting again. However, humans can relate an immediate undesirable consequence to something else that has value or is desirable in the long run and thus sidestep the problem of being controlled by immediate consequences. The extent to which this feature of language can influence behavior is almost unlimited. For example, soldiers in combat have been known to sacrifice their lives to save their fellow soldiers from death. The overarching positive and enduring value of loyalty and camaraderie trumps the highly negative short-term consequence of dying.

The behavioral analytic term for this is *self-instructional control.* Humans have the unique ability to follow symbolically derived instructions delivered by others or themselves through their own relational framing abilities. The RFT term we use for a system of instructional control relations is *rule-governed behavior*. Rule-governed behavior typically contains many individual behavioral units under instructional control, and collectively, the execution of these individual units leads to a larger, socially sanctioned outcome. Rule-governed behavior allows long behavioral sequences to be performed, without any immediate reward, in the service of obtaining desired outcomes long into the future. Human problem solving, goal-directed behavior, and complex ways of cooperating with each other are intimately tied to this type of rule governance.

Language is ultimately a social game we play together. The rules of this game require that our direct experience is no longer the most important thing; its importance is largely determined by how it is related to other things determined to be important within a larger social context. We are now capable of overriding our own wants and needs in the service of helping others: "What I really want is the best for my family"; "In my life, I play by the rules"; "I will do what is the right thing to do." We also make contact with the dark side of this powerful ability to relate anything to almost anything else.

TIPS FOR SUCCESS

Humans learn in two different ways: *contingency-based learning* through direct experience and *symbolically derived stimulus relations* created by verbal instruction.

Humans differ from animals in their widespread reliance on symbolically derived relations, because this allows vast amounts of cultural knowledge and social practices to be transmitted from generation to generation.

Once freed from the need to learn only through direct consequences, humans use language to relate anything to almost anything else and can transmit vast amounts of cultural knowledge via words.

Instructional control refers to behaviors guided by symbolically derived rules that allow humans to reduce the affective valence of short-term consequences in the service of longer-term socially sanctioned outcomes and rewards.

Rule-governed behavior refers to large sequences of behavior that are under the self-instructional control of language.

The Dark Side of Language

Self-instructional control and rule governance give humans the ability to persist with specific behaviors even when the immediate consequences of doing so are negative. This is both a blessing and a curse. We can act independently of direct consequences and go for long-term life goals and associated consequences that we have not yet experienced. This is what you did when you studied for years and years to become a psychiatrist! At the same time, this process presents considerable risk when it takes a wrong turn. *One dangerous feature of rule-governed behaviors is that they diminish the individual's "sensitivity" to the real-world results of following rules. Because of this, rule-governed behaviors are very resistant to change, even when the consequences of following them are negative.* People can ignore the consequences of maladaptive behaviors if the behaviors are under self-instructional control and rule governance. If the derived relation specifies a consequence (C) as a result of behavior (B), but what actually occurs is an unspecified (and unwanted) consequence (D), there is no guarantee the derived relationship will be modified to incorporate the discrepant result D. This phenomenon is what we mean by *context insensitivity.* In some circumstances, verbally constructed rules *prevent us* from engaging in contingency-based learning. We discuss later that, in ACT, the reason patients seek help is because they are following rules for coping and problem solving that do not actually work, but because they are largely unaware they are following rules in the first place, they engage in the same unworkable behaviors over and over again.

A system that allows us to relate anything to anything else without first having to establish the validity of that link directly carries another intrinsic risk. We can amplify our level of subjective distress by relating one distressing subjective experience to another one in the past—or to one that has yet to happen in the future. We can precipitate a full-blown panic attack by talking about a previous one or precipitate an anticipatory panic attack by imagining being in a location we associate with a previous attack, such as the supermarket. We can both trigger and amplify auditory and visual hallucinations just by talking about past experiences with them.

To give you a better idea of how this system works in real life, imagine that you and your dog are out walking on a cold winter day. You walk beside a lake that has been frozen for a few days. The ice is shining and clear. You go out onto the ice and, suddenly, it breaks, plunging you and your dog into the ice-cold water. Fear hits you like a flash of lightning; you and your dog fight for your lives. For a moment, you are under the water, and the next moment you are above the water's surface long enough to catch some air. A passerby happens to see you disappear into the water. This person calls out to some other bystanders, and they rescue you and your dog. Without this stroke of good fortune, you likely would have developed hypothermia and drowned.

If you and your dog take a walk a few weeks later to that particular place on the lake, it is reasonable to expect that you will both experience a contingency-based fear response and will be really reluctant to go out on that ice again. Whereas it would take some significant retraining to make your dog willing to walk back on the ice, you can achieve that outcome yourself just by engaging in a few basic relations, such as, "Back then, it had been freezing for only 2 days, but it's been 2 weeks of 10° temperatures, and that ice will be 6 inches thick by now."

In another way, however, the gift of language presents you with a real problem that your dog does not have. Let's assume that a few hours after you were rescued, you and your dog are sitting in front of the fireplace in your house. You have both had enough to eat and drink. What is at hand for your dog? Is your dog "remembering" the cold water and the possible brush with death? Does your dog fear that he or someone he cares about could end up there again? Nothing we know about dogs would support that. What is present for the dog, in this situation, is the warmth and satisfaction of the immediate situation. Yet it is probably not that simple for you, even though that same warmth and satisfaction are present. You begin to relate your brush with death symbolically in almost any possible way. You analyze what happened and wonder what it means in your life, looking both backward and into the future: "How did that happen? The ice looked safe enough. I've walked on ice like that many times before without problems. How could I be so stupid? Why didn't I realize the ice was too thin to walk on? This is just another time when I've sunk my own boat by acting without thinking. Dad used to tell me my carelessness would eventually come back to haunt me, and he was right." Then, you suddenly notice your daughter's shoes on the floor and remember that she and her third-grade classmates are going on a field trip to the very area where you fell into the water. "I wonder if they know how dangerous it is right now?"

Thus, humans are capable of creating two possible avenues for suffering. One is through our direct experiences and the similarities that future situations might bear to the original, just as other animals experience. The second, and more concerning, is that we can relate our own reactions to others' reactions and to other events in numerous ways, beyond the actual characteristics of the events involved. This can be helpful in some cases, for example, when using a now/then relation to put yourself above the conditioned experience of fear of the lake. However, through the power of categorization, comparison, evaluation, and prediction, you can spiral down into relating this undesirable event (almost drowning) to other things that are undesirable to you, sometimes in the distant past (being criticized by Dad, and his warning that bad things will happen to you in the future).

This feature of language is so powerful that you can generalize painful thoughts and feelings to positive situations just by relating them to some other type of unpleasant experience. Imagine you are spending time at a beautiful beach. The night is pleasantly warm, and you are sitting with some good friends and enjoying a nice meal together. People are talking and enjoying themselves, and you enjoy hearing bits and pieces of one particularly interesting conversation. The ocean is as smooth as a mirror below the large patio where you are sitting. The waiters have just delivered your favorite dinner dish. Everything is delightful; you are having a great time. Then you have the thought, "If only Ann had lived; she would have loved this."

Even good experiences can be related to bad ones. We can be transported anywhere at the speed of thought without moving. Although this provides a huge window of possibilities, it also creates a broader interface with pain and suffering. As long as pain is connected with a certain situation in the external world, we generally have the option of escaping that situation and avoiding it in future. However, where can a person run to escape from pain created simply by thinking?

As a result of their broad interface with symbolically generated pain, humans easily fall into large, organized patterns of rule-governed behaviors designed to escape from, or control, painful thoughts, emotions, and memories. Rule-governed relations supporting escape and avoidance behaviors are in the water supply of contemporary society. It is easy to understand why this would happen. When our subjective experience is painful, we naturally deal with these events in the same way we deal with external threats to our health and well-being: escape and avoidance. Being human involves the ever-present danger of making contact with subjectively unpleasant experiences.

Language and the Experience of Mind

The emergence of language and symbolic learning has created a new context for behavioral control. Thus, humans are in the unique position of having to deal with systems of behavioral control based not only in direct contingencies in the external world but also in the way we symbolically relate one thing to another in the internal world. We are so well trained in this relating that we can do it privately, without other people noticing. The private experience of receiving and reacting to these silent messages creates the experience of the *mind*. An analogy we often use is the distinction between the hardware and operating system of a computer. Our brain is the hardware, and our language system is the software—the OS-X or Windows. The mind is what the operating system shows us on the computer screen. We do not see the millions of lines of software code that form the basis of the operating system, just as we do not see relational framing at the micro level. We see the messages that are the result of relational framing.

Most people have a clear picture of what we mean when we use this analogy. The experience of mind involves an ongoing process of inner perceptual awareness (i.e., we are aware of emotions, memories, urges, thoughts, physical sensations), but we also witness on our computer screens of awareness all of the categorical, evaluative, comparative, and predictive functions of language. This means we are set up not only to be aware of ongoing perceptual experiences but also to evaluate them, compare them to the experiences of others, categorize them, or use them to predict future events or experiences. Most importantly, we experience these activities of mind in the form of an ongoing, silent inner dialogue. Whenever we stop for a moment to see if we are thinking something, we are thinking something. The human being is on the receiving end of this high-powered system, for the most part, and is powerless to stop it.

This feature of mind poses a grave danger to us, particularly when the inner dialogue of the mind functions as a form of instructional control capable of overriding the consequences of rule-following in the external environment. Even more toxic is that this instructional control can lead to patterns of rule governance that actually produce additional damaging consequences in the external world. One example is the "self-concept" generated by using language to relate anything about yourself to anything else about yourself. You can relate a historical event, such as childhood abuse, to a future outcome, such as being unable to enter into a romantic relationship because of "trust issues." Although the language relations are arbitrary and symbolically derived, the behaviors put under instructional control will be highly organized and persistent over time. Thus, although it is technically inaccurate to say childhood abuse causes "trust issues" and social isolation in adulthood, the relational system that is formed will help organize large patterns of behavior *as though* those causal relations are true. The resulting behavior patterns create the consequence specified in the self-instructional rule.

The Problem With Human Problem Solving

The evolutionary advantage of language is closely linked to the way it allows us to control or eliminate threats to survival, health, and well-being through linear, reductive analysis of their causes. By inference, when the cause of a problem is identified and removed, the problem itself will disappear. Thus, human problem solving is based in what we call *discrepancy-based reasoning*. A *discrepancy* is the difference between where you want to be and where you are. To create organized patterns of social behavior requires a near-constant stream of discrepancy-based reasoning to occur on a mass scale. Take, for example, getting to work by 8 A.M. because you have a patient scheduled. Both you and the patient have a discrepancy (problem) to be solved: namely, at 11 P.M. the night before, neither of you is at the site where the visit will take place the next morning. Your brain's problem-solving operations calculate all the steps needed to resolve that discrepancy: You must set your alarm clock for 6:30 A.M.; you have 30 minutes to shower and dress; you have another 30 minutes to eat breakfast; you must leave for the clinic by 7:30 A.M. because rush hour traffic is unpredictable and you must give yourself extra time. Each of these larger strands of problem-solving behavior involves completing many smaller actions in sequence. In ACT, we call this feature of the operating system the *problem-solving mind.* It is perpetually on the alert to identify upcoming problems and to give us the instructions needed to solve them. If you tried to cross a busy intersection without letting your problem-solving mind give you the instructions needed to do so, you would not make it very far.

THE UNWORKABLE CHANGE AGENDA

The problem-solving activities of mind are so ubiquitous and are successful on so many fronts that we automatically assume this approach will work for *every* problem we face. Remember that this feature of language probably evolved because it is able to solve virtually any problem encountered in the physical world. It is literally responsible for why we wear clothing, have a roof over our head, and have a heating and cooling system in our house. Everywhere we look, we see the trademark results of following this powerful analytical method.

If we step back for a minute and examine the parameters that the physical world imposed on our human ancestors as this feature of language evolved, we realize that two essential requirements must be met for the human problem-solving model to work. First, the identified discrepancy must be amenable to direct first-order change. Basically, this means we can undo the undesirable outcome with which we are faced if we discover and reverse the right causes. Second, any causes we identify must also be reversible or changeable. In the external world, these two requirements are easily met in the vast majority of circumstances, but what about events in the world of private experience, such as being sad, having flashbacks of a traumatic event, thinking unpleasant thoughts all the time, or experiencing back pain that persists day in and day out? Do such private events satisfy the two conditions for the human problem-solving model to work?

The short answer is no. Most private experiences not only cannot be kept from occurring but also cannot be voluntarily controlled or eliminated once they appear. Unlike the role of causation in the external world, understanding and analyzing the hypothetical causes of distressing, unwanted mental events will not make them go away. We even have a name for this process when patients carry it to extremes: "analysis paralysis." We can analyze virtually anything within our internal

Table 2–1.   Components of the unworkable change agenda

1. All discrepancies are caused; to change the discrepancy, the cause must be identified, controlled, or eliminated.
2. The reasons we give for discrepancies are good causes.
3. Thoughts, feelings, memories, urges, and sensations are good reasons; therefore, they are good causes.
4. To control the discrepancy, we must control the thoughts, feelings, memories, urges, or sensations.

world, but that will not allow us to functionally eliminate the antecedent forces that originate within our learning history. Given the overwhelming success of the human problem-solving model in almost every domain of existence, most patients (and clinicians) are simply unable to imagine another way to handle such discrepancies. We instead "bootstrap" the problem-solving model so it appears to apply equally well to unwanted discrepancies in our private world. In ACT, this ever-so-slightly modified problem-solving approach is called the *unworkable change agenda* (Table 2–1).

Our cultural allegiance to, and conviction in, the human problem-solving model is demonstrated by the fact that nearly every system of psychotherapy, as well as traditional psychiatry, incorporates the "analyze and eliminate" principle in one way or another. The psychiatrist can confidently assume that patients' efforts to address their mental health problems will follow this same basic approach. Let's say you are feeling sad, blue, and depressed much of the time. According to cultural norms with which you have been indoctrinated for most of your life, you are not supposed to feel this way. A *discrepancy* exists between the way you *should be* feeling and the way you *are* feeling. This activates the first step in the problem-solving sequence: Your poor mood can be reversed, but only if its causes are first identified. The presumption is that if the causes are identified and then reversed or neutralized, you will return to "normal." The next step is to look for reasons why you might be depressed. The problem-solving mind then comes up with some good-looking "reasons," which are then regarded as the "causes" of your mood problems (recent loss of marriage, history of abuse). If problematic thoughts ("I'm lonely"; "I just can't trust people"), feelings (boredom, loneliness), or memories (left alone and neglected as a child) arise, these "reasons" are also assumed to be "causes." The next step is eliminating or controlling their causal influence. The cause in this case is your cumulative learning history and the spontaneous appearance of emotions, thoughts, memories, and physical sensations triggered by any number of historically acquired external or internal antecedents. How do you undo, or reverse, your own learning history? How do you change the spontaneous appearance of your own emotions in the first place?

Indeed, you may even ask, "What's wrong with approaching mental health problems using this method? These disorders are abnormal, and they must be caused by something." As we have discussed, one major drawback is that cause-and-effect relationships are nowhere near as linear in the world of subjective experience; thousands of learning experiences could be seen in one analysis as contributing to suffering and dysfunction and in another as contributing to personal resiliency and positive coping abilities. The problem-solving mind inevitably will "cherry pick" the bits and pieces of learning history that share the same emotional tone. We have known for a long time that memory is incredibly mood specific. Thus, what will be dredged up in this causal analysis will be thoughts, feelings, and memories that are consistent with a patient's current mood state.

WHY UNPLEASANT PRIVATE EVENTS ARE PROBLEMS TO BE SOLVED

On many occasions in this chapter, we have referred to language as a system designed to instill social norms and ensure widespread conformity to prevailing cultural practices. We all incorporate these social norms and cultural practices as part of the ongoing process of acquiring symbolic abilities, not just the ability to use spoken language. These deeply embedded social norms create a picture of what a desirable, normal, healthy existence looks like. We are trained from early childhood on to incorporate this point of reference as a "social compass" that will both direct and regulate our behavior in innumerable life domains and social circumstances.

An unfortunate and largely overlooked reality is that a major discrepancy exists between what contemporary social training says life is like and what life *actually* is like. The culturally promoted image is that "health" means freedom from distressing, unwanted feelings, thoughts, memories, urges, or physical symptoms. The natural corollary is that to be healthy and happy is the natural "resting state" of humanity. In ACT, we call this culturally sanctioned belief the *myth of healthy normality.* Any significant deviation from this idealized state of freedom from all discomfort is therefore a discrepancy that must be addressed. When these threats to health are eliminated, we will return to a state of health and happiness. In reality, a typical human life is full of moments that produce painful, unwanted subjective experiences. People you love are going to die; you might lose a child to cancer; you might get divorced and will most certainly be involved in some painful relationship breakups; you might lose your job and retirement savings at the same time; you might be involved in a serious automobile accident. The list of uncontrollable life events goes on and on. No matter which way you turn, distressing, unwanted experiences are headed in your direction, either as a result of the history that has already transpired in your life or the history that has yet to transpire.

The problem-solving mind plays a specific role in widening the gap between the idealized view of human existence and what actually happens over the course of a human life. Everywhere we look, it seems, we receive the message that feeling bad is bad for our health, and the way to get back to our natural state of health is to get rid of anything that produces discomfort. Distressing, unwanted emotions, thoughts, memories, urges, and sensations are now problems to be solved rather than automatic, learned, immediate responses to life events as they unfold, embedded in a specific context. They are threats to your health, making contact with them is toxic, and they must be avoided, suppressed, or eliminated to protect your health. If they cannot be directly controlled or eliminated, then the next best strategy is to deny their existence, suppress them, or consciously avoid them.

The Important Role of Self-Reflective Awareness

Fortunately, relational framing also provides us with access to another mode of mind called *self-reflective awareness.* It is known by many other names in other spiritual or human growth traditions: the "observer self," "wise mind," "transcendent self," and even the "observing ego" if you are steeped in the psychoanalytic tradition. The same basic processes of language that lead to rule-following also allow us to use deictic framing to offset the regulatory effects of language. Via deictic framing, we can create a clear distinction between the ongoing experience of mind and the perspective of the one experiencing it. In this *I/you* frame, the human being is different from the mind. This way of relating to the experience of mind offers us a way to diminish the regulatory dominance of arbitrarily derived rules. We can notice we are having a dialogue with our mind. We notice that we have a mind, but we are not the same as our mind. We are the ones listening to the ongoing silent discourse of mind. This forms the basis for understanding what it means to be conscious. Language allows us to be *aware* that we exist; it gives us the experience of self. In early language training, we learn to take this kind of perspective on our own reactions largely for social communication and control purposes. However, with proper training and practice, we can extend this ability so that it helps us recognize unhelpful sequences of rule governance and self-instructional control, measure the real consequences of following rules, and make changes to existing rules or create new ones that will govern our behaviors. The growing popularity in the lay public of mindfulness practices in all their many forms is testimony to the growing recognition that cultivating self-reflexivity promotes psychological well-being. In ACT, this context of *I* as the perspective from which all our inner and outer experience unfolds is something we try to strengthen, because this allows the patient to step back and dis-identify with the contents of the mind. Unfortunately, contemporary cultural practices typically neglect or downplay the importance of self-reflective awareness, and consequently, most of us have relatively weak skills in this important area. In ACT, we assume human suffering is largely the result of failures in self-reflective awareness, leading to automatic, habitual rule governance. Thus, the focus of ACT is on teaching the patient to come back into the moment and practice self-aware behaviors such as nonjudgmental awareness, detachment, and self-compassion.

TIPS FOR SUCCESS

Rule-governed behaviors are very resistant to being changed based on their real-world consequences. Instead, they persist even when the results of following the rule are negative.

A good analogy for understanding the role of language and thought is to think of the brain as the hardware of a computer and language as the operating system. We do not typically see most language operations, just as we do not see the software code that underpins an operating system.

The relational functions of mind are habitual and ubiquitous and often are extended into matters of subjective well-being with disastrous results.

We can relate past emotional experiences or memories to future outcomes in ways that trick us into believing past experiences actually cause present-day outcomes.

Human language equips us with a problem-solving framework that is fantastically successful in the physical world but is destined to fail when applied to distressing, unwanted experiences in our private world.

Self-reflective cognition helps create the perspective of *I* and the distinction between "me" and "what I'm aware of inside of me."

Self-reflective awareness allows us to look at our own "programming" and self-instructional rules and thereby reduce their regulatory influence on behavior.

> Experiencing the distinction between yourself as an acting person on one hand, and your mind on the other, is a key factor in escaping from the regulatory influence of rule governance and is a skill that is cultivated in ACT.

The ACT Clinical Framework

We are now in a position to answer the question raised at the beginning of this chapter. How is it that bright, well-intentioned, motivated people will try the same unworkable life strategy over and over again, even though the consequences are negative and self-defeating? The answer is that their behavior is *rule governed*, and this generates an insensitivity to the negative consequences of *rule-following*. If your behavior is under instructional control, you risk continuing with that behavior regardless of the direct short-term consequences of your actions. Rule-governed behavior is often far removed from any actual contact with immediate consequences because the promised consequences of following the rule are either in the intermediate/distant future or are so abstract as to be unfalsifiable (e.g., "doing what my dad would do"). The habitual tendency to obey instructions, combined with the culturally established rules that say we must control or eliminate distressing, unwanted private experiences, sets people up to suffer.

As the old saying goes, however, it takes two to tango. Without active "buy-in" on the part of the human being, the mind's rules and mandates would simply fall on deaf ears, figuratively speaking. Thus, to understand the origins of psychopathology, we need to be aware of the processes that trap our patients in persistent, enduring patterns of unworkable behavior. In the ACT approach, three basic processes—alone or in combination—can lead to suffering and psychopathology. For visual learners, these processes are presented in Figure 2–1. In the sections that follow, we examine these toxic processes in more detail.

In popular parlance, we refer to these three toxic pathways to suffering as being *closed off, checked out,* and *disengaged.* Individuals who are suffering, including those with mental health or substance abuse concerns, are not willing to feel what they feel inside but instead are reactive, judgmental, and tend to reject any unpleasant internal experiences. Often, they have difficulty paying attention to their own experience as it unfolds in the moment and have difficulty taking perspective on themselves or the workability of their actions in the world. Their lifestyle tends to be organized not around personal values and deeply held life aspirations but rather by social rules and norms that are habitually and automatically followed. In technical terms, the three toxic processes underlying suffering and psychopathology are rule-following/context insensitivity, emotional avoidance, and behavior avoidance.

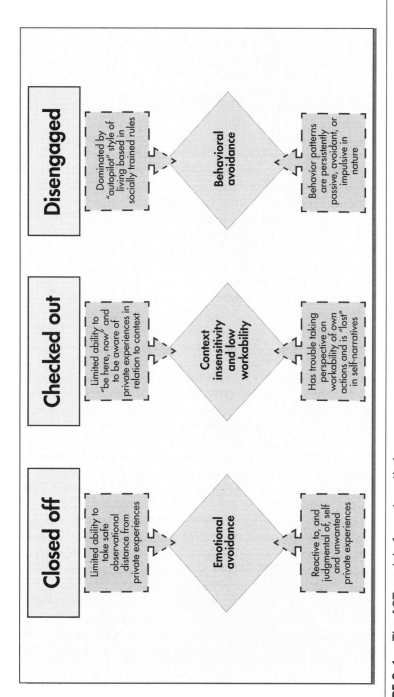

FIGURE 2–1. The ACT model of psychopathology.

Rule-Following and Context Insensitivity

In the ACT approach, rule-following and context insensitivity are at the heart of human suffering and psychopathology. *Rule-following* is problematic when it involves repeated use of rule-governed behaviors that are not serving the best interest of the human being. *Context insensitivity* means the person cannot generate the self-reflective awareness needed to foster a workable form of perspective-taking on the consequences of following a particular rule in a particular context. As we noted earlier, a cardinal feature of rule-governed behavior is that it creates insensitivity to the actual consequences of following a specified rule, and as a result, unworkable rules do not get changed and patterns of unworkable behavior persist despite negative consequences. When combined with low levels of reflective self-awareness, rule-following results in an over-identification with products of mind, such that the distinction between the human and the mind is lost. In many instances, people trapped in this process are not aware they are following rules, nor do they understand what rules they are following. Furthermore, failure to separate oneself from the processes of the mind (e.g., emotions, memories, intrusive thoughts, sensations), a cardinal feature of deficient self-reflective awareness, severely limits our perspective-taking abilities. Thus, rule-following with deficient self-reflective cognition is a prerequisite for 1) believing that a distressing, unwanted private experience is a threat to one's health; 2) believing that the immediate goal is to suppress, control, or eliminate such experiences rather than make room for them; and 3) continuing persistent use of avoidance strategies that paradoxically make the avoided experience more intrusive and psychologically distressing. The resulting context insensitivity produced by rule-following and deficient self-reflective awareness prevents the individual from recognizing the futility of this system of rule governance, thus reducing the likelihood that new, workable strategies will be implemented.

For a clinical example of the basic problem of rule-following and context insensitivity, consider the problem of rumination and worry, both cardinal features of mood and anxiety disorders. In most cases, the patient has repeatedly analyzed and "thought through" a particular problem but has not achieved the hoped-for consequence of feeling less depressed or anxious. Still, the patient continues to ruminate because a rule is being followed that says, "If you think about this long and hard enough, you'll eventually discover why you're not happy, and then you can fix it." When rumination gets really bad, it can dominate a person's behavior to the extent of completely blocking important life pursuits; the direct consequence—no change in mood, blocking of life pursuits—does not affect the behavior of ruminating. The problem is that the rule-governed relation is able to change the meaning of these immediate consequences by creating a new relation ("just keep at it; it takes time, and you'll eventually unlock the secret that will let you feel better"). Now rumination is no longer evaluated based on its immediate impact on one's mood or sense of life vitality, it is about "doing the right thing" and "what I must do to solve my problem in the long run."

Emotional and Behavioral Avoidance

Ultimately, as we pointed out earlier, attempts to suppress, control, or eliminate distressing private experiences are not just destined to fail; they actually make matters worse. Most private experiences are historically learned and automatically triggered responses that cannot be controlled voluntarily. We think what we think, we feel what we feel, we remember what we remember, and no amount of cognitive effort is going to reverse that reality. Instead, persistent attempts to suppress, control, or eliminate distressing, unwanted experiences have the paradoxical effect of increasing our level of subjective distress. Research within both experimental psychopathology and emotion science clearly demonstrates that efforts at suppression and avoidance result in a *rebound effect* (Flynn et al. 2010; Wegner et al. 1987). This means that when thoughts, feelings, memories, or urges are suppressed, they soon rebound back into awareness in a far more intrusive way and are experienced as more aversive and uncontrollable. In ACT, we have a quite pedestrian way of saying this: "If you're not willing to have it, you'll get more of it."

When direct attempts to control or eliminate unwanted private experiences backfire, we have a fallback position. If the distressing experience cannot be controlled or eliminated directly, the next best option is to avoid making direct contact with it. This unwillingness to make direct psychological contact with distressing, unwanted private experiences is called *emotional avoidance*. Although people avoid experiences other than unpleasant emotions (e.g., traumatic memories, uncomfortable urges, intrusive negative thoughts, painful sensations), the common pathway shared by all these experiences is that they create negative affect. In the end, private experiences are avoided because of the emotional discomfort they create when experienced directly. In some scientific circles, the term used to describe this general tendency to avoid any kind of unpleasant internal experience is *experiential avoidance*. High levels of experiential avoidance have been associated with almost every conceivable kind of mental or addictive disorder as well as with high levels of psychological distress in nonclinical populations (Hayes et al. 1996).

In this book, we use the term *emotional avoidance* as a synonym for *experiential avoidance*, because most often negative emotional experiences or the eminent threat of having them is what drives rule-governed avoidance behaviors. Indeed, lowered levels of present-moment awareness might serve a protective function, if the goal is to keep from making experiential contact with distressing, unwanted experiences. However, "checking out" (e.g., reduced perspective-taking ability, exaggerated rule-following, context insensitivity) to support a strategy of emotional avoidance also has a cost. Patients practice experiential avoidance by verbally regulated means, such as refusal to talk about their private experiences, distraction, deliberate self-instructions to think about something else, changing the topic when they come close to making contact with unwanted experience, daydreaming, or chronic worrying.

An effective way to pursue emotional avoidance is by meticulously identifying and avoiding real-life situations, events, or interactions that might trigger distressing, unwanted private experiences. Alternatively, some people use impulsive, self-defeating behaviors that effectively result in their expulsion from social contexts that might trigger unwanted private experiences. This pattern of isolation, withdrawal, or impulsive reactivity is called *behavioral avoidance*. Behavioral avoidance is toxic because those life situations that matter the most are precisely the situations most likely to produce painful and unwanted private experiences. You cannot fall in love if you are not willing to have the feelings associated with falling out of love. Anything that really matters in life is also capable of inflicting painful emotional consequences. In fact, it is fair to say that what makes these life pursuits so important is that failure, disappointment, or setback is a distinct possibility. Being willing to subject ourselves to the pain of loss, disappointment, or failure legitimizes our striving. Avoidance behaviors rapidly generalize and can quickly become the dominant feature of a person's lifestyle, such that contact is lost with basic life aspirations and goals. Life itself becomes organized around the need to avoid specific kinds of private experiences. As is true for emotional avoidance, behavioral avoidance does not make things better; it makes things worse. Ignoring a major marital problem because of the fear of rejection or divorce does not make the marital issue go away; it will continue unabated, and remaining silent may actually add to those marital problems.

Patients often come for psychiatric care after they have been in distress for years and their ways of coping have failed. They may feel alone, defective, lacking purpose, and unable to live the kind of life they believe other people are living—fundamentally, their sense of life vitality is going downhill. Their avoidance of distressing emotions and the real-world experiences that might produce them (e.g., relationships, social roles, activities) has resulted in a variety of powerful and distressing cognitive, emotional, and physical reactions. In ACT, these reactions are conceptualized as the logical and necessary results of avoidance, and they cannot be understood in a functional sense without understanding the exterior and interior contexts in which they are embedded. Normally, a patient will be following a rule that relates "health and happiness" to "freedom from emotional distress" and a companion rule that specifies "to achieve health, I must get rid of my emotional distress." Following this rule opens a Pandora's box of unworkable, rigid, and unchanging patterns of avoidance behavior. As long as the rules remain silent, unrecognized, or unquestioned, these behavior patterns will persist regardless of how intelligent, well-intentioned, and motivated the person might be. For these reasons, in ACT, a core mantra reflects this alternative approach to human suffering: *People are not broken; they are only trapped.*

Before we discuss the ACT treatment approach, remember that rule-following/context insensitivity and emotional and behavioral avoidance are the natural results of our hardwiring and social training. All of us are trained to follow rules that encourage the use of emotional and behavioral avoidance strategies, and we do so even though these strategies do not really work. Thus, from an ACT perspective, no clear dividing line exists between the dilemmas of daily living that we all face and the issues that people with "mental health problems" are facing. With one twist of fate, the tables could easily be reversed so that you become the patient and the patient becomes the psychiatrist. The dividing line, if one exists that actually matters, is the extent to which emotional and behavioral avoidance are functioning as barriers to living a life worth living. ACT does not deny that other variables may contribute to clinical problems (e.g., genetic, biological, sociocultural), but the culturally promoted practice of emotional and behavioral avoidance is assumed to be of central importance in every case, regardless of the type of diagnosis present.

TIPS FOR SUCCESS

Rule-following can result in a dysfunctional self-instructional control designed to regulate, eliminate, or suppress distressing, unwanted private experiences.

Rule-following produces *context insensitivity*, or the reduced ability to appraise the real-world consequences of avoidance strategies, such that those unworkable strategies continue to be used.

Low levels of self-reflective (present-moment) awareness make people more prone to following rules, without being aware they are doing so.

Low levels of awareness also can be part of an array of emotional avoidance strategies.

Emotional avoidance is the unwillingness to make direct, undefended contact with emotionally distressing, unwanted private experiences.

Emotional avoidance paradoxically increases the intensity and invasiveness of distressing, unwanted private events.

Behavioral avoidance involves systematic attempts to avoid life events, situations, or interactions that might trigger feared and unwanted private experiences.

Persistent patterns of behavioral avoidance activate emotional feedback loops that create "symptoms" of distress that result in help-seeking behaviors.

Humans are "hard wired" to follow mental rules that encourage various kinds of emotional and behavioral avoidance. Thus, all humans are set up to experience the emotional consequences of these toxic processes.

The ACT Treatment Framework

The ACT treatment framework consists of three therapeutic mechanisms specifically designed to reverse each of the three toxic processes that produce suffering. For each process that leads to psychological rigidity and suffering, a corollary ACT process leads instead to psychological flexibility and a sense of vital, purposeful living. One important implication of this approach is that psychopathology and psychological health are underpinned by the same basic processes, defined on a continuum ranging from deficit to strength. This approach is directly analogous to theories of circuit-based or biochemical mechanisms involved in mental disorders—the same circuit or neurotransmitter is implicated in mental health and mental illness. The same pathways and means are implicated in both brain function and in dysfunction. Figure 2–2 presents the ACT model of psychological resilience.

In basic terms, the answer to being closed off, checked out, and disengaged is to foster openness to internal experience, promote context sensitivity via reflective self-awareness, and encourage values-based life engagement. As shown in Figure 2–2, cultivating self-reflective awareness, because of its beneficial impact on the problem of automatic rule-following and context insensitivity, underpins all of the therapeutic mechanisms of ACT. For this reason, being self-aware is often called the "center pillar" of the ACT model. Just as the windshield wiper on a car sweeps left and right to keep the visual field clear for the driver, self-reflective awareness sweeps to the left to help us stay detached and nonjudgmental about our internal experiences and then sweeps to the right to produce clarity about our personal values, life aspirations, and behavioral intentions. All the while, self-reflective awareness keeps us from lapsing into rule-following and falling prey to the context insensi-

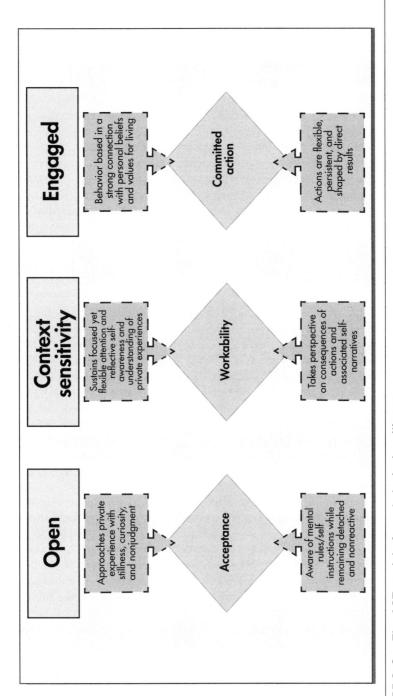

FIGURE 2–2. The ACT model of psychological resilience.

tivity that rule-following produces. It also creates a positive form of self perspective-taking. An important part of perspective-taking involves moving beyond the immediacy of distressing private experiences and looking at the "bigger picture" of life. This type of perspective-taking brings the individual into contact with personal values such that they can function as a new form of self-instructional control.

Self-reflective awareness thus plays a key role in helping the individual discriminate between life contexts in which rule-following is both appropriate and workable and life contexts in which contingency-based learning is more likely to be a workable approach. This central role explains why ACT employs so many different kinds of attention-control interventions, such as controlled breathing, relaxation training, guided imagery, exposure, experiential processing exercises, mindfulness exercises, and metaphors. All of these interventions are designed to teach the patient how to stay in the moment, practice acceptance of what shows up, and engage in more workable, values-based strategies.

The Three Mechanisms of ACT Treatment

Apart from maintaining a relentless focus on helping patients get present and focus self-reflective attention in the moment, what should you, the psychiatric clinician, do to increase the probability they will break loose from rule-following and act in a more flexible way? Three basic principles guide all ACT treatment decisions. They are not necessarily applied in any particular order but are to be considered more as parallel features of the therapeutic process; they appear and reappear from one session to the next. Indeed, the ability to fluidly move between these principles heightens the impact of the clinical conversation in ACT. For ease of understanding, we pull apart and describe each principle separately, with the caveat that the ability to move fluidly between these principles is the cornerstone of ACT.

CONTEXT SENSITIVITY (WORKABILITY)

As we have already noted, context sensitivity is a process by which patients use self-reflective awareness to identify patterns of rule-governed behavior, examine their real-world results, and choose whether to use the same strategies again or try new ones. Another clinical term used is *workability*. Workability is the essential metric to which the ACT clinician keeps returning over and over again. After all, the goal of treatment is to help patients determine which life strategies are working and which are not. We are, in effect, teaching patients to discriminate between the situations in which it is useful to follow the instructions of mind and situations in which those instructions are likely to backfire and make things worse. Most importantly, conversations about workability implicitly suggest an alternative to the definition of what is "workable," other than whether a particular strategy helps us control or eliminate distressing unwanted emotions: this new metric is whether a particular strategy moves you in the direction of living a valued life, regardless of its impact on distressing private experiences. Workability turns the clinical conversation from finding new and better ways to control or eliminate distressing private experiences to seeking valued directions in life. The patient comes to understand that this necessarily involves being willing to have distressing private experiences show up as a direct result of engaging in a valued action.

It is fair to say that establishing workability as the "yardstick" of success in life is the first big acceptance move patients must make in ACT. Although patients usually have lots of direct experience with the results of avoidance, they usually have significantly less with the results of living according to their values. We cannot engage in both approach and avoidance behaviors at the same time, so something has to give: Patients first have to stop using unworkable strategies before they can discover more workable ones. Furthermore, patients can, and do, become quite invested in being "right" about the need to follow avoidance rules that often have been repeatedly socially reinforced.

Using workability as the new metric, we essentially create new rule-governed relationships to counter patients' older, more well-practiced avoidance rules. One new rule is to stop doing things that do not work. Another is that for a strategy to be considered successful, it must promote patients' *longer-term interests* as they relate to the patients' unfolding *best* interests, given the patients' life context. Indeed, some avoidance strategies actually work well to promote patients' *short-term interests*, if those interests primarily hinge on controlling or eliminating distressing private experiences (e.g., drinking, using drugs, purging, lashing out, self-harming behaviors). These strategies usually fail to pass the test of intermediate- or longer-term workability. For drugs or alcohol to work as emotional-control strategies, the patient has to take drugs or drink more and more often and consume greater and greater amounts until a second big problem called addiction develops. In truth, most of the fast-acting avoidance strategies that work in the short run share one common feature: You must keep doing them more and more frequently over time in order for them to continue working, and they will eventually have a life-diminishing effect.

The main way to elicit this type of recognition is to analyze examples of situations the patient finds distressing or troubling, with the clinician and patient working together to identify antecedent factors (A) to the patient's behavior (B) and the resulting consequences (C). The goal is to help patients make experiential contact with the paradoxical results of avoidance to discover which types of events, situations, and interactions create distressing, unwanted internal experiences and trigger avoidance-based self-instructions. Often, self-reflective awareness, and the perspective-taking ability it engenders, will come into the conversation as the psychiatrist and patient attempt to gauge whether the consequences ensuing from avoidance strategies are "worth it." If not, a discussion of what alternatives to avoidance are available will often lead to the second ACT mechanism: openness.

OPENNESS

In ACT, we pose an alternative to emotional avoidance: *openness.* One key aspect of this behavioral strategy is *acceptance,* or the "A" in ACT. Acceptance means taking a detached, nonreactive, and nonjudgmental stance toward what shows up in awareness. Struggling with or trying to control or change what one is thinking, feeling, remembering, or sensing is unnecessary. Indeed, no action is necessary at all.

Practicing acceptance is very difficult if we cannot keep an observational distance between ourselves and what shows up in awareness. This tension connects back to the critical role self-reflective awareness plays in promoting the ability to take perspective on our responses or reactions. The behavioral repertoire underlying acceptance is the ability to take perspective, to make a distinction between oneself as an acting person and whatever shows up in one's awareness. For acceptance to occur, we must drive a wedge between simple awareness of whatever is present and the products of mentation. The closer we get to the symbolic activity of the mind, the harder it becomes to recognize that we are not the same as our thoughts, feelings, memories, or urges. Lack of such observational distance leads to overidentification with the literal meaning of our private experiences, and those evaluations in turn trigger control- and avoidance-oriented self-instructions. Thus, practicing openness allows patients to use self-reflective awareness to detach from the literal meaning of their private experiences. Having a thought called "I am a loser" is not the same as *being* a loser. When this distinction is lost, rules take over, and the ability to respond flexibly is lost.

Overidentification with the *content* of mentation is the typical state of affairs when patients enter therapy. Most patients do not even know that they are hooked by and following mental self-instructions until they are asked, "What does your mind tell you to do when sadness (the voices, anxiety, guilt, shame, loneliness, the urge to drink or do drugs) shows up?" Thus, the problem is not only that they are following a mental rule that does not work but also that they are not aware of the presence of mental instructions that encourage avoidance.

The first skill is to help patients dis-identify with the content of mental experiences and simply notice that these mental products (i.e., distressing thoughts, feelings, memories, urges, or sensations) are present. Developing the ability to establish an observational distance from one's reactions in situations where these reactions arise (what we feel, think, sense, and remember) is absolutely essential if one is to escape the regulatory influence of avoidance-based rule-following. The products of mentation in the moment (i.e., feelings, thoughts, memories, urges) are to be noticed and recognized as part of immediate perceptual experience but are not to be taken "literally." One can learn to just notice mental events and activities in the moment and to establish an observational distance from them as they occur.

Another way to describe this essential skill and its helpfulness is to say that we can take a nonreactive, nonjudgmental stance toward the contents of mind. A popular term for this in lay culture is to practice *detachment*, or letting go, of any urge to react to or struggle with what has shown up in awareness. We can have thoughts, feelings, and memories show up, notice them, and then choose what to do next, including doing nothing at all. Detachment introduces a kind of distance or skepticism about mental events, including emotions and the literal meaning attached to lived experiences. This aspect of ACT may seem paradoxical to some, because many therapies, particularly traditional cognitive-behavioral therapy, actually encourage patients to actively engage their distressing experiences with the aim of changing their meaning, in the belief that doing so will change their emotional reactions from mostly negative to mostly positive. This "fork in the road" reveals the essential difference between a *content*-oriented therapy and a *context*-oriented approach. In the contextual approach, the content or form of private experiences does not need to be changed; we only need to recognize the distinction between the private experience and the person having the private experience. As we discussed earlier in this chapter, the instructional control of the problem-solving mind only works if we "react" to and "attach" significance to the content of the messages in order to control or eliminate distressing content. Practicing nonjudgment means just what it says: we do not judge the truth or falsehood of anything that appears in awareness, including instructions coming from the mind. In contrast, making judgments about the "meaning" of private experiences necessitates taking actions based on those judgments. The culturally transmitted rules about what to do about painful emotions are full of judgments about what is good and bad for us and equally strong judgments about what we must do to protect our health. In the silent mental space created by being nonreactive and nonjudgmental, none of this cultural training matters. The rules coming from the problem-solving mind are just strings of words that, if said over and over very rapidly, would quickly disintegrate into incomprehensible guttural sounds.

This critical aspect of ACT work had its foundations in the repeated use of the workability metric described in the previous section. This teaches patients to use a specific kind of self-reflective analysis, of noticing that "this is something I think/feel/remember" and then that "this is what I did in response to what I was thinking/feeling/remembering." We can use the approach of openness, of establishing an observational distance, when coming into contact with the content of spontaneously aroused thoughts, feelings, or memories. Naming those private experiences is analytically important for understanding which aspects of a situation tend to trigger avoidance behaviors, but the focus is not on judging whether a private experience is justified. In ACT, everything is "real" at the perceptual level; you *did* have a thought, a feeling, or a sensation in your body. You can be a witness to those private experiences, and describe them quite accurately, without using any evaluations or judgments at all.

Another consequence of using this skill is that it increases ongoing contact with, and awareness of, private experiences as they unfold from moment to moment. It allows us to have a clean interface with moment-to-moment experience, thus allowing us to better "connect the dots" between events outside and inside of us. If your sadness or anxiety is not a sign of psychopathology, then what does it signify? Perhaps your emotional responses are telling you that something important to you is at stake in this situation.

In the practice of ACT, psychiatrists will quite frequently, out of genuine caring and curiosity, ask patients things such as, "What is showing up for you right now as we talk about this? Can you just let yourself touch that in your mind's eye and notice if it has a texture, a shape, a color, a temperature, a smell?" Alternatively, they might ask, "Are you with me right now? Are you here in the room, or are you somewhere else? Can you bring yourself back into the room with me?" This aspect of self-reflective awareness, or taking perspective on our own responding, allows us to transcend the provocative and evocative pull of distressing private experiences. If we are going to make any judgments about ongoing and distressing private experiences, it is that they are small matters on a cosmic scale, destined to change with the passage of time. In addition, any painful internal experiences are a shared feature of humanity and link us to other humans, rather than putting us on an island separate from others, as our mind would like us to believe. This allows us to remain in contact with distressing internal experiences and yet not get absorbed in their painful nature.

Engagement

Thus far, we have focused on the many problems that can arise because of the language-based ability to interact with, evaluate, and respond in self-defeating ways to our internal experiences. Language is in many ways a double-edged sword. Rely on it too heavily, and you suffer. Rely on it too lightly, and you suffer. In our quest to avoid suffering, we must not overlook the fact that the ability to interact with our own responses is an asset to be mobilized for positive clinical purposes. A distinct advantage may be gained from being able to follow self-supplied instructions, when those instructions are applied to the right purpose.

In ACT, we help patients develop new rule-governed relations that help them rise above the desire to feel good now and engage in their longer-term best interests as framed by their deeply held values and aspirations in life. Although the ultimate goal is to help patients engage in workable behaviors situated in a dynamic life context, the principle of engagement is also realized in the act of valuing itself. In ACT, we want patients to engage with these deeply held beliefs and life aspirations because doing so is inherently uplifting and brings out the best in each of us. Patients can set a destination in life for which they are willing to endure pain and discomfort now and keep moving toward their destination. In ACT, these positive, forward-looking instructional control relations are called *values.* Values are the underlying principles that we want to live by and for, and they function as motivational fuel for moving toward vitality-producing life pursuits. Values can never be reached in the literal sense, because the ends they refer to involve a never-ending quest. If you value being a loving, devoted, passionate life partner, no matter how good you were at doing that today, you still have to do more of it tomorrow. You do not achieve being a loving, devoted, passionate partner; you can only aspire to be that kind of person throughout your life. Only human beings can aspire to exemplify certain abstract qualities such as compassion, love, loyalty, and altruism. These are the most complex symbolic activities language has to offer.

For many patients, engaging in actions based in their values occurs more or less automatically once they have learned to accept, rather than avoid, their distressing, unwanted experiences. If you no longer let yourself be inhibited or controlled by everything that is automatically aroused in you and instead just notice what is there in a nonjudgmental way, what will your next step be? What is important to you in this situation? If avoidance-based rule-following no longer has you in its grasp, where will you go? What active steps can you now take that are consistent with your values?

If patients take new concrete steps in a valued direction, the memories, thoughts, feelings, and physical sensations that functioned as barriers in the past likely will be triggered once more. In that moment, the problem-solving mind will automatically produce the avoidance rule and warn of the dire consequences of not following it. Using the skills of nonreactivity, nonjudgment, and present-moment awareness, patients simply notice what is displayed on the computer screen of awareness.

Once freed from the need to obey the instructions of the problem-solving mind, patients reach a *choice point.* A choice point is a moment in time when we are free to move in one of two directions: toward avoidance and control of unwanted private experiences or toward valued life ends. This is not a decision based in an elaborate pro/con analysis. Rather, it is a choice based in values, which exert a different kind of self-instruction control, called *appetitive control.* Appetitive control means a behavior is under the control of previously experienced or predicted positive reinforcement. The patient engages in a new response because that response has been mentally assigned a positive valence or tropism; it is something the patient believes in and is drawn toward. A new world order is thus established in the rule-governed relation: "Going after what matters to me in my life is more important than controlling how I feel along the way." This new form of self-instructional control essentially incorporates older avoidance rules by reference and thus overrides their dominance in the patient's response hierarchy. The result is greater behavioral variability and flexibility in life situations that require them.

In ACT, we call this form of values-based responding *committed action,* the "C" in ACT. Committed action involves the conscious intention to act in values-consistent ways in specific situations, despite the emotional discomfort such actions may arouse. A kindling effect occurs as patients learn that the health-producing effects of committed actions clearly outweigh the health-promoting effects of avoidance. These new language relations spill over into other valued areas and quickly generalize as the new way to organize daily behavior. Even when avoidance behaviors prevail and values are not lived up to, a new value surfaces that states when commitments are not followed, the next step is recommitting to the committed action. There is no such thing as failure, only choices that are values consistent and choices that are not. By employing values as the framework for organizing and guiding daily routines and behavioral choices, we are taking the best feature that human language has to offer—the ability to persist over long periods of time—and turning it into a powerful clinical mechanism.

TIPS FOR SUCCESS

A ubiquitous focus of ACT is strengthening patients' self-reflective awareness and perspective-taking ability, with the goal of helping them establish observational distance from their own private responses.

Three basic therapeutic processes underpin the ACT treatment approach: *context sensitivity/workability*, *openness*, and *engagement*.

Context sensitivity/workability requires psychiatrists to help patients learn to discriminate between situations in which it is useful to engage in control-based strategies and those in which acceptance is the best course of action.

Workability offsets the pernicious effects of avoidance-based rule-following by helping patients make direct experiential contact with the costs of avoidance, thus increasing their reliance on contingency-based learning.

Openness requires psychiatrists to help patients learn to create observational distance from, and practice acceptance of, distressing and unwanted emotions, thoughts, memories, cognitive experiences, urges, or sensations. Openness decreases the likelihood patients will use emotional avoidance strategies.

Engagement requires psychiatrists to help patients develop new flexible rules that help them rise above the desire to feel good now and instead act in the service of personal values and life aspirations. Engagement decreases the likelihood that patients will use behavioral avoidance strategies.

Summary

In this chapter, we introduced the most basic elements of the ACT approach, ranging from its basic science origins to the fully evolved present-day model of psychopathology and clinical intervention. Along the way, we touched upon one of the most paradoxical features of human evolution: language. Language is the crown jewel of humanity, but it is also responsible for the worst that humanity has to offer. The unlimited relational power of language has been extended into areas in which it does not belong, but we have been relatively powerless as a species to stop this negative evolutionary process. ACT is a clinical model that actively attempts to undermine the dominance of language by teaching the owners of this powerful operating system to see it for what it is, not what it appears to be. Only by driving a wedge between the human and the human's mind can we allow other forms of human intelligence (e.g., intuition, prophecy, inspiration, compassion) to play an equally important role in how we live our lives. Interventions designed to promote heightened context sensitivity, perspective-taking on the workability of one's actions, openness to immediate experience, and engagement in values-based actions are central to the practice of ACT. All of these therapeutic principles lead to psychological flexibility and the ability to respond to new life challenges with new strategies, particularly when the old strategies no longer work. Personal values and life aspirations now function as the new framework for organizing and guiding daily life and behavioral choices. In doing so, we are taking advantage of the defining feature of rule-governed behavior and transforming it into a powerful clinical methodology. In essence, we use the most basic evolutionary advantage of language (i.e., the ability to follow workable self-instructions) to offset its most damaging effects (i.e., the ability to follow unworkable self-instructions)! In essence, we have to fight fire with fire without getting burned.

The Essentials

- Language is at the heart of all human suffering and psychopathology.
- Language is a system for relating one thing to another thing, anchored in a surprisingly limited number of relations.
- The ability to relate anything to anything else also broadens our interface with painful experiences.
- At the social organization level, language functions as a powerful system of regulatory control.
- At the individual human level, language regulates behavior via a process known as self-instructional control, or silently stated mental rules for how to behave in a specific context.
- Some socially sanctioned mental rules see distressing, unwanted internal experiences as harmful to our health, triggering futile attempts to control, eliminate, or avoid those experiences.
- Overidentifying with avoidance self-instructions leads to ever-widening, unworkable patterns of emotional and behavioral avoidance.
- Patients develop symptoms of distress in response to widening patterns of emotional and behavioral avoidance but seldom realize their behavior is under the control of mental rules.
- ACT helps patients develop and strengthen their self-reflective awareness and perspective-taking skills. These abilities allow patients to create a safe observational distance from the mental mandates of the mind.
- ACT encourages patients to be open to their uncomfortable internal experiences while remaining nonjudgmental, nonreactive, and self-compassionate.
- ACT seeks to bring patients into contact with their closely held values, or aspirations for a life well lived, and to intentionally live in accordance with those values.

Suggested Readings

Costa J, Pinto-Gouveia J: The mediation effect of experiential avoidance between coping and psychopathology in chronic pain. Clin Psychol Psychother 18(1):34–47, 2011

Fledderus M, Bohlmeijer ET, Pieterse ME: Does experiential avoidance mediate the effects of maladaptive coping styles on psychopathology and mental health? Behav Modif 34(6):503–519, 2010

Fledderus M, Ernst T, Bohlmeijer ET, et al: The role of psychological flexibility in a self-help acceptance and commitment therapy intervention for psychological distress in a randomized controlled trial. Behav Res Ther 51(3):142–151, 2013

Gloster AT, Meyer A, Lieb R: Psychological flexibility as a malleable public health target: evidence from a representative sample. J Contextual Behav Sci 6(2):166–171, 2017

Hayes SC, Strosahl K, Wilson KG: Acceptance and Commitment Therapy: The Process and Practice of Mindful Change, 2nd Edition. New York, Guilford, 2011

Kashdan TB, Rottenberg J: Psychological flexibility as a fundamental aspect of health. Clin Psychol Rev 30(7):865–878, 2010

Levin M, MacLane C, Daflos S, et al: Examining psychological inflexibility as a transdiagnostic process across psychological disorders. J Contextual Behav Sci 3(3):155–163, 2014

Meyer EC, Kotte A, Kimbrel NA, et al: Predictors of lower-than-expected posttraumatic symptom severity in war veterans: the influence of personality, self-reported trait resilience, and psychological flexibility. Behav Res Ther 113:1–8, 2019

Törneke N: Learning RFT: An Introduction to Relational Frame Theory and Its Clinical Application. Oakland, CA, New Harbinger, 2010

References

Flynn J, Hollenstein T, Mackey A: The effect of suppressing and not accepting emotions on depressive symptoms: is suppression different for men and women? Pers Individ Dif 49:582–586, 2010

Hayes SC, Wilson KG, Gifford EV, et al: Experimental avoidance and behavioral disorders: a functional dimensional approach to diagnosis and treatment. J Consult Clin Psychol 64(6):1152–1168, 1996 8991302

Hayes SC, Barnes-Holmes D, Roche B (eds): Relational Frame Theory: A Post-Skinnerian Account of Human Language and Cognition. New York, Kluwer Academic/Plenum, 2001

Ramnerö J, Torneke N: The ABCs of Human Behavior: Behavioral Principles for Practicing Clinicians. Oakland, CA, New Harbinger, 2011

Törneke N: Learning RFT: An Introduction to Relational Frame Theory and Its Clinical Application. Oakland, CA, New Harbinger, 2010

Wegner DM, Schneider DJ, Carter SR 3rd, et al: Paradoxical effects of thought suppression. J Pers Soc Psychol 53(1):5–13, 1987 3612492

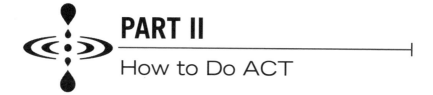

PART II

How to Do ACT

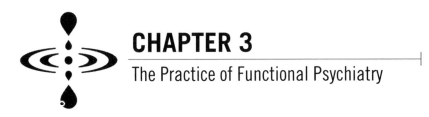

CHAPTER 3

The Practice of Functional Psychiatry

Accept that some days you're the pigeon, and some days you're the statue.

—*Roger C. Anderson*

In Part I, we described some of the core benefits of adopting the ACT approach in psychiatric practice and presented a broad overview of the ACT framework. We examined the basic science foundations of the ACT model and presented a transdiagnostic clinical theory of both psychopathology and human resilience. This theory holds that two highly toxic forms of behavior have been empirically linked to psychopathology and behavior dysfunction: emotional and behavioral avoidance. We also examined an underlying, potentially destructive feature of language that enables unworkable patterns of avoidance: the unwitting tendency of people to follow socially conditioned self-instructional rules that encourage the use of emotional and behavior avoidance strategies. The tendency to follow mental rules is heightened in the presence of low levels of self-reflective awareness and a reduced ability to take perspective on the consequences of one's own actions. We introduced a set of basic clinical intervention principles that, when applied in practice, promote three core psychological processes that foster engagement with values-consistent behaviors and collectively offset the tendency to engage in rule-following and avoidance: 1) openness to and acceptance of distressing inner experiences; 2) awareness and perspective-taking that lead to better objective assessment of the workability of behaviors; and 3) strengthening the connection between personal values and action tendencies in the world.

In Part II, we provide you with a step-by-step approach to adopting ACT principles into your psychiatric practice. This chapter describes the principles and practices of functional psychiatry, which can be thought of as the starting point for adopting ACT-consistent theoretical concepts and core interviewing and case conceptualization strategies into ongoing psychiatric evaluation and management activities. Chapter 4 provides you with an easy-to-follow algorithm for structuring treatment sessions so the stage is set to optimize the likelihood of behavior change. Chapter 5 introduces you to specific ACT interventions you can use to increase openness, promote a stance of workability, and foster a sense of values-based engagement within the patient's life context. Chapter 6 creates a framework for blending the use of medications and ACT interventions in a way that is consistent with the overall mission of functional psychiatry. By the time you are finished with these four chapters, you will have a very detailed "mental map" of how to apply ACT in your psychiatric practice.

After finishing Part I, you may be asking, "How does all of this affect my clinical practice activities when I'm in the room with a patient?" In this chapter, we attempt to identify areas in which a traditional psychiatric approach might be augmented by some basic functional concepts derived from the ACT approach. The potential impacts of integrating ACT into a psychiatric evaluation are described at all stages of the process: what the psychiatrist is looking for in the evaluation process, how information obtained from the patient is condensed and interpreted for treatment planning purposes, how "findings" are communicated to patients, and how targets are selected for psychiatric intervention.

Before we start, it is important to realize that our medical and psychiatric training teaches us to "filter" the information given to us by patients and then tells us how to help them based upon the "meaning" of the information garnered. If your psychiatry residency took place in a psychoanalytically oriented environment, you will be interested in acquiring certain kinds of information, and your interview and case conceptualization methods will fit that approach. If your residency occurred in a biologically oriented training environment, you likely will be interested in collecting very different kinds of information using another distinctive set of data collection and interpretation strategies.

Every trained mental health clinician receives some type of "filter" during training. We often refer to these filters as "schools of thought," and they abound not only in psychiatry but also in many other professions. The filter installed by a school of thought tells you what is important and what is not. It lets you bypass certain types of information while focusing heavily on other kinds of information. The key thing to remember is that every clinician has a filtering system in place. Nothing is inherently bad about that reality, as long as you recognize that no definitive "right" or "wrong" filtering system exists, no matter how strong your allegiance is to your particular school of thought. From the functional psychiatry perspective, a filtering system is "right" when it supports the optimal well-being and best interests of your patient, and it is "wrong" when it does not.

The question, then, is what are the best interests of the patient? What do we mean by that phrase? The answer to this question is really at the heart of any school of thought, because each approach has a somewhat distinctive theory of illness/suffering (i.e., how people experience suffering or dysfunction) and theory of cure (i.e., what is needed to help people out of their suffering or dysfunction). In most cases, the theory of illness leads more or less logically to the theory of cure, so the best interests of the patient are closely tied to how human suffering and dysfunction are explained within a school of thought. Here, we run into an unresolvable dilemma. Each school of thought has its own definition of what patients' best interests are, because each has its own theory of psychopathology and theory of cure. Therefore, functional psychiatry is a school of thought, just as biological psychiatry is a school of thought or psychodynamic psychiatry is a school of thought. We want to be clear about our underlying assumptions and recognize that these assumptions sometimes lead to very different answers to the core questions that confront psychiatrists from the beginning to the end of the treatment process.

In this chapter, we examine the core assumptions and clinical implications of the functional psychiatry approach and review some of the research evidence supporting this framework. We introduce a structured interviewing approach designed to elicit the information the functional psychiatrist is most interested in. We include case dialogues to demonstrate how the core concepts of the functional psychiatry approach are explained to patients during a psychiatric interview. Finally, we introduce some brief, useful, empirically validated self-report measures designed to assess the core psychological processes articulated in the ACT model. As we expand upon the core principles and practices of functional psychiatry, we think it will be useful to compare and contrast the implications of this approach with those of other areas of psychiatry. The only resources you need in order to try this approach are an open mind, a willingness to reflect on your current practice, the courage to try new skills, and the patience and resolve to make room for the initial discomfort of trying something new. You will notice that through simple practice you can quickly become more comfortable using these effective, evidence-based practices to help your patients.

Functional Psychiatry: The Meaning of Symptoms

Recall that one of the two major components of a school of thought is the *theory of illness*. In the daily practice of psychiatry, patients come to see us because they are in a heightened state of emotional distress. We call the various elements of this state of distress "symptoms." Symptoms may have cognitive, affective, behavioral, or physical aspects. By definition, symptoms always have a subjective dimension, and they differ from clinical signs that are, by definition, directly observable. Symptoms generate some form of discomfort experientially.

Most psychiatrists have received little exposure or training related to a functional analytic approach to symptoms. Because the functional approach is a cornerstone of ACT, we examine it more closely.

SYMPTOMS HAVE MULTIPLE FUNCTIONS

First, recognize that human beings have evolved neurologically, physiologically, and biologically to "react" to the world that surrounds them. These reactions can be seen as points of contact between the human organism and the surrounding world. A significant percentage of these reactions involve distressing and unwanted private content, because the world is not always a fun place to be. The function of distressing internal emotional responses is to "get our attention" and motivate adaptive behavior change. Indeed, the Latin root of the word *emotion* literally means "movement." Distressing emotions function at the interface between the human and the demands of the external world. These emotions create a feedback loop, and if the person fails to adapt behavior successfully in response to the message contained in the feedback loop, that loop will continue unabated. It may even worsen if the possible consequences associated with nonadaptation grow in significance. Symptoms will arise as a result.

Symptoms thus may serve multiple adaptive functions, almost in the way the "check engine" light on a car's dashboard serves an adaptive function. When the warning light comes on, we do not know for sure what is wrong with the engine; we just know something, or many things, could be wrong. The light is telling us to do something to figure it out. If we consider that symptoms are often nested within a social or cultural context, we can thus conceive that they also serve an adaptive social function. In the sections that follow, we delve more deeply into these functions, but the immediate list of functional meanings might include

- *The symptom signals that an important discrepancy exists between what the individual is seeking and what he is receiving.* When you want to have a relationship with someone you love and instead that person tells you your relationship is over, the discrepancy triggers a wide array of uncomfortable experiences. In ACT, we call this "clean pain" because it is a natural response to a legitimately painful life situation.
- *The symptom functions to help the individual avoid, eliminate, or suppress another distressing and unwanted private experience.* Depression is an

excellent example of this. People with depression often describe their emotional state as "numb." What are they numb to? Usually, some life problem is producing feelings of sadness, disappointment, guilt, or loss. The haze of depression keeps the patient from making direct experiential contact with uncomfortable emotions.

- *The symptom provides a socially acceptable justification for undesirable performance.* Again, people with depression or anxiety frequently use their symptoms to explain deficits in socially expected behavior. For example, a patient with depression says, "I was too depressed to get dressed and go to work." This statement implies that the experience of depression itself is causing the patient's inability to perform in a socially accepted way, and therefore she is not to blame for what happened.
- *The symptom results in being relieved of socially required duties or responsibilities.* The people surrounding a person who is symptomatic will normally begin to adjust their behavior around the functional deficits exhibited by that person. For example, a person with chronic pain is not asked to go on a family outing because, in the past, going on such outings has resulted in a worsening of the chronic pain.
- *The symptom is a direct result of a destructive coping process, such as suppression or avoidance, that results in a paradoxical increase in the frequency and intensity of feared or avoided experiences.* In ACT, it is understood that pain is unavoidable. Accepting and tolerating pain associated with living one's life is seen as a health-producing strategy, whereas repeated experiences of pain due to suppression or behavioral avoidance are not. An excellent example is a patient who engages in compulsive hand-washing or germ-detecting behaviors. These behaviors are designed to control the emotional discomfort associated with images of loved ones contracting diseases, but the compulsive rituals themselves become a trigger for the recurrence of these images. The image of loved ones being infected with disease and dying is not pleasant, but in and of itself, it would not lead to psychopathology; the unwillingness to have this experience results in the symptoms that define OCD.

CENTRAL TENETS OF FUNCTIONAL PSYCHIATRY

Functional psychiatry is the study of how human behavior functions to help a person adapt more effectively to his surrounding context. The task of adapting to the world as context requires continuous "read and react" adaptation. The human being is literally being challenged to respond effectively on a minute-by-minute, hour-by-hour basis. As noted in the previous chapter, people live not only in the physical world surrounding them but also in their heads. By "heads," we mean a couple of things. First is that inside the head of any person is a collection of private events, such as thoughts, feelings, memories, and physical sensations. These are learned automatic responses to challenges originating in the external environment, but they can also be responses to events within the private world of mind. This means that humans not only react to external events but also react and respond to their private experiences.

Second, within the interior world of the patient is the experience of mind as an "inner advisor" (often more of an inner critic) that constantly issues mandates and directives on how to behave in response to the appearance of both external life circumstances and associated internal reactions. The experience of being an "observer" of the activities of the mind is another, although this psychological function is a "weak link" for most people who are in a state of duress. This lack of observational distance makes people highly susceptible to the self-instructional regulatory functions of the mind.

The problem is that many of these regulatory functions are extrapolations of a threat detection and resolution program that evolved long ago to protect us from what were then almost exclusively physical threats in the external world. The minds that evolved in our early ancestors functioned optimally by developing a singular focus on finding food and not being eaten by predators—with avoiding predators being all important. As outlined in Chapter 2, this survival and procreation-based system is hard wired to produce physiological arousal, leading to a hyperfocus on the most salient external or internal threat cues to the exclusion of other salient information and an equally strong hard-wired tendency to avoid threats to well-being. Whereas our threat avoidance system certainly helps us not step in front of cars, the same program, when transferred into the context of private internal experiences, paradoxically increases the intensity and intrusiveness of the distressing private events we are trying to avoid. This simple, empirically supported observation underpins several important principles of functional psychiatry.

SYMPTOMS MAKE US HUMAN

A key principle of functional psychiatry is that to be "symptomatic" is to be "human." Being alive means being in contact with the challenges of the world around us, and being in contact with those challenges means we will perpetually have symptoms that compel us to change adaptive strategies. This ability to rapidly and effectively change adaptive behavior in response to symptoms of distress is what is called *psychological flexibility*. Flexible individuals are able to vary their behavior in response to inner experiences that signal whether a particular behavioral adaptation is working or not and are thus more resilient in challenging environments. They use private events to help guide new and more effective ways of responding to the challenges of the surrounding world.

AVOIDANCE OF DISTRESS, NOT DISTRESS, IS THE ENEMY

Another key principle of functional psychiatry is that the presence of distressing, unwanted private events is not the "problem," per se; instead, the patient's attempts to suppress awareness of, control, or eliminate these experiences are what lead to destructive results (Hayes et al. 2011). Not only are we hard-wired to experience distressing private experiences, but they are, for the most part, involuntary, habitual, historically learned ways of reacting. The urge to avoid, resist, control, or eliminate them originates in overidentification with the threat appraisals of the inner advisor and an inability to establish a safe observational distance from its regulatory influence. This ultimately leads to repeated failed attempts to suppress awareness of, control, or eliminate distressing internal experience. When efforts to control or eliminate the private experience become the dominant focus of individuals' attempts to adapt, their ability to flexibly adapt behaviors to address the original challenge drops to below threshold. The challenge is thus not met, and the resulting negative consequences further trigger the feedback system. Until those challenges are met, the individual will continue to be symptomatic (Gloster et al. 2017).

SYMPTOMS ARE NOT SIGNALS OF LATENT ILLNESS

This leads to another very important premise of functional psychiatry. Patients are not broken in the sense of being ill or constitutionally defective; rather, they are trapped in a cycle of unworkable avoidance behaviors that paradoxically increase levels of symptom distress. Thus, the primary goal of intervention is to undermine the use of avoidance strategies, such that patients are carefully and gently put back in contact with their unpleasant, unwanted private events while learning to notice and handle them more effectively. This approach, in turn, directs the patient's attention and motivational energy back to the task of adapting to meet the current environmental challenge.

SYMPTOMS MOTIVATE ADAPTIVE RESPONDING

Another key principle of the functional approach is that symptoms, unless avoided, function as powerful motivational forces that promote personal growth and, in some cases, psychological healing. Symptoms, even distressing ones, are not the "enemy within"; instead, they are valuable pieces of information about what is important to the patient in her life context. As we noted earlier in this chapter, symptom distress can increase when a discrepancy arises between what the patient wants in life and what she is getting. The discomfort associated with being symptomatic will motivate the person to do something different to resolve the discrepancy, a positive behavioral adaptation. If we focus only on controlling or eliminating distressing symptoms, we might inadvertently allow the patient to lose contact with the deeply held personal values that produce symptom distress in the first place. Thus, the last thing a functional psychiatrist would seek to do is to numb out, eliminate, or unduly regulate the patient's contact with those distressing private events!

What Does "Better" Look Like?

What does "better" look like? The answer to this key question leads us to the second component of any school of thought: the theory of cure. How do we know when the patient is "better" and can be discharged from a particular phase of treatment? In functional psychiatry, "better" is not the control or elimination of distressing symptoms; "better" is living a valued life and making room for the inevitable discomforts that arise as part of doing so. In the functional approach, patients' best interests are determined with sole reference to their wants, needs, and aspirations in life. Failure to realize those wants, needs, and aspirations leads to the distressing, unwanted private events that patients then try to avoid. Rather than seeking to control their emotional distress, functional psychiatrists reorient patients' attention back to those things that matter in life. From a functional perspective, any interventions, regardless of their makeup, that enable patients to actively approach life situations that matter to them and to act in a values-consistent way in those situations are functionally "true." Interventions that effectively remove the patient from making experiential or behavioral contact with life pursuits that matter are functionally "false."

For several decades, the traditional approach to psychiatry has adopted a phenomenological or topographical approach to the analysis of symptoms. The underlying theory of illness here is that symptoms are signals or signs of a latent disease process. Taxonomic classification systems such as DSM-5 (American Psychiatric Association 2013) are based in the assumption that discernibly different symptom clusters signal the presence of unique underlying psychiatric syndromes. Thus, one logical central goal of traditional psychiatric practice is to use interviewing methods that allow the psychiatrist to match the patient's symptom reports with the appropriate constellation of symptoms in the diagnostic taxonomy. That match, if it occurs, leads to assigning a specific diagnosis to the patient, which in turn should lead to a specific treatment or remedy being applied.

Similarly, if symptoms are a sign of underlying illness, then the theory of cure would quite logically hold that the reduction or elimination of symptoms signals that the underlying illness or condition has been cured. Thus, one aspect of the topographical approach is the explicit goal of decreasing the intensity or frequency of painful or otherwise unwelcome symptoms. Basic research in the neurosciences has focused on illuminating the mechanisms of brain function and dysfunction, with the hope that such mechanistic explanations will lead to improved treatments and better the lives of people living with mental disorders. Such an approach naturally leads to the use of interventions that may reduce the frequency, intensity, or presence of symptoms. Indeed, intervention outcome measures often used in research on psychiatric disorders focus on pre- and postintervention evaluations of the qualitative and quantitative dimensions of the specific symptom constellation thought to be definitive of the underlying illness being studied. Reductions in symptom scores below a certain threshold are assumed to indicate that the underlying latent illness has been controlled or cured.

ACT is fundamentally different in its intention. Reducing the burden and pain of certain life experiences—some of which may be understood as symptoms—takes a "back seat" to helping the patient move toward a full and vital life. ACT recognizes that certain experiences that often result in patients seeking professional care, such as unpleasant emotions, may in fact be key motivators of adaptive behavior. In such cases, treatments designed to numb patients out or to reduce symptom distress could very well end up damaging their best interests. By closing the door on the motivating effects of symptom distress, we might inadvertently help patients maintain an avoidance-based lifestyle that will eventually lead to another mental health crisis.

ACT provides therapeutic strategies that may be readily integrated into usual psychiatric practice, and it offers a positive path forward in the care of patients who present with longstanding and seemingly intractable mental health concerns. Many of these patients will never be completely symptom free, yet the inclusion of ACT techniques can do much to support their sense of vitality, purpose, and meaning in life.

Combining ACT with psychopharmacological interventions can be immensely helpful and can play an important role in the practice of functional psychiatry. Medication-based interventions generally work, in a functional sense, by taking the edge off the uncomfortable feelings of anxiety or depression, helping to control cyclic mood disorders by improving sleep, decreasing impulsivity, and distancing patients from voices or fearful beliefs. These changes in turn allow patients to function more fully in important life areas that have been collaboratively identified by the patients and their psychiatrists.

The functional approach works synergistically with psychopharmacological interventions, helping psychiatrists and patients determine how much of which specific medications might help the patients engage more fully in their lives while paying attention to common unwanted effects that might obstruct functioning, such as sedation, weight gain, sexual effects, emotional numbness, physiological dependence, or cognitive issues. Even when a chosen medication does a good job of reducing or controlling a patient's level of symptom distress, if the unwanted effects of the medication result in severe reductions in motivation or cloud cognitive abilities so the patient cannot function properly in important life contexts, then that medication is not "effective." *Effective* does not mean symptom control or elimination; it means the medication is helping the patient realize important life goals and aspirations.

TIPS FOR SUCCESS

Symptoms of emotional distress are ubiquitous in both the general and clinical population; to be human means to have symptoms.

Symptoms serve multiple private and social functions and are not simply a sign of underlying mental illness.

Symptoms function as a motivational feedback loop and stimulate adaptive responding.

The goal of psychiatric treatment is to help patients utilize their symptoms rather than numb out awareness of, eliminate, or control them.

Getting "better" is not being symptom free but, rather, being able to function in accordance with one's values, aspirations, and goals in important life contexts.

Treatments that eliminate symptoms but do not promote adaptive, values-based functioning in the patient are not "effective."

A Tool Kit for Functional Psychiatric Practice

Now we can return to the original question: "What does this new approach look like in practice? How do I change my practice if I want to add in the functional approach?" In this section, we describe a set of practice tools and strategies that will support you in making this transition, one that we believe will actually speed up clinical change, even if a little more up-front work is required. First, we address the challenge of deeply understanding the internal experiences of our patients—their private events. We then describe an interview protocol that will help you better understand the patient's life context and the significance of his distressing symptoms in relation to that context. Next, we describe a method called the Four Quadrant Case Analysis that will help you interpret the data you have gathered from your patient and allow you to develop a specific treatment plan based in functional principles. Along the way, we use some sample psychiatrist–patient dialogues to demonstrate the "language" of functional psychiatry. Finally, we introduce various self-report surveys that measure processes of central significance in the functional approach.

TEAMS: AN APPROACH TO UNDERSTANDING PRIVATE EVENTS

Although the practice of psychiatry involves working in the private world of language and internal experiences, we do not tend to think of these processes with the same degree of precision as we do, for example, clusters of symptoms. The TEAMS approach helps clinicians isolate the individual components of distressing private experiences reported by clients (Robinson et al. 2011). After all, if we cannot isolate which component of a private experience is stressing our patient, it will be very hard to target the intervention. TEAMS is an acronym for the five distinct forms of internal experience:

- Thoughts
- Emotions
- Action tendencies (urges)
- Memories
- Sensations in the body

Another discovery over years of clinical training is that most clinicians have a "blind spot" for certain private experiences. They might be capable of identifying distressing emotions but fail to recognize the even more unsettling physical sensations the patient is experiencing at the same time. Also, we must understand the phenomenology of distressing private events. For most patients, these events do not come into awareness in nice, tight, clean packages. Instead, they come into awareness all at once and seem hopelessly intermingled. When this happens, the level of threat posed by an unpleasant experience skyrockets, creating strong urges to avoid, suppress, or escape. Thus, the ability to create a TEAMS profile for each patient is highly beneficial: 1) The psychiatrist knows that individual TEAMS elements are the most distressing for the patient and thus can direct interventions in a more precise manner; and 2) The TEAMS approach creates a pathway for helping the patient make important discriminations among a bundle of different internal experiences, thus promoting beneficial effects on emotion processing and an ability to be open to immediate internal experiences.

Table 3–1 provides a simple framework for recording and analyzing TEAMS reported by, or observed in, a patient in session. We encourage

Table 3–1.   TEAMS analysis worksheet

Private event	
Thoughts	
Emotions	
Action tendencies	
Memories	
Sensations in body	

you to practice using the TEAMS approach with a few patients or perhaps to complete a self-assessment of your own TEAMS in response to an unsatisfying interaction with a challenging patient! This will help foster a deeper appreciation of how "busy" the world between our ears can get and how easy it is to get lost in private experiences.

The Contextual Interview: Love, Work, Play, and Health

As we have noted, symptoms of distress do not arise in a vacuum. The functional model assumes a close relationship between how things are working in the patient's life context and her symptoms. Thus, the first order of business in the functional psychiatric interview is to learn more about the patient's life space. The initial set of questions do not really focus on the patient's symptom profile; instead they focus on the important areas of living that define the quality of life for most of us. We call this the "Love, Work, Play, and Health Interview" (Table 3–2).

 Clinical Tool 1: Life Context: Love, Work, Play, and Health Interview
Clinical Tool 2: Approach-Avoidance Analysis Worksheet

As can be seen in the way the questions are phrased, this interview is both very casual and conversational in nature. The fact that the psy-

Table 3–2. Love, work, play, and health interview

1. Who do you live with? Where do you live (in your home or someone else's home, an apartment, dormitory, or homeless)? Do you get along with the people you live with? Do you like where you live?

2. Are you single, divorced, or in a relationship? If in a relationship, partner's name, how long, and how are things going? If unattached, are you dating or interested in meeting someone? If divorced, how long ago? Who divorced whom? How did the divorce affect you?

3. Do you have kids? If so, how old are they? Are they all from your current partner? How are they doing at home, with peers, at school? How do you feel about your role as a parent? Are you satisfied, unhappy?

4. How do you support yourself? Do you work, are you a student, or on disability of some kind? If working, how do you like your job? Do you get along with peers at work? If a student, how is school going? What are your future plans once you graduate?

5. Do you have friends or other meaningful social connections? How often do you catch up? What stuff do you do together? When was the last time you got together with a friend or friends?

6. Do you have some connections in your community? Membership in clubs, charities, volunteer work, church, or church-related activities?

7. Family relationships: siblings, parents, uncles, aunts, grandparents, or other family? Do they play an important role in your life? When was the last time you talked with them or visited?

8. How do you spend your leisure time? What do you do for fun (e.g., watching movies, playing video games, outdoor activities)? Do you have hobbies or other interests that promote your personal growth or inspire you? What do you like to do during your leisure time? When was the last time you did any of these things?

9. Do you have a spiritual life? Are you religious? Of what faith, if any? Do you have a self-guided spiritual practice such as meditation, chanting, reading the Bible, writing poetry? Does it play an important role in your life?

10. Do you get any exercise, walk, ride, run? In the past? Team sports, now or were you ever into any? When was the last time you exercised?

11. Do you use alcohol or recreational drugs? How often? How much do you consume? Do you have any concerns about your pattern of use?

12. Do you smoke, chew, or vape? How often? How long? Any interest in quitting or cutting down?

13. Are you sleeping okay? If not, what kind of sleep problems are you having? When did they start? Do you have problems with nightmares or night terrors?

14. Are you eating well? Do you eat nutritious foods? Skip meals? Take supplements of any kind?

chiatrist is asking so many questions about the patient's life context conveys a sense of genuine interest and curiosity. This helps reduce any defensiveness or stigma the patient may be experiencing and is likely to make him feel more comfortable discussing difficult issues that might surface during the interview. Some psychiatrists find it useful to keep session notes in real time using the ACT Approach-Avoidance Behaviors Worksheet, which makes it possible to see the "big picture" of the patient's approach and avoidance tendencies nested in his life context. The session dialogue that follows is an example of how the psychiatrist might introduce the contextual interview:

> Psychiatrist: You're probably a little anxious about coming to meet a stranger, me, to talk about personal things—which is quite natural, of course. I'll be aware of that and will structure things in our conversation over the next hour [50 minutes, 30 minutes, whatever is available] or so to ensure that you can get your difficulties across adequately. I want to get an overall sense of you as a person, and particularly what is *working* in your life, as well as what is *not working* so well, so that we might come up with a couple of strategies to have things *work a bit better.* Does that sound like a plan?
>
> Gary: Yeah, I guess that would give you a better handle on where my life is at right now.
>
> Psychiatrist: The perspective I bring to meeting all of my patients, indeed, to everyone I meet, is that *suffering is normal* [emphasized]. Our difficult thoughts and feelings are part of our reactions to important life events or challenges, which can certainly get in the way of climbing our mountains of life. We've done the surveys and find that as many as 20%–30% of people report problems with anxiety and 10%–20% report problems with depression, and these numbers are growing. Likewise, with problems with alcohol and substance use. Add in relationship difficulties, overwork, and the ongoing daily stresses we face, and that's *everybody,* me included! It's not as though I'm at the top of my mountain of life with all of my own personal challenges sorted out. I'm still struggling away as I climb my mountain, and now I'm meeting you struggling to climb your mountain. [Motions with arms, emphasizing the two mountains.] When people get stuck on their climb, they naturally want help, so they come along to see me. Once I get a sense of how you're stuck, I can share with you a few things I've learned about mountain climbing. My role is to be more like a coach, to help you get unstuck so you can climb your mountain a little more freely. I think you'll find that the skills that I will coach you in will work in all kinds of life situations as you continue your climb. Does that make sense?
>
> Gary: This is very different than what I thought would happen when I finally decided I needed some help, but it's kind of a relief to know there isn't something really wrong with me.

The contextual assessment can take up a fair amount of the session. Often, in fact almost always, important information that might play a role in making an accurate functional diagnosis will just spontaneously appear inside the interview itself as the patient and psychiatrist get to know one another.

Conducting a Functional Analysis: The "Three Ts"

At a certain point in the interview process, the psychiatrist will have gathered enough information about the patient's life context and will want to "shift gears" and begin to look at her symptom complaints as they are nested, or situated, in her life context. As mentioned previously, symptoms are feedback loops that arise when discrepancies between desired life and actual life outcomes arise in one or more of these important life domains. These domains are generally nested within a social context, which makes it very important that the psychiatrist examine the "problem" from many different angles.

CASE EXAMPLE: MARY

Mary, a mother with two teenage sons, presents because of increasingly severe depression. One of the teenage children is into street drugs, and Mary both feels guilty about not raising her kid "right" and struggles with wanting to help but being powerless to stop the drug use. Her strategy for coping with all this is to not let herself think about her son's problems, because when she does, her anxiety and worry escalate, and she cannot stop the bad images of him being dead from an overdose from coming into her head. She has also ignored her other son's attempts to engage her about his brother's problem, and an unwritten rule has developed in the house that the subject of drug addiction is not to be raised. Her other son is quite angry about this "cone of silence" and has stopped relating to his mother about a lot of things. This distancing has not been lost on Mary, who interprets this as yet another indication that she is failing as a parent.

As this brief case example illustrates, actions nested in a social context can create layers and layers of cause-and-effect relationships that are overwhelming to the patient.

A central objective of the functional analytic interview is to help patients and psychiatrists understand these cause-and-effect relationships as clearly as possible. We want to know what patients are doing in response to these feedback loops, how those responses are working, and how these responses are in turn impacting other responses and feedback loops. A functional analysis is also commonly referred to as A-B-C analysis. This method was described in Chapter 2, but it bears repeating here because of the central importance this analytic method plays in functional psychiatric practice. A-B-C is an acronym for the process by which behaviors are learned, shaped, and maintained:

A: Antecedent events that serve as triggering stimuli
B: Behaviors, public or private, emitted in response to the antecedent
C: Consequences following appearance of the behavior, both negative and positive, that increase or diminish the likelihood of that behavior being used in the same or similar situations in the future

In the functional approach, the assumption is that the relationship between A, B, and C is producing a cycle of unworkable results for the patient. Basically, the usual problem is that the short-term consequences (C; temporary relief from distressing private events) of avoidance behaviors (B) maintain those behaviors, even though the long-term result is to create more emotional distress and to trigger more challenging life events, situations, or interactions (A). As highlighted by the example of Mary, strategies that turn out to be self-defeating in the long run might be powerfully reinforcing in the short run. In Mary's case, her strategies of not allowing herself to think about her son's problems and encouraging others in her family to do the same protects her from the aversive experience of worrying, being anxious, and having terrifying images of her son lying dead from an overdose. Her avoidance strategies are being powerfully reinforced in the short run. In the long run, those same avoidance strategies are having a destructive impact on her relationship with her other son, creating yet another source of symptom distress for her to deal with. Therefore, the psychiatrist wants to understand how this cycle works, both in the short term and in the longer term. The behavior analytic approach allows the psychiatrist to understand specific instances of clinically relevant behavior, situated in the context that gives that behavior its functional meaning, and gauge the ways the patient's maladaptive behaviors are being shaped and maintained.

Some models of functional analysis are quite complex and can be way too time consuming to be feasible in a time-limited psychiatric interview. To make the process simpler and more straightforward, we recommend using the "Three Ts" approach (Robinson et al. 2011), which is a streamlined way to conduct a quick functional analysis of the patient's presenting complaints. The Three Ts stand for

- **Time:** Analysis of the recent chronology of the problem and possible contextual shifts that are now bringing the problem into clear focus
- **Trigger:** Analysis of antecedents, responses, and consequences that are maintaining the problem behavior
- **Trajectory:** Analysis of changes in the topographical or functional features of the problem behavior over time

Clinical Tool 3: Problem Context: The Three Ts

Table 3–3. The "Three Ts" interview

Time	When did this problem start?
	How often does it happen?
	What happens before/after the problem?
	Why do you think it is a problem now?
	Has anything changed or shifted in your life context that is making the problem more serious?
Trigger	Does anything—a situation or a person—seem to set it off?
	Are there internal triggers that show up?
	What happens after you react the way you do?
	How do you feel about yourself afterward?
	How do other people around you react to your behavior?
Trajectory	What's this problem been like over time? When did it first come up in your life? Have there been times when it was less of a concern?
	When it was less of a concern, what were you doing differently?
	Have there been times when it was more of a concern? Is there anything you've done that made it worse?
	How has it been recently? Does it seem to be getting worse, better, or about the same as before?

In Table 3–3, we present an interview protocol for conducting a Three Ts analysis. Recall from Chapter 2 that a primary therapeutic goal of ACT is to help patients enter a state of self-reflective awareness in which they can objectively determine the unworkable nature of avoidance strategies. In effect, the psychiatrist repeatedly will use the Three Ts interview to teach patients how to analyze their own adaptive responses without self-criticism to promote context sensitivity and foster contingency-based learning rather than automatic, habitual rule-following.

Most patients do not think about their problems in such behavior-analytic terms. Their efforts to problem-solve are over-focused on eliminating distressing experiences and negative cognitions, unworkable strategies influenced by the invisible self-instructional rules of language. Thus, the act of stepping back and studying behaviors and their consequences is a good way to bring patients to a state of self-reflective awareness and help them assess the workability of their actions in context. This approach helps patients discover firsthand the effects of following self-instructional rules that promote unworkable patterns of avoidance.

The overarching goal is to help them make direct contact with the actual results of rule-following, not the results specified in the rule, per se. Being sensitive to context requires patients to take perspective on their own responses, assess the workability of those responses in relation to expressed values and life aspirations, and change strategies based upon actual results. The simple analytical framework of the A-B-C approach supports this cornerstone feature of ACT.

CASE EXAMPLE: MIKE

Mike is a 41-year-old married man who presents for evaluation and management of mixed depression and anxiety. He worked part-time as a college course instructor until a couple of years ago, when funding cuts resulted in his contract not being renewed. Since then, he has relied on a consulting business to pay his bills, but that business has been slowly shrinking. He has been looking for work for 6 months without success and has been struggling with handling both the role change from breadwinner and the tightened finances at home. He and his wife were unable to have children, and currently the marriage is strained. His primary care physician prescribed a trial of citalopram for anxiety and depression, but the medication was stopped after Mike experienced an onset of suicidal thoughts. He recently told his wife, Gina, that at times he wishes she were not around so that he could run away or take his own life.

During the contextual interview, Mike reveals that he tends to hide in his office and avoid talking with his wife about their marital issues and financial difficulties. They are no longer sexually intimate and sleep in different bedrooms. He believes she is deeply disappointed in him as a breadwinner and as a husband. He blames his depression and anxiety for his inability to take the steps necessary to get a job. He also reports problems with sleep onset at night; he tends to lie in bed and ruminate about his problems and about why he cannot be successful like other people. He has been drinking two or three glasses of wine in the evening because this helps him calm down.

Psychiatrist: It might seem unusual that we've spent so much time talking about this stuff about your life. I do this on purpose, because this is what is *most important* [emphasized]—what you want your life to be about. Right now, you're not getting what you want out of life.

Mike [nodding]: Yes, I agree, that sure is the most important stuff, and I don't know what to do about it. [He looks sad but also a bit relieved and validated.]

Psychiatrist: My understanding is that you had this big change in your career 2 years ago when your contract expired. Is that when you started to struggle with your mood, or did you have problems like this earlier in your life?

Mike: I think I had problems even earlier, like when Gina and I learned that we couldn't have children because it turns out I'm infertile. We decided not to adopt if we couldn't have one of our own. That was a pretty low point for me. That was maybe 10 years ago, I guess.

Psychiatrist: Since then, 10 years ago, would you say these problems for the most part disappeared until 2 years ago, or have they been ongoing?

Mike: I would say that they kind of went dormant until I lost my job.

Psychiatrist: Okay. Then over the past 2 years, would you say your mood problems have worsened, gotten better, or stayed about the same?

Mike: I think they've worsened, especially since it became obvious to me that my consulting business isn't going to make it.

Psychiatrist: You talked about you and Gina sort of drifting apart, such that you are no longer having sex or doing intimate things together. Was that happening in parallel with the job problems, or is it on its own track?

Mike: Well, now that you mention it, I think they're related. I think we were kind of bouncing along trying to adjust to being married without any kids. We were still able to enjoy sex, and we often did things together. I wouldn't say we were healed, but I think we were heading in the right direction until I lost my job at the college. She had to go back to work at a local department store to help us make ends meet. I could tell she was unhappy about that. I felt it was really my fault; I should have been preparing to either move up to a regular faculty position or look for faculty positions elsewhere. I didn't do that. I took the easy money of the year-to-year contract teaching position instead. That was a big mistake.

Psychiatrist: I want to make sure I've got this right. You're saying that your mood problems get triggered when you run into really big life challenges, like having your career stall out, learning you can't be a father, or sensing that Gina is unhappy with you and drifting away. Those would be difficult pills for anyone to swallow. I mean, I can see that you would certainly be sad about not having children and about watching your life partner pull away from you. You have very good reasons to be anxious here. Your career is up in the air; you have to pay your bills with no job in sight. I mean, I would be very sad and anxious if I were in that situation.

Mike: Yeah, that about says it. At least you understand where I'm coming from.

Psychiatrist: These problems are very hard emotionally on you, I can tell. It seems as though you spend a lot time just trying to deal with all these thoughts and feelings that come up.

Mike: Yeah, if I can't get this depression and all this anxiety under control, I'm not able to do much of anything else.

Psychiatrist: It sounds like your approach is that, to stop this tailspin you're in, you first have to gain some measure of control over your anxiety and depression. How do you do that? What have you tried?

Mike: Well, I go to my office and try to compose myself. When I'm about to write a letter of application or make a call, I remind myself to just be positive, even if I feel negative. I do spend a lot of time thinking about the past mistakes I've made; maybe if I learn from those mistakes, I'll feel more confident inside. And I guess interacting with Gina face-to-face is a huge trigger for me, because I know she is disappointed in me as a husband.

In this exchange, the psychiatrist uses the Three Ts approach to help Mike "connect the dots" between his distressing emotional experiences and the unmet challenges he is facing in his life. His emotions are not a problem to be solved. They are signals that he needs to listen to rather than attempt to avoid or eliminate them. Thus far, most of his strategies seem focused on achieving freedom from his emotional distress through various escape and avoidance behaviors.

Assessing Workability: Eliciting Patient Values and Avoidance Strategies

Another important assessment activity interwoven within the Three Ts conversation is to pose a series of questions designed to get patients to articulate deeply held values about living while revealing the unworkable results of avoidance strategies they have been using. This sequence of interviewing is often referred to as the *clinical focusing questions* (Strosahl et al. 2012). These questions are designed to engage patients in a discussion about their values in life, what they are seeking in important life domains, and whether their current avoidance strategies are promoting progress toward those valued life outcomes. Table 3–4 presents a broad template for implementing the workability assessment sequence, which can surface spontaneously during the Love, Work, Play, and Health Interview and the Three Ts assessment processes. The first and foremost important component of a workability assessment is to know who and what matters to the patient. The second major component is to determine the extent to which the patient's current behaviors are moving him toward or away from those valued life pursuits. Creating a dynamic and ongoing tension between what the patient wants in life versus what the patient is getting by using avoidance strategies is a core dynamic in ACT. Thus, the patient's behaviors are working when they move her toward valued life ends, and they are not working when they move her away from those valued life ends. The psychiatrist is thus freed from having to argue with, convince, or cajole the patient into agreeing that avoidance behaviors are not working. The psychiatrist can usually just ask the workability question and let the patient come up with the answers.

When compiling the results of the workability assessment, a written framework, such as the Workability Assessment Summary worksheet, may be useful. This allows the psychiatrist to quickly summarize infor-

Table 3–4. Clinical focusing questions

1. What would tell you that you were doing better?	"If you got everything you wanted out of our meeting today, what would be different when you left here? What would you do differently in your life?"
2. What have you tried so far to make that happen in your life?	"Most people try several different strategies to be different, the way you just described. Can you tell me some of the things you've tried?"
3. How have those strategies worked?	"I can tell you've put a lot of effort into these strategies. Would you say that the issue is better/same/worse now?"
	"It seems as though you are in some kind of strange loop here. On the one hand, you hear your mind saying that these things will work. On the other hand, you tell me that your actual experience is that things are no better, or even worse than before. Is it possible that, despite what your mental advisor is telling you, these strategies actually make things worse, not better?"
4. What kind of life would you choose, if you were free to choose?	"Let's imagine you were free to choose the kind of life you would like to be living. Furthermore, imagine that the problems we've been talking about are no longer getting in the way of you living that kind of life. What would that life look like? What would you be doing that you are not doing now?"
5. What has been the cost of avoidance on being able to live the life you would like to be living?	"Thinking about the kind of life you told me you would like to be living, and thinking about how your life is going right now, would you say the strategies you are using right now are moving you in the direction of a valued life, or are they pushing you in the other direction?"
	"What stands out for you as the most important thing in life that you are losing out on?"
	"Is it possible that the strategies you described are cutting you off from the type of life you want to live?"

mation garnered in the interview so it is available for all the questions contained in the workability interview sequence.

 ## Clinical Tool 4: Workability Assessment Summary Worksheet

Once the psychiatrist helps Mike see the immediate connection between his distressing symptoms and the life challenges he is facing, the stage is set to help him discover the destructive effect his avoidance-based coping strategies are having on the things that matter to him most in life. The psychiatrist will now focus the interview to help bring Mike into direct contact with the unworkable results of his escape and avoidance strategies and the impact they are having on his sense of life direction and vitality.

Psychiatrist: Tell me, if a miracle happened here today and everything you could wish for happened as a result of us meeting today, what would that look like? What would be different in your life?

Mike: Well, as I said before, I would feel better inside. I wouldn't be so depressed and anxious.

Psychiatrist: If you weren't depressed or anxious anymore, what would you be doing differently in your life?

Mike: I'd probably be able to land a job, and Gina and I might spend more time together, and we would get closer.

Psychiatrist: So, looking at all of these things you've been doing to get control of your anxiety and depression—and it sounds like you've been hard at it the past 6 months in particular—and thinking about your depression, your anxiety, and these thoughts that you are to blame and are a disappointment to Gina, would you say these problems are better now than they were before, are they about the same, or are they actually worse now?

Mike: Well, I certainly don't think they are better. I wouldn't have come in to see you if they were. I actually think they're worse.

Psychiatrist: Let's come back to that in a moment, because maybe some strange kind of trick is being played on you here. I wonder, if you could live the kind of life you want to live here and now—and let's imagine that you're free to choose that life—what would that look like in terms of these important life areas we've talked about?

Mike: Well, I guess the most important thing is I would have a strong bond with Gina. We would take this on together. I do love her and want to protect and provide for her. I want us to be intimate—not just sex, but sharing moments of being together. I want to do something meaningful in my career. Something that helps people. I love teaching others what I know. I think I would have a broader friendship network. I would like to see Gina get back into some of the outdoor activities we really enjoy.

Psychiatrist: When you think about this life you've just described to me, and then the strategies you've been using to gain control of your negative thoughts and feelings—coping behaviors like hiding out in your office, avoiding interactions with Gina so you don't have to feel guilty, drinking a fair amount of wine at bedtime, sleeping in a different bed than Gina—do you think these strategies are moving you toward the kind of life you want to live, or are they moving you away from your dreams?

Mike: Definitely not toward…definitely not toward at all. It feels like I'm losing my grip on the things that are important to me.

Psychiatrist: Losing your grip is a nice way to think about this, because when we lose our grip on a glass or something like that, we naturally squeeze harder, and that actually makes us lose our grip faster. If we relaxed our grip at exactly that moment, the glass might have more of an interface with our hand and might not slip out. So, some of the things you've tried to help you get on top of your problems seem pretty natural to me, and your experience is telling you these things are not working. You could squeeze harder here and do what you've been doing even more than before; what's your sense of that?

Mike: It's not going to work. I can see that pretty clearly.

Psychiatrist: So, what would loosening your grip look like if you took that approach in this situation?

In this brief exchange, the psychiatrist uses the sequence of focusing questions to help Mike make contact with the fact that his control and avoidance strategies not only are failing to control anything (things are actually worsening in terms of his mood problems, rumination, and self-criticism) but also are actually undermining the things that really matter to him in his life: nurturing his marriage, being a teacher, having more friends, and spending more leisure time with his wife. In many situations, simply bringing the patient into direct contact with the destructive effects of avoidance strategies is enough to stimulate a change in approach. Building self-reflective perspective-taking on the workability of one's own actions is often all that is needed to trigger new adaptive responses.

TIPS FOR SUCCESS

The TEAMS assessment method allows psychiatrists to more accurately profile patients' specific distressing internal experiences.

The Love, Work, Play, and Health Interview, also known as the contextual interview, is a systematic, casual, effective way for getting to know patients and communicating a sincere interest in, and curiosity about, the life areas that really matter to them.

The contextual interview is often the first component of the functional psychiatric interview sequence.

The Three Ts interview uses the A-B-C model of functional analysis to help psychiatrists and patients identify unworkable patterns of adaptive behavior.

Unworkable patterns of adaptive behavior usually involve escape and avoidance strategies that are immediately reinforced by their positive short-term impact on emotional distress but have iatrogenic long-term results.

The focusing question sequence is designed to get patients into direct contact with the unworkable longer-term consequences of escape and avoidance strategies.

Often, using functionally oriented interview techniques to foster self-reflective perspective-taking on the workability of emotional and behavioral avoidance strategies will produce an immediate change in patients' approach.

Case Formulation and Treatment Planning Using the Four Quadrant Method

At a certain point in the interview process, the psychiatrist must convert the information obtained in the initial interview into a clinically useful case analysis and formulation. This formulation might include a DSM-5 diagnostic impression, if that is required by private insurance companies or government-run health programs. The data must be transformed into a practical and clinically usable functionally oriented case formulation that immediately tells the psychiatrist what to target in treatment. What intervention should the psychiatrist use to help the patient? To help distill and make sense of the information garnered in the functional contextual interview, we suggest psychiatrists use a time-tested behavioral analytic method known as a four-quadrant analysis. Several variations of this approach have been clinically adapted by ACT practitioners. The four-quadrant concept is a time-tested behavioral analytic method that can be used for both case conceptualization and treatment planning purposes. A variety of case conceptualization systems have been described in the ACT literature that follow the conceptual framework of this method. We examine one such variant here called the ACT Four Quadrant Case Analysis (Strosahl et al. 2012). In Chapter 4, we examine another well-known variant called the ACT Matrix.

📝 Clinical Tool 5: ACT Four Quadrant Case Analysis

In the Four Quadrant Case Analysis, each quadrant contains data directly relevant to understanding the patient's predicament and potential sources of helpful intervention. On the X axis we analyze "behavior." Here, we make an important distinction between behavior that occurs in the context of *public actions* and the person's *private events.* Public actions are things the person does or does not do in the external world. These behaviors are observable to others, even if done secretively so no one will see them (e.g., drinking alone in the garage to avoid detection by a family member is still an "action"). Private events are experiences "between the ears" and typically involve aspects of covert experience such as thoughts, feelings, memories, urges, or sensations. These experiences can be verbally reported to others, but others cannot actually see these events as they unfold in consciousness.

On the Y axis, we attempt to gauge the workability of actions or private events. Here we distinguish between behaviors that are *not working* and behaviors that *are working* to promote the patient's personally chosen values and goals in life. Thus, we have four basic quadrants in which to condense the specific results of the contextual and workability assessment interviews:

- Q1 (upper left): Actions or behaviors that are not working
- Q2 (lower left): Private events that function to promote unworkable actions
- Q3 (lower right): Private events that could facilitate workable actions
- Q4 (upper right): Actions or behaviors that are working

Figure 3–1 presents an analysis of information obtained from Mike during his interview, using the four-quadrant method. In general, items that end up in Q1 and Q2 surface during the clinical analysis of behavioral (Q1) and emotional (Q2) avoidance. As shown in the figure, the Q1 and Q2 quadrants are full of both actions and mental processes that drive Mike toward avoidance. He is actively avoiding certain types of emotional experiences (e.g., being anxious, feeling like a failure in Gina's eyes), and to aid him in this quest for emotional control, he is following self-instructional rules that are guaranteed to fail (e.g., avoids talking with Gina to escape feeling like a failure). The ongoing experience of failing to control these distressing experiences paradoxically escalates his hypervigilance to symptoms while decreasing his sense of self-efficacy. Because he cannot directly control his painful emotions and self-critical thoughts, the next best strategy is opting out of life situations that might trigger them. The cost, however, is that his marriage is steadily weaken-

Workability

	Not Working	Working
Public actions context	**Q1** Very disengaged and avoidant Hangs out in office Avoids discussions with Gina about their marriage, intimacy, finances Sleeps apart from Gina Fails to complete job applications Drinks two or three glasses of wine to calm down	**Q4** Is willing to seek psychiatric care ? Connect values about marriage to specific actions involving approaching Gina (leisure activity together, sleeping together, discussing career options) ? Focus job-seeking activities on teaching positions to increase follow through
Private events context	**Q2** Rule-following and emotional avoidance: "Can't perform if I feel depressed or anxious" "Need to get control of this stuff" Suicidality as form of escape Fusion with self-critical narrative: "I'm to blame for all of this" "I'm a disappointment to Gina" Ruminates about "What ifs?" and "Why can't I?"	**Q3** Able to connect with values about marriage, career, wanting friends, wanting to spend more time doing leisure activities with Gina ? Accept presence of sadness, anxiety as valid indicators of what matters to him ? Practice self-compassion instead of self-punishment to allow him to make contact with his narrative and not be pushed around by it

FIGURE 3–1. Four-quadrant analysis of Mike's case information.

ing, he is not able to get a job to solve his financial issues, and he cannot make a career-changing move such as applying for a faculty position in another city or state. The catastrophic impact of Q1 behaviors is usually what "turns the tide" and convinces patients to seek psychiatric help. Similarly, items that end up in Q3 and Q4 represent opportunities for treatment planning and picking a specific intervention.

In contrast to the problem analysis focus of the first two quadrants, entries in Q3 and Q4 allow the psychiatrist to summarize a patient's current strengths and suggest potential avenues for intervention. The psychiatrist can now begin thinking about what changes might be needed in either or both of these quadrants so that the patient is willing to engage in values-based approach behaviors. Notice the convention we use in Figure 3–1 of putting a question mark (?) in front of an entry. This means that, if implemented correctly, a new self-instructional rule might help improve Mike's ability to behave according to personal values and life aspirations. For example, he has overidentified with a self-narrative that he is to blame for all the problems that have fallen on his family and that he is a disappointment to Gina. It is clear he values his marriage and wants to reestablish closeness with Gina. What if we could get Mike to treat himself with kindness even while acknowledging that he, like all humans, can make mistakes? That might increase the chances he would engage in behaviors designed to approach Gina and strengthen their marriage. As it now stands, the very sight of Gina sets off his harsh self-criticisms, which trigger avoidance behaviors designed to ease the emotional distress associated with those self-criticisms.

Treatment Planning Using the Four Quadrant Case Analysis

Two broad classes of interventions "leak out" of the Four Quadrant Case Analysis: strengthening interventions and establishing interventions. A *strengthening intervention* takes a strength the patient already exhibits and deliberately attempts to increase it. The strength may be manifest at the level of private experience or in the action's context. In Mike's case, note that one Q3 attribute is his ability to articulate several basic values that are important to him. Note, however, that these values are not being realized in the workable actions context (Q4). This immediately suggests a possible strengthening intervention designed to connect Mike's values to specific approach behaviors he will try with Gina or in relation to his job seeking.

An *establishing intervention* is designed to create an entirely new self-instructional rule or overwrite an existing rule that previously promoted unworkable avoidance strategies such that it now promotes workable action. We are, in effect, establishing a new rule that the patient will follow. An establishing intervention may challenge an existing rule, such as "you will feel and act better if you can control depression and anxiety and think positive, even when you believe you're to blame and are a disappointment." Alternatively, we can pose a new formulation of the old rule and demonstrate experientially that it works better in terms of the patient's optimal well-being and best interests: "The fact that you are sad and anxious about this situation shows you care about your family, your marriage to Gina, and your ability to support your family. You have nothing to be ashamed of for being sad or anxious when things that really matter to you are not working out the way you want them to."

TIPS FOR SUCCESS

Behaviorally focused case formulation is an important step in the functional psychiatric interview process, allowing for more precise treatment selection.

The four-quadrant model of case analysis allows the psychiatrist to use interview data to identify specific self-instructional processes and associated behaviors that are, and are not, working for the patient.

Effective treatment planning usually involves selecting interventions that reinforce workable self-instructional rules (strengthening interventions) or create new, more viable rules to replace or override unworkable ones (establishing interventions).

Several variations of the four-quadrant approach are used in ACT, some of which can be used collaboratively with patients.

The Use of Patient- and Clinician-Based Measures in Functional Psychiatry

Not surprisingly, the self-report surveys used by functional psychiatrists differ quite dramatically from the symptom-based measures that characterize the more conventional, disorder-oriented psychiatric approach, in which the focus is on reducing symptom frequency and severity; the tools of the trade thus measure those features of a patient's presenting problem. In functional psychiatry, we take distressing symptoms as a given and instead focus on the patient's ability to function in effective, valued ways even when distressing symptoms are present.

In this section, we briefly introduce three specific measures helpful for routine functional psychiatric care: the Acceptance and Action Ques-

Table 3–5. The Acceptance and Action Questionnaire–II

1. My painful experiences and memories make it difficult for me to live a life that I would value.
2. I'm afraid of my feelings.
3. I worry about not being able to control my worries and feelings.
4. My painful memories prevent me from having a fulfilling life.
5. Emotions cause problems in my life.
6. It seems like most people are handling their lives better than I am.
7. Worries get in the way of my success.

tionnaire–II (AAQ-II; Bond et al. 2011), the Cognitive Fusion Questionnaire (CFQ; Gillanders et al. 2014), and the Valuing Questionnaire (VQ; Smout et al. 2014). We like these measures because they are short, easy to administer, easy to score, and easy to integrate into the opening moments of the psychiatric interview. All three measures use a simple Likert 1–7 rating scale for each item. Here, we briefly describe the item content for each scale to demonstrate how the focus of interest shifts from measuring the intensity and frequency of symptoms to measuring patients' relationship to symptoms and functional capacity when symptoms are present.

THE ACCEPTANCE AND ACTION QUESTIONNAIRE–II

The AAQ-II (Table 3–5) is one of the original, psychometrically sound measures of experiential avoidance, and up to now it has been the measure most frequently used in studies of ACT. The AAQ-II has proven to be broadly useful in predicting positive clinical outcomes. Changes in AAQ-II scores in the "right" direction have been shown to predict a positive response to ACT. In other words, in keeping with the tenets of the ACT framework, weakening avoidance and strengthening values-based approach behavior is one of the active mechanisms of change. The AAQ-II is brief and very easy to administer, readminister, and score.

 Clinical Tool 6: Acceptance and Action Questionnaire–II (AAQ-II)

THE COGNITIVE FUSION QUESTIONNAIRE

The CFQ (Table 3–6) is a brief and psychometrically sound measure of cognitive fusion that can also be used at intervals to track therapeutic progress. It is useful in a wide range of settings, such as mental health, physical health, guidance, and coaching as well as training settings. Similar to the AAQ-II, the CFQ is brief and easy to score and interpret. It can be used on a session-by-session basis to help patients see changes in their openness to inner experiences.

Table 3–6. The Cognitive Fusion Questionnaire

1. My thoughts cause me distress or emotional pain.
2. I get so caught up in my thoughts that I am unable to do the things that I most want to do.
3. I overanalyze situations to the point where it's unhelpful to me.
4. I struggle with my thoughts.
5. I get upset with myself for having certain thoughts.
6. I tend to get very entangled in my thoughts.
7. It's such a struggle to let go of upsetting thoughts even when I know that letting go would be helpful.

 Clinical Tool 7: Cognitive Fusion Questionnaire

THE VALUING QUESTIONNAIRE

The VQ (Table 3–7) is another brief, psychometrically sound measure that assesses values-based processes in daily living (Smout et al. 2014). It can be used to track patients' progress from week to week. Validation studies have shown the utility of this measure with various clinical problems.

 Clinical Tool 8: Valuing Questionnaire

ADDITIONAL ACT-CONSISTENT MEASURES FOR CLINICAL PRACTICE

Obviously, other ACT-consistent self-report measures are available that the psychiatric clinician may be interested in using. One is the Five Facet Mindfulness Questionnaire, Short Form (FFMQ-SF; Bohlmeijer et al. 2011), a 24-item measure of five core mindfulness skills that have been shown to change in a positive way in response to mindfulness-based training and interventions. The FFMQ-SF can be useful in situations in which the psychiatrist wants to formally assess the strengths and weaknesses of patients' mindfulness skills. It can be completed multiple times over the course of treatment to see if clinical interventions are strengthening.

Table 3–7. The Valuing Questionnaire

1.	I spend a lot of time thinking about the past or future rather than being engaged in activities that matter to me.
2.	I am basically on "autopilot" most of the time.
3.	I work toward my goals even if I don't feel motivated to.
4.	I am proud about how I have lived my life.
5.	I have made progress in the areas of my life I care most about.
6.	Difficult thoughts, feelings, or memories get in the way of what I really want to do.
7.	I continue to get better at being the kind of person I want to be.
8.	When things don't go according to plan, I give up easily.
9.	I feel like I have a purpose in life.
10.	It seems like I am just "going through the motions" rather than focusing on what is important to me.

 Clinical Tool 9: Five Facet Mindfulness Questionnaire: Short-Form (FFMQ-SF)

Another clinically useful tool is The Flourishing Measure, a short quality-of-life survey of patients' level of satisfaction with many of the life areas that are the focus of the contextual interview assessment (Vander-Weele 2017). It could easily be implemented as a functionally oriented outcome measure in lieu of or in addition to measuring changes in symptom severity.

 Clinical Tool 10: The Flourishing Project Measure

Another easy to use in-session assessment is the Flexibility and Alliance Session Tool, nicknamed FAST. FAST is a "quick and dirty" assessment of the "pillars" of psychological resilience we discussed in Chapter 2, in which patients rate the extent to which their behaviors in-between therapy sessions have been promoting psychological and emotional resilience. This allows the psychiatrist to quickly see what has been going right and what has been going wrong for patients since the last therapy session.

Clinical Tool 11: Flexibility and Alliance Session Tool (FAST)

Another in-session measure that directly maps onto the emotional resilience framework is the Pillars Assessment Tool (PAT; Robinson et al. 2011). This tool can be completed by the psychiatrist singly or in collaboration with patients. The PAT helps identify areas on "pillar strength" and "pillar weakness" and thus can be used "on the fly" to direct ACT interventions to the appropriate target. Some ACT practitioners like to use scaling techniques to quantify the strength of each pillar, where 1=extremely weak and 10=extremely strong. The PAT can then be used as a type of treatment progress measure, assuming ACT interventions should improve skill level of each of the three pillars.

 Clinical Tool 12: ACT Pillars Assessment Tool (PAT)

How to Integrate Self-Report Surveys and Functional Psychiatry Concepts

You will see that, by their very content, functionally oriented self-report surveys begin helping patients take a more practical, less judgmental perspective on the meaning of their symptoms of distress. Thus, engaging the patient in completing these brief surveys opens the door for the psychiatrist to introduce important functional concepts early in the initial interview process. Because most patients have been exposed repeatedly to "illness" theories of emotional distress on television, they will sometimes ask the psychiatrist directly about the focus of the questions contained in these surveys. As the following brief clinical dialogue demonstrates, the patient's curiosity presents the psychiatrist with an ideal opportunity to offer a different perspective on the meaning of distressing symptoms.

CASE EXAMPLE: CAROL

Carol [handing completed surveys to psychiatrist]: These questions are kind of weird. They don't seem that concerned about how bad I'm feeling inside. I thought that was the reason people get help: because they're feeling bad and need to feel better?

Psychiatrist: Well, helping you get better at handling those difficult feelings is the goal, of course, but in kind of a different way. Let me look at this stuff first for just a little bit. [He pauses to scan the surveys.] Okay, so I looked at a few of your answers, and I think I've got a better understanding of some of the issues that might be getting in the way of living your life the way you want to live it. Before we go into more detail about your current life situation and struggles, let's discuss these survey results a little bit, so you can better understand why those questions are so important, okay?

Carol: Okay with me.

Psychiatrist: All of us have difficult emotional moments in the course of living a normal life. Sometimes we get caught up in our worries, anxieties, frustrations, low moods, anger, and pain and have trouble letting go of them. The type of challenging emotions we struggle with is unique to each of us, depending on our genetic makeup, temperaments, cultures, and personal lived histories. Does that make sense?

Carol: Yeah, there sure are a lot of people with problems out there.

Psychiatrist: You might be more susceptible to having some of these emotional challenges show up due to the stresses in your current life situation. As we go through our lives, stressful things happen—relationship issues, educational or work problems, health problems—and when stress happens, we can get more caught up in our reactions. We get tangled up in those very natural but difficult thoughts and feelings that go along with being stressed, and those thoughts and feelings can get in the way of living our lives effectively, of being the kind of person we want to be in our relationships, of being able to learn and work effectively, and of simply having fun and, naturally, in regard to our health. We get stuck. If you think about it, these questions are asking whether that is happening to you in your current life situation. Really, the key issue isn't whether you have life situations that stress you out; that happens to just about everyone! The key issue is whether you get tangled up in your emotional responses to the extent that you can't do the things that matter to you in those situations. Does that make sense?

Carol: Yes, now that you put it that way, I can see how that would be important.

Psychiatrist: So yes, we'll certainly be keeping track of how you're feeling inside, and we'll try to improve on that as well. I know this is a very superficial first glance, but does it speak to how things have been with you? That some types of feelings are harder to go through without struggling with them and making them worse, and that sometimes we lose sight of what really matters to us in life? That's why I had you complete the survey that asked you about your values in life.

Carol: Well, I do feel like I spend more time reacting to my emotional issues than enjoying being alive.

As the preceding dialogue demonstrates, even something as simple as completing a few carefully chosen self-report surveys can spark a patient's curiosity and openness to seeking a new perspective on old, ongoing problems.

Summary

We hope this chapter helped you develop a clear sense of how the functional contextual approach can enliven each clinical encounter and each day of working as a psychiatrist. This emphasis on *function*—the patient's optimal well-being and best interests—allows the practicing psychiatrist to shift gears, particularly when a more limited symptom-elimination approach is not yielding positive results or when the patient's symptoms have indeed improved, but the patient still does not seem to be engaging in valued life pursuits. The functional approach allows the psychiatrist to adopt a flexible, vital, life-oriented way of working. Most importantly, the values that brought most of us into the practice of medicine and psychiatry were to help patients overcome or at least cope better with their suffering and experience the joy of living. In the functional psychiatry approach, these values are mobilized within each clinical encounter and, in a fashion, are empirically demonstrated to benefit patients both quickly and over the long term. The World Health Organization (2014) defined *health* not merely as the absence of disease but as "a state of well-being in which every individual realizes his or her potential, can cope with the normal stresses of life, can work productively and fruitfully, and is able to make a contribution to her or his community." This definition is right out of the functional psychiatry playbook!

The Essentials

- The functional psychiatry approach holds that symptoms of emotional distress are signals that the patient's life is out of balance in some important way, rather than signs of a latent underlying mental illness.
- The goal of functional psychiatric intervention is not so much symptom elimination or control as it is teaching patients how to accept the presence of emotional distress and use it as motivation to implement more workable life strategies based on personal values.
- The functional psychiatrist seeks to help patients develop the self-reflective awareness and perspective-taking abilities to assess the workability of their adaptive responses.

- Medications are useful to the extent they promote positive changes in patients' ability to engage with, and function effectively in, the life areas that matter to them.
- The functional psychiatric interview process seeks to identify patients' strengths and weaknesses in functional capacity in the life areas most important to them, as well as analyze specific life situations that trigger unworkable avoidance strategies.
- The key activities in functional psychiatric case formulation involve identifying patterns of workable and unworkable responses, both in the public actions context and the internal context of mental rules and self-instructions.

Suggested Readings

Fledderus M, Oude Voshaar MA, Ten Klooster PM, et al: Further evaluation of the psychometric properties of the Acceptance and Action Questionnaire-II. Psychol Assess 24(4):925–936, 2012

Ramnero J, Törneke N: The ABCs of Human Behavior: Behavioral Principles for the Practicing Clinician. Oakland, CA, New Harbinger, 2008

Wyder M, Kisely S, Meurk C, et al: The language we use: the effect of writing mental health care plans in the first person. Australas Psychiatry 26(5):496–502, 2018

References

American Psychiatric Association: Diagnostic and Statistical Manual of Mental Disorders, 5th Edition. Arlington, VA, American Psychiatric Association, 2013

Bohlmeijer E, Ten Klooster P, Fledderus M, et al: Psychometric properties of the Five Facet Mindfulness Questionnaire in depressed adults and development of a short form. Assessment 18(3):308–320, 2011

Bond FW, Hayes SC, Baer RA, et al: Preliminary psychometric properties of the Acceptance and Action Questionnaire-II: a revised measure of psychological inflexibility and experiential avoidance. Behav Ther 42(4):676–688, 2011 22035996

Gillanders DT, Bolderston H, Bond FW, et al: The development and initial validation of the cognitive fusion questionnaire. Behav Ther 45(1):83–101, 2014 24411117

Gloster AT, Klotsche J, Ciarrochi J, et al: Increasing valued behaviors precedes reduction in suffering: findings from a randomized controlled trial using ACT. Behav Res Ther 91:64–71, 2017 28160720

Hayes S, Strosahl K, Wilson K: Acceptance and Commitment Therapy: The Process and Practice of Mindful Change. New York, Guilford, 2011

Robinson P, Gould D, Strosahl K: Real Behavior Change in Primary Care: Improving Patient Outcomes and Increasing Job Satisfaction. Oakland, CA, New Harbinger, 2011

Smout M, Davies M, Burns N, et al: Development of the Valuing Questionnaire (VQ). J Contextual Behav Sci 3(3):164–172, 2014

Strosahl K, Robinson P, Gustavsson T: Brief Interventions for Radical Change: Principles and Practice of Focused Acceptance and Commitment Therapy. Oakland, CA, New Harbinger, 2012

VanderWeele TJ: On the promotion of human flourishing. Proc Natl Acad Sci USA 31:8148–8156, 2017

World Health Organization: Mental Health: A State of Well-Being. Geneva, Switzerland, World Health Organization, 2014. Available at: https://www.who.int/features/factfiles/mental_health/en. Accessed December 17, 2018.

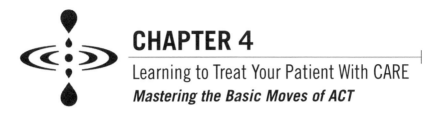

CHAPTER 4

Learning to Treat Your Patient With CARE
Mastering the Basic Moves of ACT

How can we know the dancer from the dance?

—*William Butler Yeats*

In Chapter 3, we discussed the guiding principles of functional contextual psychiatry. Those principles form the basis of the ACT intervention framework, which views symptoms, and what to do about them, in a very different way. The functional psychiatrist creates a new definition of what doing "better" means and what the goals of the session will be. The psychiatrist wants to help the patient open up to distressing, unwanted internal experiences and use a flexible, values-based approach to making needed adaptations. Painful private experiences are now seen as a natural, honorable result of the patient pursuing basic hopes, aspirations, and personal values. There is something very uplifting about engaging a patient in a conversation that helps him move from a stance of emotional and behavioral avoidance to one of openness to inner experiences and a newfound willingness to experiment with behaviors grounded in personal values.

ACT helps patients shift how they frame and address their problematic inner experiences, and significant qualitative change can sometimes be achieved in a single clinical encounter. This makes ACT a potentially beneficial approach to use when the number of contacts you have with a patient will be limited or spread very far apart in time or when the patient will be seen for very short sessions. Okay, you say, it sounds good, but isn't this complicated? Aren't the clinicians who do this like master salsa dancers? Yes, sometimes they are, but *every* salsa dancer starts by learning the basic count: quick, quick, slow; quick, quick, slow. You learn by paying attention to the basic count and continue until it becomes second nature. You cannot spin and do other, more advanced salsa moves until you have the basic cadence down. You may not look as cool as a master dancer, but as we like to say in ACT, you can only start from where you are, not where you would like to be! Once you get out on the dance floor, you will begin to sense the rhythm inside the dance of change and become more and more skilled at making advanced ACT moves over time. It just takes practice.

In this chapter, we offer each different type of learner a special way to learn basic ACT moves. For those who learn by watching, we have integrated a series of instructional videos into a detailed discussion of the CARE approach. In the last section of this chapter, we introduce and demonstrate how to use the ACT Matrix, a clinical technique that has steadily grown in popularity with ACT practitioners across the globe. In each case, the video demonstrations have been organized in a step-by-step fashion, so we recommend watching them in the appropriate sequence. Allow yourself about an hour just to work your way through the video tutorials. Jumping around is not recommended!

For those who learn by reading, later in this chapter we go into a detailed clinical dialogue that shows how the CARE approach and ACT Matrix are "unpacked" over the course of a clinical interview. We offer commentary about how to make the appropriate "reads" of salient clinical behaviors and then how to "react" to those behaviors using ACT-consistent language and interventions.

For those who learn by doing, we offer access to new, online clinical practice support tools that will support your efforts to use the CARE approach or to intervene using the ACT Matrix. We provided quite a few such tools in the preceding chapter, but more are still to come! We want to emphasize that combining these educational methods may produce the best results of all. Being flexible, curious, and persistent is a very good formula for learning ACT.

Learning to CARE: A Basic Approach to ACT

What can the psychiatrist do to help patients shift from actively avoiding distressing, unwanted private experiences and the life situations that trigger them to seeking valued life ends, even if doing so results in considerable emotional discomfort? The basic dance of ACT is to help patients realize that emotional discomfort is not the enemy of vital living but is rather an integral part of living according to one's values. Each contact the psychiatrist has with a patient is an opportunity to create this "a-ha" recognition within that patient. The natural rhythm of the clinical conversation and overall flow of an ACT session are organized around a set of principles known as CARE. CARE is based in the principles of the Four Quadrant Case Analysis approach we introduced in Chapter 3. Similar to that approach, each letter of the CARE acronym stands for a specific clinical task the psychiatrist will want to accomplish, often in sequence, during the course of a session. If the CARE interview sequence is done correctly, the psychiatrist will be able to take the information from the interview and put it directly into a Four Quadrant Case Analysis! Figure 4–1 presents an overview of each of these four tasks and their positioning in the treatment session.

In the sections that follow, we look at each of these crucial clinical in-session tasks in more detail.

C: Assess Context Sensitivity and Workability

The first important principle of the ACT model is that symptoms of distress, whatever form they take, are always embedded in a life context. We cannot understand the meaning of a patient's symptoms without also understanding the basic features of her life space. Thus, the psychiatrist will want to engage the patient in a conversation about what is (and is not) happening in her life. This means examining her central relationships (i.e., intimate partners, parenting, family, friends), work life, how she spends time when not working, and what she does for fun and to relax, as well as her health habits, spiritual life, and ways of cultivating self-growth. This process of getting to know the patient instantly communicates that the psychiatrist is both interested in and cares about her psychological health.

🎥 Video 1: Brief Contextual Assessment

Another central feature of the contextual assessment is to address the workability of the patient's current behavior patterns, because unworkable behavior patterns produce symptoms of distress. These symptoms are a signal that his life context is not working in some important way. As discussed in Chapter 2, workability is always assessed with reference to the patient's underlying values in the same life areas that the contextual interviewing is targeting. The best way to get into the patient's network of avoidance behaviors is to go "digging for pain" (Strosahl et al. 2012). The psychiatrist wants to elicit, in as much detail as possible, the life situations and contexts that produce emotional discomfort for the patient, so that he will begin to react in session the way he reacts in similar real-life situations. This strategy can be a little unsettling for the patient, but it usually produces lots of clinically relevant material and quickly builds the therapeutic alliance.

🎥 Video 2: "A-B-C" Analysis of an Emotionally Charged Situation

---

Assessment tasks	Intervention tasks
C: Context Assess context sensitivity/workability • Determine the degree of patient's functional status and participation in major life areas • Locate the main sources of emotional and behavioral avoidance in patient's life context • Determine the extent to which patient is "sensitive" to the unworkable consequences of avoidance	**E: Experiment** Experiment with new behaviors • Try new approach behaviors patient will implement in context • Ensure patient accepts that new behaviors are likely to trigger previously avoided private experiences • Augment "meaning" of new behaviors by linking them to patient's values
A: Avoidance Assess avoidance rules and functions • Discover which private experiences (thoughts, emotions, memories, urges, sensations), situated in context, "trigger" avoidance self-instructions • Help patient verbally articulate the avoidance rules that are being followed • Determine patient's ability to "be present" when emotionally challenging material appears in session	**R: Reformulate** Reformulate self-instructional rules • Change patient's awareness of, and mental relationship to, avoidance rules such that they lose their regulatory power • "Overwrite" existing avoidance rules such that they function as approach rules • Introduce new "superordinate" rules that override the self-instructional avoidance functions of old rules (values)

Public actions context | Private events context

FIGURE 4–1.   Essential clinical tasks in the CARE intervention sequence.

From an ACT perspective, a patient comes in for help because a discrepancy exists between what she is seeking in life and what she is getting. Thus, the psychiatrist wants to engage her in a discussion about her values in order to "frame" this dynamic: the discrepancy between what she would like to be doing in life and what she *is* doing in life "turns on" symptoms of distress. This is the shift from trying to eradicate uncomfortable internal events to looking at the patient's behaviors in context. From a contextual perspective, behaviors are not automatically bad or good; the values context within which the behavior is nested creates its emotional significance and personal meaning. Thus, the most important question is how well specific behaviors are working to help the patient move toward who she wants to be in her life. The bigger and more numerous the discrepancies are, the more deeply distressed and symptomatic the patient will be. ACT practitioners can quickly get at the issue of patient values in a multitude of ways, ranging from written self-report exercises such as the Valued Living Questionnaire (discussed in Chapter 3) to more experientially based assessments such as the Bullseye Values Exercise. Whatever specific techniques you use, be sure to start the conversation about the patient's values early on in the interview sequence.

Clinical Tool 13: Bullseye Action Plan
Clinical Tool 14: Bullseye Action Plan Instruction Worksheet

Video 3: The Bullseye Values Exercise

A: Articulate Avoidance Rules and Functions

In the ACT model, the root cause of suffering of all kinds is engaging in unworkable patterns of emotional and behavioral avoidance as a result of rule-following. As discussed in Chapter 2, the self-instructional rules that support emotional and behavioral avoidance tend to generalize and spread very rapidly because almost anything a patient does in life can potentially trigger a distressing, unwanted thought, memory, feeling, urge, or physical sensation.

Remember that in human language, anything can be related to anything else, without restriction. Thus, most patients over time develop multiple types of avoidance behaviors, including distraction, suppression, or relying on external means (e.g., drugs, alcohol, food) to control or mute their distressing, unwanted private experiences. Most patients are not even aware that are following rules that do not work; the self-awareness and perspective-taking needed to create this recognition has to be cultivated in session. Most patients just assume that the goal for everyone is to avoid painful, unwanted emotions or to demand "magic pill" solutions that will quickly eliminate their discomfort. For most patients, avoidance is a given, a normal thing everyone does—and they are right! Avoidance behaviors of all kinds are pervasive in our culture. The good news is that because patients will see the need to avoid as a given, they feel no shame in talking about these behaviors.

Often, patients will assertively declare that they are just doing what they are supposed to do. Their almost complete naiveté about the paradoxically negative effects of avoidance means that they feel no stigma associated with discussing it in session. This is a huge advantage for the psychiatrist, who, to capitalize on this opportunity, will have to refrain from condescending to, lecturing, or cajoling patients about the unworkable consequences of avoidance.

Instead, the psychiatrist will want to paraphrase what a patient is saying and try to accurately construct a picture of his life context and the challenges he is facing in that context. The psychiatrist will gently help the patient "discover" that avoidance is a core strategy he has been using to control or eliminate unwanted private experiences. At the same time, the psychiatrist will help him discover the paradox of avoidance behaviors: although the self-instructional rules that promote avoidance specify that this practice will help him feel better, he actually feels worse inside. His life problems are not getting better; they are getting worse. The emotions the patient is experiencing are not going down in intensity; they are going up. In this phase of the CARE interview sequence, the psychiatrist helps the patient recognize the avoidance behaviors he has been using, links these back to the problem of workability, and begins to implicitly undermine the patient's conviction in the workability of avoidance strategies.

📹 Video 4: Analyzing Avoidance

At this point in a CARE interview, the problematic results of following avoidance rules have been made apparent to the patient via genuine curiosity and guided discovery. The psychiatrist has asked questions in a nonjudgmental and curious way. The patient's answers to these questions have required her to increase her level of self-reflective awareness and perspective-taking. Often, if the interview had to end at this point due to time constraints, the patient probably would begin to spontaneously implement new strategies. Just becoming aware of the presence of these destructive self-instructional rules is sometimes all patients need to escape their regulatory power. The psychiatrist could gently suggest the patient experiment with "holding still" and not engaging in avoidance behaviors in some situations that previously have triggered her, just to see what happens. Their end-of-session agreement could be that the next time they meet, they could look at some alternative strategies she might want to experiment with. For now, the agreement is that she will stop doing what does not work and see what shows up in the void created by this nonaction.

R: Reformulate Self-Instructional Rules (Reframing)

Something we stated in Chapter 2 bears repeating here. *All* human behavior is rule governed and under the influence of self-instructional control. Thus, the main clinical question is not whether patients are engaged in rule-following but rather, what rules are they following? The transition from the more problem-focused aspects of the CARE sequence to the strengths-based or solution-focused aspects of the interview occurs as psychiatrist and patient begin to negotiate a new, more workable set of rules that the patient will follow. The goal is to create a new definition of the "problem" such that the patient can solve it in a direct fashion. Keep in mind that he has been attempting to solve this problem by trying to control or eliminate these experiences, and this has only served to worsen the problem. He has become progressively more mired in the very experiences that are supposed to be "solved" by using control and elimination strategies. When patients enter treatment, they usually feel "stuck." The psychiatrist's goal is to get the patient to use a different strategy, but the patient must first embrace the new problem definition before he can begin to change his strategy.

These new self-instructional relationships can be created in two basic ways. One is by introducing a new relationship that has not previously been accounted for in the existing self-instructional rules that promote avoidance. A good example is deliberately forming a link between the patient's pain and the patient's values. Often, this can be a quick exchange that captures the patient's attention. Linking personal values with emotional distress in a positive way enables a new potential rule: "Behaving according to your values is more important than controlling how you feel, because your emotional distress is a sign that you care, not that you are broken." This new relation references the old relation ("painful feelings are bad for you and need to be eliminated") but then is placed above the old rule in the chain of self-instructional influence. We call this a *superordinate rule*. Its behavioral regulatory influence supersedes that of the old rule. Patients must understand that the old rule will most certainly show up again, but when it does, the new rule will show up with it.

Video 5: Linking Emotional Pain to What Matters

Another way to reformulate and reframe avoidance functions is to test both the response and the consequence specified in the existing rule by practicing a response that conflicts with that self-instructional command. In essence, the psychiatrist helps the patient disobey the existing rule and try something different. A lot is at stake here for the patient, because the existing rule promises bad things will happen if the avoidance behavior is not performed. The psychiatrist must be both sensitive to and respectful of the patient's desire to avoid harm. However, when this act of disobedience to the mind is successfully completed, the new *contingency-based* (i.e., directly learned by an experiential test of workability) rule changes the nature of the patient's A-B-C relationship to the unwanted, distressing experience. Instead of running away from it, the patient holds still and simply lets it be there, practicing nonreactivity and acceptance instead of avoidance.

All of this can be written in a single sentence, but it actually involves linking several new rules together and equipping patients with the skills needed to conform to this new way of relating to disturbing content. First, patients must learn to "hold still" and "be present" when threatening content shows up. Many variations of present-moment awareness and attention-control skill-building exercises are available to help patients become observers of, rather than participants in, inner experience. Most ACT practitioners have a favorite present-moment exercise that works particularly well when they use it in therapy.

📹 Video 6: Eliciting Simple Awareness of Experience

ACT uses a wide range of metaphors and analogies, because these nonliteral forms of communication naturally lead to broader, more durable and workable forms of self-instructional control. In other words, reformulating self-instructional rules becomes easier when those new rules are "carried" in physical or psychological metaphors and analogies. In addition to its heavy reliance on nonliteral forms of communication, ACT uses language in many other "odd" ways that principally are designed to destabilize patients' confidence in the linear reasoning of the problem-solving mind. One common strategy is to treat private experiences such as thoughts, feelings, memories, or urges as entities with their own designs and intentions that are not necessarily "friendly" to the individual. Making mental events into entities both creates and solidifies the distinction between *you* (thought, emotion, memory, urge) and *me* (the human receiving these experiences). This practice also allows patients to begin to "see" the act of mental experiencing as a process rather than as reality.

📹 Video 7: Promoting a Sense of Self as Separate From Inner Experiences

Metaphors and analogies are powerful forms of self-instruction because they sidestep literal, linear forms of self-instructional control. Remember that language is ultimately a social game, played on the basis of agreed-upon rules. Metaphors and analogies violate these rules and install new rules that relax the requirement for literal correspondence. Exercises such as the Bullseye are not what they appear to be, by mutual agreement. The patient and psychiatrist know that the Bullseye is not about marksmanship with darts or bows and arrows. It refers to another topic—being true to one's values—that normally would never be discussed in these terms. Metaphors allow the psychiatrist and patient to suspend the need for literal truth in their communications. This short-circuits self-instructional rules that are linked to literal, socially installed rules about handling private experience. In clinical terms, these nonliteral forms of communication make it less likely the patient will be unwilling to engage in some new approach or acceptance behavior in session. Using metaphor as a nonthreatening psychological space allows previously avoided content to be experienced in a different way.

Being open to and accepting of what shows up in the mind's eye is really just a different way of relating to private content. It does not require the content to be changed or evaluated in any way; no struggle is necessary. In essence, an acceptance self-instruction is the exact opposite of an instruction to eliminate, change, or control an unwanted experience. Giving patients the opportunity to practice and strengthen openness skills is thus a prerequisite for effective ACT treatment. Again, this openness can be practiced in a multitude of ways within the treatment session. Openness interventions are typically not gauged by how much time they consume but by their qualitative impact on the patient.

Video 8: Promoting Observational Distance From Distressing Inner Experience

---

E: Experiment With New Behaviors

In Chapter 2, we noted that rule-governed behaviors, by their very nature, have a repertoire-narrowing effect on human behavior. Put another way, the problem of context insensitivity means the patient is unable or unwilling to try new behaviors in situations in which existing behaviors do not work. The final piece of the CARE interview sequence is to get the patient to agree to try something different, to add new behaviors to her existing repertoire. After all, up to now, we have simply been intervening in the interior world of the patient's avoidance behaviors and rule-following. If nothing different happens outside the psychiatrist's office, then the therapy has failed. Thus, the job of the psychiatrist is to "seal the deal" with the patient so she will vary her response in at least one important life domain. To achieve this result, the psychiatrist will need to circle back around to the patient's stated values and reactivate the dynamic tension between avoidance behaviors and living a valued life. Although this conversation was started in the opening minutes of the interview, it will not be finished until it is revisited in the context of helping the patient choose to try something different. If the psychiatrist has only a vague sense of the specific values-based behaviors the patient would engage in if freed from the domination of the inner advisor, then the first step is to pose this question to the patient.

📹 Video 9: Analyzing Barriers to Valued Living

The "C" in ACT stands for *commitment*, and the verb tense of this concept is *committed action*. Committed action involves patients choosing to engage in values-consistent behavior, situated in a life context that matters to them, with full knowledge that doing so may well trigger unpleasant, distressing private experiences. To do this requires patients to be willing to expose themselves to the threatening situation, to get in contact with and take a stance of openness toward immediate private experiences and the avoidance self-instructions triggered by those experiences, and to choose to remain in the threatening situation and "do what matters." Metaphorical and experiential exercises that teach openness and acceptance in session can be thought of as miniature versions of the same processes that will happen in the patient's life outside of therapy. Committed action is a more complex behavioral task than simply learning to write thoughts down on a piece of paper or holding sticky notes in one's lap. This is the "real deal" for patients, because it will unfold over longer stretches of time, and their life context is far more chaotic and unpredictable than the test-tube environment of the psychiatrist's office. Physical metaphors that require patients to move around and operate in space are particularly useful, because such kinesthetic experiences can function as nonliteral representations of the patients' intended actions. Metaphors referring to journeying or to staying on course while navigating treacherous or unclear terrain or waters are particularly useful. Again, many, many ACT-consistent metaphors for willingness and committed action have been developed over the years.

📹 Video 10: Passengers on the Bus Metaphor

Because of the qualitative change process of ACT, the psychiatrist must help patients devise a highly focused, circumscribed new behavior to use rather than engage in a broad, heroic (and probably unsuccessful) plan to change multiple behaviors at once. Selecting smaller, targeted goals is a better clinical strategy because it is more likely to succeed. This can be a deceptively difficult task, because any behavioral experiment must be situated in patients' life contexts such that they can practice new, meaningful responses without being overwhelmed by the force of the situation. By approaching this task verbally and logically, the psychiatrist may fall into the trap of teaching patients more avoidance behaviors. Experientially based metaphorical exercises involving directionality, such as the Life Path Exercise, are very effective in helping patients identify and isolate small, values-based behaviors they can practice within their life context.

 Clinical Tool 15: The Life Path Exercise
Clinical Tool 16: The Life Path Exercise Instructions

 Video 11: Life Path Goal Setting Exercise

Said another way, teaching the patient how to vary his behavior is more important than what behavior is varied. Small variations in behavior are still variations. Subjectively speaking, the patient will notice that this new behavior, even though it is small, is different from what he has done in this situation in the past. The cardinal rule of behavior experiments is to prevent the patient from failing, from feeling like a failure, at all costs. Once they devise a behavioral experiment, the psychiatrist will want to ask the patient about any expected or unexpected barriers he thinks he might encounter that would prevent the experiment from happening. Also, the psychiatrist will want to check the patient's "confidence level" about actually being able to execute the experiment as planned, usually on a 1–10 scale. Last, the psychiatrist will negotiate an interval of time before the patient will return for a follow-up visit to share the results of his experiment.

TIPS FOR SUCCESS

In every treatment session, the psychiatrist wants to both organize and direct the therapeutic conversation so it naturally ends with the patient ready to try something different.

The CARE interview gives the psychiatrist specific clinical interviewing tasks that, if executed properly, will set the stage for powerful and lasting clinical change.

Each letter in the CARE acronym stands for a specific clinical task:

- **C**onduct a contextual assessment
- **A**ssess and undermine avoidance rules and behavior
- **R**eformulate and reframe self-instructional rules
- **E**xperiment with new behaviors to increase adaptive skills

Clinical Applications of the CARE Approach

Although the steps of the CARE approach have been described sequentially, they may not roll out that way in any particular session. The ability to use them fluidly and flexibly will come as the psychiatrist gains experience with the model. In this section, we use a case example to show how to apply the CARE approach in a typical 20-minute medication consult appointment.

CASE EXAMPLE: JANET

Janet is a 40-year-old married woman who has been seeing her psychiatrist for the past 3 years. She has had persistent low-grade depression for many years. She is seen quarterly for a 20-minute "med check" to refill her antidepressant medications. Prior to this visit, the focus of treatment had been on medication, with only modest results. Janet generally rates her depression as an 8 on a 10-point scale. She adequately attends to activities of daily living yet has chronic passive suicidal ideation. She sleeps well but reports low energy and anhedonia. She has a good appetite and has been increasing her weight by about 5 pounds per year. She is concerned about developing diabetes, which runs in her family. Janet has tried several antidepressants and augmentations with lithium, T4, and various antipsychotics, all of which were ineffective or poorly tolerated due to weight gain and oversedation. Current psychotropic medications are bupropion XL 300 mg/day and venlafaxine ER 300 mg/day, which Janet feels are somewhat helpful and does not want changed.

The psychiatrist has tried to get Janet to participate in various forms of therapy and psychoeducational skill building, with limited success. Janet had agreed to see a therapist but quit after a couple of sessions, stating that she "didn't feel like we connected." She had also agreed to take a mindfulness-based stress reduction course but never followed through. The psychiatrist has tried to refer Janet back to her primary care physician for medications, but Janet has resisted this, reporting that the meetings with him are "helpful," and she does not want to stop. The psychiatrist is concerned Janet might see ending their treatment relationship as yet another example of being rejected. During the 20-minute schedule slot allotted for a medication check, the psychiatrist decides to try the CARE interview sequence to see if it can change Janet's perspective on her long-term struggles with depression.

C: Assess Context Sensitivity and Workability

The psychiatrist starts out with the "C" of the CARE acronym and tries to help Janet place her behavior in a different context designed to increase her self-reflective awareness and perspective-taking abilities. This will shift the focus of the conversation from Janet's long-term goal of "feeling less depressed" to beginning to understand the ongoing contextual triggers for her depression.

> Psychiatrist: Janet, I was wondering if we could talk more about what's going on in your life right now and if what we've been trying is moving you in the direction you want to go.
> Janet: What do you mean?
> Psychiatrist: Well, first of all, I want to be sure I'm clear about when your depression started and the direction it's been going. We've been meeting for 3 years. Remind me when your depression started.
> Janet: I remember being depressed when my mother died, especially that first year, but then I did better; I was 22. Of course, I missed my mother, but Brian was different back then, more attentive, and I managed. Then the kids were born, and I was so busy. I loved being a mom, especially when they were little. Our block had a lot of small children; our boys were part of that gang, and I made friends with the other moms. I always liked to bake and to have my sons and their friends come over for fresh cookies. I was happy.
> Psychiatrist: That sounds like a nice time. When did things change?
> Janet: I've been depressed really since we moved here; it's almost 12 years now. We moved because of Brian's work; it wasn't my idea. I don't have any friends here.

The issues of wanting friends, of feeling better when behavior is organized around goals, and resenting Brian are details the psychiatrist mentally files away as possibly helpful for later.

> Psychiatrist: Has the depression changed over time? We've discussed how the medications maybe have helped a little, and you didn't think the therapist was helpful. What else have you tried to feel better, and did it help?

The psychiatrist is beginning to contextualize the depression and set it in the context of unworkable avoidance behaviors.

> Janet: Nothing has made it better. I try to stay busy around the house to keep my mind off of how unhappy I am. I force

myself to go to my kids' school events, thinking I'll meet some people I like, but it never works out that way. I tell myself to quit being a crybaby and get used to my new life. I thought about registering for a jewelry-making class at the arts center, but I just can't get myself to do it. I would probably stop going soon after starting it, and that would just make me feel worse, something else I don't follow through with. I'm more depressed the longer I live here. I think the medications are helping, but I'm not sure.

The psychiatrist now has a picture of the trajectory of the depression and some of the elements that likely are keeping it in place. The psychiatrist will now conduct a contextual interview focusing on the patient's work life, primary relationships, leisure, recreational and self-growth pursuits, and health-protective lifestyle behaviors.

Psychiatrist: If it's okay with you, can we take a few minutes to review what's going on in your life right now so I'm up to speed? You've told me your husband is out of town for work a lot, and you feel isolated in this town. Do you stay in touch with any of your old friends from where you used to live?

Janet: I feel like I'm all alone. I've lost contact with my old friends, and I haven't made any friends in this town. That's the problem—no one is friendly. Brian works out of town a lot, and he pays more attention to the newspaper or his phone when he's around. We talk on the phone every day, but mostly it's a quick check-in about the house or the kids. I feel like he's checking me off his to-do list. It's been even worse since my oldest son left for college last September. He would have his friends over, and I'd bake for them. My younger son isn't the social butterfly my oldest is; he's into video games and spends most of his time with his gamer friends at their homes. Now I'm mostly alone at home. If it weren't for my dog, Andy, I'm not sure I'd get out most days. Walking Andy is just about the only exercise I get, and that's the best part of my day. When I'm alone at home, he sits by me or sometimes will sit on the sofa with me while I'm reading.

Psychiatrist: Before you had your kids, did you have a career or a job you liked?

Janet: I had a natural talent for math and studied accounting and bookkeeping in college. I was an "A" student, too. I got a job right out of college. I actually really liked my job, but it just wasn't in the cards for me to keep working after I had my kids. Brian promised that he'd support us and that I wouldn't need to go back to work. Now I've been out of work for so many years, I don't know if I'd be able to get a good bookkeeping job. So, I have to get my money from

Brian. He never says anything bad about me not working, but he doesn't seem to care one way or the other about how I'm doing.

At this juncture, Janet's "depression" makes much more sense. She has experienced the loss of many close friends, feels at least somewhat neglected by her husband, is dealing with the departure of her oldest son to college, and feels alone much of the time. The psychiatrist will now help Janet look at her current behaviors in terms of what she is seeking in her life versus what she is getting in life.

Psychiatrist: I'm wondering how feeling anxious and depressed has affected your ability to go for what you want in life. If you were feeling better, if we discovered the magic pill that would take away your depression and give you your energy back, what would you be doing differently?

Janet: I don't know. I just feel stuck about what to do.

When someone has been stuck in unworkable behaviors, it sometimes takes some mutual brainstorming to move them forward.

Psychiatrist: Could we take a minute to think about how your life might look different if you were feeling better? You mentioned you were doing fine in your life before you moved here. What things did you do back then? Are there things you were doing more of or less of? Are there new activities you might start, or things you might try, if you didn't have to worry about feeling sad or worried or rejected? You mentioned thinking about taking a jewelry class, for example. You also really seemed to enjoy working as a bookkeeper. You mentioned being disappointed that you and Brian are not spending as much quality time together.

Janet: Oh. Yes, if I wasn't so depressed, I would probably be taking some type of art class. I've also thought about looking for a part-time job to get out of the house, but I don't want to leave Andy alone. If I wasn't so angry at Brian, I might try to cook more, like he wants me to. I thought about joining a book club at the library, too; that might get me around people who I might be interested in.

Psychiatrist: That sounds like a lot of ideas. So on the one hand, there's the prospect of doing these things [puts a hand out in front of her, like a bowl], such as taking a jewelry class at the art center, joining a book club to see if you could make friends there, finding a part-time bookkeeping job, and trying to make your relationship with Brian be more like you'd want it to be. On the other hand [holds out other hand next to first], there's the life you've been living. You stay home most of the time, you avoid people, you don't talk to Brian about feeling neglected, you think about getting involved in hobbies or going back to work but back off because you feel tired. Which of these strategies—getting involved or avoiding things so you won't feel more hurt—is more likely to work to give you the life you want, a life that feels rich and satisfying to you?

Janet: Well, I would get out more, I guess, and try to meet some people. But I've tried to be friendly. When I first moved here, I tried to be friendly, but it didn't work. That's why I don't try anymore.

Psychiatrist: It sounds like your mind is telling you the best way to protect yourself from rejection is to withdraw. I'm wondering: What does your experience tell you?

Janet: When I look at it that way, staying at home and avoiding people hasn't helped, but I don't know what else to do.

A: Articulate and Undermine Avoidance Rules and Behaviors

The psychiatrist now moves to the second step in the CARE acronym, namely, to call out the avoidance strategies the patient is using and help her question their usefulness. In this step, the psychiatrist wants to help Janet become aware of and describe the self-instructional rules that are producing unworkable avoidance behaviors. The psychiatrist knows that helping Janet accept her unpleasant and distressing emotional experiences will give her more flexibility in choosing how she responds to them, with the eventual goal of allowing her to choose more workable behaviors.

Psychiatrist: My concern is that we've been focusing on helping you feel less depressed, but maybe your depression is a signal things are out of balance in your life right now—actually, going back many years, it sounds like. The neat thing is, you seem to have a lot of ideas about doing things differently, but you're still having a hard time doing the things that might help life feel like the life you want. Can we talk about what's getting in the way? Can you notice any thoughts, feelings, memories, or urges that come up when you think about doing something different?

Janet: It's that this town is terrible. I'll never be happy here, and there's no use in even trying anymore.

Psychiatrist: Yes, I've noticed that thought comes up for you again and again. Can you just notice it as a rule your mind is producing?

Janet: But it's true!

Psychiatrist: Right now, the goal isn't to judge if a thought is true or not, but just to notice the instructions your mind is giving you when you think about building a better life for yourself. Can you keep doing just what you are doing? Maybe say to yourself, "I notice I'm having the thought that this town is terrible, I'll never be happy here, and there's no use in even trying anymore." And notice having the thought that *that* thought is true. Some people have other thoughts or mental rules show up, such as, "looking at my thoughts is a stupid thing to do" or "how is this going to help me?" Are you having those thoughts?

Janet: I'm not thinking that, but I am wondering why we're talking about this now?

Psychiatrist: Great question. We all have busy minds that are always generating thoughts, feelings, and memories, making us worry about the future or feel sad about something in the past. It's impossible to get our minds to turn off and stop giving us instructions about what to do. Being able to observe your mind's chatter, without judging it or trying to stop it, might help you feel a little less hopeless about your situation. After all, if it's literally true that this town is terrible and you'll never be happy, what options do you have in life? This thought rules out the possibility of you ever building a better life. If I had a truth like that to deal with, I probably would be doing exactly the same thing you're doing—shutting down emotionally and withdrawing from everything that matters. Noticing your mind's chatter *as chatter* gives you more options. Can you just notice, when you think about signing up for the jewelry class, what comes up for you? What makes it harder for you to pedal the bike in that direction?

Janet: Well, now that you ask, if I think about signing up for the class, I get the thought that "everyone is unfriendly." Then I start feeling anxious, almost humiliated, imagining being in class and everyone ignoring me. [She stares at her lap and begins to tear up.]

Psychiatrist: That sounds like a hard thought to have, if you took it literally. I could imagine it *would* be hard to sign up for that class if that's what comes up for you every time you think about it. So then you don't sign up?

Janet: Yes, and then I'm upset with myself that I haven't signed up. I feel like I'm stuck here, and the years are just passing by. Like you said, it makes sense that I feel depressed.

Psychiatrist: I'm guessing you've tried a lot of things over the years to help you get rid of these uncomfortable thoughts and feelings. I know we've tried medications, and they've helped some but not enough. What else have you tried?

Janet: I distract myself.

Psychiatrist: Does it work to distract yourself?

Janet: Sometimes for a while, but no. Then I feel like I'm wasting my life away watching TV. I enjoy baking, but there's no one left in the house to bake for, and thinking about that makes me feel worse. I've tried thinking more positive thoughts, but I'm not really Ms. Happy Sunshine, so that just makes me feel more hopeless.

Psychiatrist: Yeah, most of us are not really successful at getting rid of uncomfortable thoughts; it's just not how our minds work. If someone hung Andy over the side of the Morrison Bridge and told you they would drop him unless you stopped feeling anxious—do you think you could do it?

Janet: Probably not.

Psychiatrist: What if they asked you to dance like a chicken and sing "Yankee Doodle Dandy" or they would drop him?

Janet [smiling]: I'm not much of a singer, but I'd give it my best shot.

Psychiatrist: What else have you tried to feel better?

Janet: I don't know.

Psychiatrist: Some people just try to opt out of everything.

Janet: Yes. I isolate myself. That's my main thing. If Andy wasn't around, I might stay in bed all day.

Psychiatrist: Has that helped you get rid of the uncomfortable thoughts or stop feeling unhappy or anxious?

Janet: No. When you say it like that, it probably makes it worse.

Psychiatrist: What else have you tried to help get rid of these thoughts or to feel better? Some people try to think their way out of feeling bad, decide if their thoughts are true or not, analyze why they continue to have these unwanted thoughts, or talk themselves out of having the thoughts. Have you found yourself using any of those strategies?

Janet: I don't usually argue with my thoughts. It feels like it's true that this town is unfriendly. But I guess I analyze my childhood—my parents died before the kids were born—and I think I wouldn't be so depressed if that hadn't happened.

Psychiatrist: Has analyzing your childhood and the impact of your parents dying led you to any new, useful insights? Sometimes that kind of self-reflection can be very helpful.

Janet: It helps me to think about my mom and cry sometimes, but it hasn't helped me move on with feeling better now. I just feel stuck.

R: Reformulate Self-Instructional Rules

The psychiatrist has now developed a good understanding of how the patient's avoidance strategies are creating a vicious circle of increasing depression and decreasing life involvement. The psychiatrist wants to reframe the "problem" for Janet, not as one involving chronic depression as the culprit, but rather as one in which she is not being open to the signal her depression is giving her.

Psychiatrist: Today we've been talking about the gap between what you'd be doing if you were living the life that feels true to who you are, in your heart of hearts, and what you're doing now. My concern is that we've been focusing on helping you feel less depressed, but maybe your depres-

sion is a sign things are out of balance in your life right now
and actually going back many years, it sounds like.

Janet: What is it saying to me?

Psychiatrist: Well, it could be telling you that many of the emotional reactions you're having are due to this disconnect
between what you want in your life and what you're getting. The pain you're feeling inside is a reflection of your
values not being met in a lot of important areas in your life.
You can try to suppress that pain, but taking that approach
requires you to check out of your life. Right now, would
you agree you're pretty checked out of your life?

Janet: Well, that's an odd way to put it, but I think I am checked
out. I don't feel much of anything inside except this terrible sense of aloneness.

Psychiatrist: I want to help you check back in, to get back in
touch with what matters to you and to begin building that
kind of life.

Janet: That's kind of scary. My first image was of all of the disappointments that are coming my way.

Psychiatrist: The fact that disappointment is a possibility for you
also tells me these things you've told me are important in
your life really do matter to you. If something matters to
you, it's always possible that it won't work out the way
you planned. You might even say the risk of failure is what
makes these basic life aspirations so important. The feelings we've been talking about, like feeling alone, missing
your old friends, feeling abandoned by Brian, fearing rejection by people you might be interested in befriending,
these are all the natural results of caring about being connected to others. Just as a plant needs water to thrive, most
humans need intimacy and a sense of social belonging.
When you don't have those connections, your emotions
are going to kick into gear and tell you to do something different.

Janet: Almost everything I'm unhappy about involves feeling
lonely.

Psychiatrist: Sometimes it's helpful to think of living according
to your values as like shooting an arrow at a target on the
archery range. The goal, of course, is to put that arrow in
the center of the target, the bullseye. Although it would be
nice to land an arrow in the center of the target, what
makes the game of archery fun is the fact that you are doing your best to hit the bullseye. That is what to do with
values; you aim your behaviors in the direction of your
personal bullseyes. Think about what's important for you,
who you want to be if you look back in 20 years and see
yourself as you move forward with things. For example,
in the area of relationships, what would the bullseye look
like for you?

Janet: I'd like to have at least one friend. I'd like Brian to be nicer to me. I'd like my oldest son to move back to town and go to college here so I can be near him.

Psychiatrist: Those are great goals. My only concern is they rely on other people, so you may be setting yourself up for disappointment. Regardless of what other people do or don't do, what values could help you be the person you want to be with respect to the important relationships in your life?

Janet: I don't know what you mean.

Psychiatrist: For example, you might say, "I have the value of being open to getting to know people in this town and plan to try some behaviors that move me in that direction. I value forming relationships more than I value protecting myself from rejection, setback, or failure."

Janet: Oh, you want me to dance like a chicken and sing "Yankee Doodle Dandy" even though I'll have anxiety. [She smiles.]

Psychiatrist: Exactly. As another example, we've discussed your goal of taking a class at the art center. What value does your love of art reflect? Being creative? Learning something new in life?

Janet: Yes. I have a value of…having fun and being creative.

Psychiatrist: A lot of times, the things that are important to us make us feel more anxious *because* they're important to us. Is this true for you? Which makes you more anxious, buying dog food for Andy or signing up for the jewelry class?

Janet: The jewelry class. You're right, because…because it means something to me.

Psychiatrist: Right. For many of us, doing things that are important to us, or new for us, brings up anxiety. [He extends his hand, palm up.] If we want to have a life that includes openness to friendships [turns hand upside down], we've got to assume feelings of anxiety and thoughts of "it's not going to work" are going to take a ride on the back of the hand. You might not be able to have one without the other.

Janet: I never thought about it like that. I've been waiting to feel better before I sign up for that class. You're saying I might never feel better?

Psychiatrist: I'm suggesting you might never feel better if you don't pursue what matters to you in your life. If you pursue those things, you have a chance to experience the entire range of human emotions, not just the dark ones you're now avoiding. I'm saying that having thoughts and feelings, including uncomfortable thoughts and feelings, is a normal human thing our minds do. Waiting for our minds to go silent before we start behaviors that reflect our deeply held values—well, that doesn't seem to work for most of us. Avoiding living your life according to your values, according to what is important for you, creates suffering. That's what your depression is telling you.

Janet: I'm confused. So, what am I supposed to do?

E: Experiment With New Behaviors

The psychiatrist has succeeded in getting Janet to entertain a different definition of her "problems" so that controlling how she feels is no longer the prime directive of her self-instructional rule set. The psychiatrist has, in effect, helped her formulate a new self-instructional rule powerful enough to offset the behavior-regulatory influence of her existing avoidance rules. This creates an opportunity for them to explore alternative strategies that are not anchored in the need to control or avoid the way she feels inside but rather are based in her valued life aspirations and pursuits.

> Psychiatrist: What about spending some time between now and the next time we meet doing the noticing exercise we talked about? Paying attention to what your senses are noticing and what thoughts and feelings come up for you, even if they're uncomfortable thoughts and feelings? Practicing curiosity about what comes up and being kind to yourself. Not letting yourself get flooded with the thoughts, but not struggling to push them away—just noticing them and letting them go. Some people like to practice this grounding/noticing exercise for a longer time; others like to do it for shorter times, maybe only 30 seconds or up to 5 or 10 minutes a few times a day, like when they're stressed, or when they wake up and when they go to sleep. Is this something you could experiment with?
>
> Janet: Yes. But I might forget.
>
> Psychiatrist: If you forget, just notice that you forgot and return to your practice. Does your mind try to beat you up for forgetting? Was there a reason it was hard to do? Were you trying to do it to be calm? Sometimes it helps you be calmer, but expecting it to make you feel better isn't the goal. You might get calmer, you might not. The goal is to just notice whatever shows up and practice nonjudgment. There's no way to do it wrong. Would you be willing to experiment with spending a few minutes a day doing this? Is there a time of day that would work for you?
>
> Janet: It's quiet in the mornings.
>
> Psychiatrist: Like when you first get up?
>
> Janet: Maybe, or after my shower.
>
> Psychiatrist: On a scale of 1–10, how likely are you to experiment with noticing your thoughts when you first wake up or after you take a shower?
>
> Janet: I think that would be a 10. I have a lot of time on my hands. I think I can do this every day.
>
> Psychiatrist: Every day would be great, but if you forget to do it, can you notice what your mind says to you before and afterward?
>
> Janet: What do you mean?

Psychiatrist: Well, if your mind is like most of our minds, it might try to bully you for not being perfect, like saying, "You can't even remember to practice noticing. You're such a loser. You're hopeless." Or something like that.

Janet: Oh. Yeah. [She smiles.] I think I'll call to see if I can get registered for that jewelry class. That would get me out of the house and maybe meet some interesting people.

Psychiatrist: On that same 10-point scale, can you tell me how confident you are that you'll register for the jewelry class and attend it?

Janet: I think that's a 9. I've wanted to do this for a long time, and it's something I'm interested in.

Psychiatrist: Before we stop today, how helpful was this session for you today—also on that same 10-point scale?

Janet: I think an 8.

Psychiatrist: What makes it an 8? What was helpful, and what could I do better?

Janet: It was really helpful for you to talk to me about what the medications can and can't do. I realize I've been waiting to feel better so I can get on with my life, and now I need to think about this. I'm sort of disappointed that there's no "magic pill," but it's good for me to know. I hope you don't mind me saying this, but sometimes you talked too much, and I sort of got lost.

Psychiatrist: I appreciate your feedback. Thank you.

Janet: You didn't mind me saying that? Brian says I'm too opinionated, and that's why I don't have friends.

Psychiatrist: No, it's helpful for me. We're about out of time; what I'd like to do today is renew your medications but not change them. Usually we meet every 3 months, but I'd like to see you back in about a month so we can see how your noticing practice and jewelry class are going. Would that be okay with you?

Janet: Yes. I'd like to use a follow-up session with you to keep me honest!

In this session, the psychiatrist successfully moved through all four components of the CARE interview sequence. Sometimes, the time available or level of patient distress will limit movement to only one or two of the CARE components. In addition, the phases of the clinical conversation often are not linear, and it will be necessary to jump back and forth between components based on the patient's responses. This is natural in the CARE approach. However, many practitioners find that this framework helps them remember the four major pieces of the interview, particularly when they are feeling anxious because they are just starting out! When first practicing CARE, be kind to yourself. You will make mistakes. You need to continue to stretch yourself and remain flexible and self-compassionate—learning how to fit this into the existing approach you use will take time. You may find yourself thinking, "I'm going to stick to psychopharmacology, it's what I know." If this happens, you may want to ask yourself whether medications alone are providing the patient outcomes you are trying to achieve. Remember, we are all merely human, and most of us have that "inner critic" to take along with us whenever we try something new.

Learning the ACT Matrix

In this section, we both describe and demonstrate the essential features of a powerful clinical method known as the ACT Matrix, or "the matrix" for short. This a relatively new way of delivering ACT that incorporates essential clinical activities of the CARE approach while making it more transparent for practitioners and patients alike (Polk and Schoendorff 2014). In this section, we present a brief overview of the ACT Matrix, outline key concepts that guide matrix work, and demonstrate its use with a patient. For readers interested in learning the intricacies of matrix-style work, we supply a couple of recommended readings at the end of this chapter. Throughout this section, you can also watch brief instructional video segments that demonstrate how matrix work looks "boots on the ground" and access and download useful clinical practice tools to use as you develop your skills with the ACT Matrix approach. Working through the instructional video will take about 30 minutes of your time. We recommend watching the videos in sequence and in one sitting so you can get a real sense of how the matrix unfolds in a typical patient interview.

BASIC OVERVIEW OF THE ACT MATRIX

The ACT Matrix is really a patient-centered version of the Four Quadrant Case Analysis we described in Chapter 3. What makes the matrix unique is that it is primarily an intervention tool designed to be used in collaboration with the patient. The matrix boils ACT down to two basic forms of discrimination training: 1) noticing the difference between the patient's actions in the outside world and the internal or mental experiences that precede or follow them; and 2) noticing the difference between how it feels to move toward people and things the patient cares about or away from unwanted thoughts and feelings. At the center of these two processes is "me noticing," which can help the patient become more aware of ongoing influences on her behavior, as well as the function of her behaviors. A component of "me choosing" emphasizes that sources of behavioral influence are not automatic; the patient has to attach meaning and purpose to them to give them their regulatory power.

Normally, matrix work is started after the psychiatrist has assembled a fairly complete picture of the patient's life context, including areas that seem to be working well and areas that are not working. This information will be reformulated within the matrix format, with active involvement and participation of the patient. Each aspect of the ACT Matrix can be used to initiate a discussion of either decreasing unworkable private or public behaviors or increasing workable private or public behaviors. In this sense, the ACT Matrix is very similar to the Four Quadrant Case Analysis, although the terms used to describe each sector of the matrix are quite different.

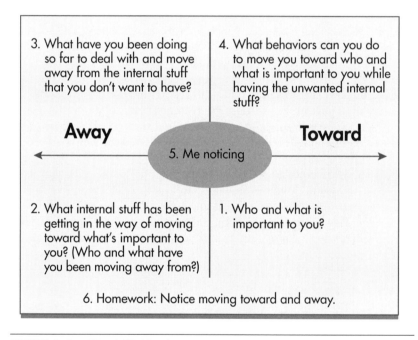

FIGURE 4–2. The ACT Matrix.

  Clinical Tool 17: The ACT Matrix Template

INTRODUCING THE ACT MATRIX TO THE PATIENT

A pictorial view of the ACT Matrix is presented in Figure 4–2. The actual exercise can be conducted using a preprinted blank matrix form, which the patient and psychiatrist can complete together and then return to over time. The patient must first understand the matrix as a task consisting of the six core steps seen in the figure. You may find it helpful to give the patient an educational handout. Handouts for adults and youth will obviously vary in terms of how the basic matrix concepts are represented. Adults are generally comfortable working with more abstract verbal concepts, whereas children and adolescents respond better to simple visual images. When describing the visual space of the matrix, the horizontal axis is usually the initial focal point because it teaches the patient to notice and name his *toward moves* (values-based approach behaviors and being open and accepting) and *away moves* (emotional and behavioral avoidance strategies) in everyday activities. These terms will later be used to cue both self-reflective awareness of and perspective-taking on the patient's workable and unworkable behaviors. The vertical axis teaches him to notice the difference between "mental activities"—the world inside the skin—and "behaviors in the world" outside the skin that can be seen and heard by others.

 Clinical Tool 18: ACT Matrix Patient Education Handout for Adults
Clinical Tool 19: ACT Matrix Patient Education Handout for Children and Adolescents

---

 Video 12: Introducing the ACT Matrix Model

ASSESSING PATIENT VALUES: WHO AND WHAT MATTERS?

In keeping with the tenets of the CARE approach, an immediate goal of matrix work is to have patients identify who and what matters to them in their current life. *Who matters* are the people who are important to the patient, including spouse or partner, immediate and extended family, friends, and colleagues. *What matters* are life activities and undertakings that are important to the patient and can include work, hobbies, social or political activism, spirituality, and so on. The initial focus on patient values creates an immediate positive tone to matrix work and will help the patient stay engaged when the conversation turns to more difficult personal issues. Throughout the process, the psychiatrist must be willing to self-disclose about who and what matters in his or her own life, so as to create a sense of shared journey through life. To whatever extent possible, the psychiatrist should try to keep the conversation casual and model a friendly, curious, open attitude.

 Video 13: The Matrix—Assessing Values

ASSESSING INTERNAL OBSTACLES

As noted earlier, the term *away move* is used to describe emotional and behavioral avoidance because it moves the patient away from unpleasant or unwanted thoughts and feelings. The psychiatrist must normalize both kinds of avoidance as things that "everyone does, even me." The initial focus will be on the patient's unwanted thoughts and feelings, listed in the lower left hand quadrant. These are the private experiences, including thoughts, feelings, mood states, memories, urges, or physical sensations that can sometimes function as barriers to moving toward who and what matters. A key feature is establishing that the patient is the one who notices these experiences and chooses how to relate to them when they show up. The perspective of "me noticing" can be construed as criticism by some patients, so the psychiatrist should simply point out that "someone" is aware of these experiences and "someone's" behavior is being affected by them. There is no pressure to have patients engage in a different response at this juncture.

🎥 **Video 14: The Matrix—Difficult Thoughts and Feelings: What Gets in the Way?**

ASSESSING BEHAVIORAL AVOIDANCE

In keeping with the core tenets of the CARE approach, the end result of internal experiences triggering emotional avoidance is that it creates behavioral avoidance. Now, the patient is exhibiting away moves that other people can see and respond to. These away moves can have a negative impact on the patient's ability to move toward who and what matters. As such, he may experience negative consequences in response to these away moves. The psychiatrist might even point out that the precipitating event for seeking professional help has been the persistence of these uncomfortable consequences.

🎥 **Video 15: The Matrix—Assessing Behavioral Avoidance: Away Moves**

DISCUSSING VALUED ACTIONS

Few, if any, patients engage only in away moves. For most of us, daily living is composed of a mixture of toward and away moves. At this point in matrix work, the psychiatrist turns back to exploring the patient's values-consistent behaviors. This not only puts the finishing touch on the initial phase of matrix work but also returns to the positive affect associated with values-based actions. It allows the psychiatrist to portray the patient's intentions in a positive frame while pointing out that all of us get hooked by, or caught up in, internal experiences that make us turn away from who and what matters. Most importantly, the dynamic tension between away and toward moves never stops for any of us. Thus, it is important to be connected to the "me noticing" process itself, because this is one sure way to short-circuit automatic, mindless away moves.

📹 Video 16: The Matrix—Assessing Valued Actions: Toward Moves

---

DISCUSSING THE SHORT- AND LONG-TERM WORKABILITY OF AWAY MOVES

The reinforcing power of emotional and behavioral avoidance strategies is due to the fact that these strategies often work in the short run to alleviate distressing, unwanted states of mind or to allow patients to escape from uncomfortable events, situations, or interactions in the external world. As mentioned, the problem is that avoidance behaviors often backfire in the long run. They can generate additional negative inner experiences and lead to problems in the patient's life context. In matrix work, the psychiatrist generally should focus first on the short-term consequences of away moves, because these may, in fact, be positive. Only after examining short-term results in detail should the conversation turn to examining long-term results. By contrasting the often seemingly positive short-term results of away moves with the generally negative long-term results, the psychiatrist can reinforce contingency-based learning for the patient as opposed to automatic rule-following.

📹 Video 17: The Matrix—Assessing Away Moves: Effectiveness Short Term
Video 18: The Matrix—Assessing Away Moves: Effectiveness Long Term

---

STUCK LOOPS: ANALYZING RECURRING PATTERNS OF AWAY MOVES

Because of the inordinate amount of detail generated in matrix work, the patient and psychiatrist have ample opportunity to focus on how to increase the patient's toward moves while decreasing her away moves. This begins to give the patient a better understanding of how her away moves reinforce themselves and create downward spirals of negative mental experience and disappointing life results. The psychiatrist should use the visual space of the ACT Matrix in interesting ways, such as by drawing concentric arrows between one quadrant and another to show how the downward spiral of avoidance works.

 Video 19: The Matrix—Identify Core Avoidance Behaviors: Stuck Loops!

USING METAPHORICAL INTERVENTIONS IN MATRIX WORK

ACT is rich in its use of metaphors and, similarly, matrix work is ideally suited for the use of metaphors. Indeed, the ACT Matrix itself is a big-picture metaphor for the things that cause us to get stuck in life and the things that help us get unstuck. The mental experiences that populate the lower left quadrant can never be eliminated, so the most powerful root metaphors will be those that create the possibility of "carrying" internal obstacles even as one steadily achieves a life rich in toward moves. Visual metaphors, such as drawing a ladder between the lower left and upper right quadrants and then asking the patient to imagine climbing the ladder step by step, can be a perfect vehicle for examining the "pull" of internal obstacles. Time-tested ACT metaphors such as the "person in the hole" highlight both the inevitability of life challenges and the need to give up on unworkable patterns of away moves in order to address those challenges. In this metaphor, the patient is asked to imagine she is walking blindfolded on the field of life and inadvertently falls into a deep hole. She then discovers the only tool in her possession is a shovel. Shovels are not very good tools for getting out of deep holes, but if it is the only tool she has, she might be tempted to keep using it even though it does not work. This metaphor conveys a simple but important self-instruction about letting go of strategies that move her away from who and what matters to her.

Video 20: The Matrix—Person in the Hole Metaphor and Choosing Toward Moves

---

In the following case example, we present an unfolding clinical dialogue to demonstrate how the psychiatrist used the ACT Matrix with Mike, the patient we introduced in Chapter 3. Table 4–1 describes the five central questions the psychiatrist wants to help the patient answer, using the matrix as a guide. Notice that these questions are very similar to the clinical focusing questions we also introduced in Chapter 3.

Table 4–1. Five central questions to ask when using the ACT Matrix

1. Who and what are important to you?

2. What are some of the difficult thoughts and feelings that can show up and get in the way of moving toward who or what is important?

3. Who is the one choosing who and what are important, and who is the one noticing what shows up and gets in the way?

4. What are some things I can see you doing when you are hooked by, or trying to move away from, these difficult thoughts and feelings?

5. What are some simple things you can be seen doing, or that you could do, to move you toward who and what is important to you?

CASE EXAMPLE: MIKE

Psychiatrist: If it's okay, I'd like to show you a model, a point of view, that many people find helpful to enable them to move toward the people and things they care about even in the presence of obstacles such as difficult thoughts and feelings. Now, this doesn't claim to be the *only* model; it doesn't claim to be the *true* model, or even to represent reality; it's simply a model, or a point of view, that many people find helpful to do what matters to them even in the presence of obstacles. Would that be okay, or is there some other way you'd like us to use our remaining time together today?

Mike: No, I'm fine with learning more about your approach.

Psychiatrist [places blank sheet of paper in front of Mike]: Now, I believe you have a dog in your life named Rex?

Mike [smiles]: Yes.

Psychiatrist: When all creatures of the world do things, including humans and dogs, we either do them to move *toward* things we like [draws an arrow on the right end of the horizonal line and writes "TOWARD" atop the right-hand side], which for Rex might be a bowl of food, or you if he's taking you for a walk, yes?

Mike [smiling at the connection to his dog]: Yes!

Psychiatrist: *Or,* all animals, including humans, do things to move *away* from things we don't like, which for a dog like Rex is always something in the moment, such as thunder or lightning or perhaps a bigger, scarier dog, yes? [He draws an arrow on the left end of the horizontal line and writes "AWAY" atop the left-hand side.]

Mike: Yes, Rex really doesn't like thunder!

Psychiatrist: Notice that right here in the middle of everything, I'm drawing this little circle; we'll call this, "me noticing." This means you are the centerpiece of all of this. You are the one who notices whether you're moving toward people and things you care about or away from difficult thoughts and feelings. You are the one who is aware of your actions.

Mike: Okay, I like the word "aware," because I don't always feel I have control over my actions.

Psychiatrist [draws dotted line upward and downward from central circle]: Yes, that's something I hear quite often from people I work with. You know, humans are different: we can move *toward* things that are not there in the moment and cannot be seen by others. You've spent many a lovely day inside working on relatively tedious things when you could have been doing more fun things outside, in the service of longer-term goals like studying for a degree, for better work, doing work for money to live more freely—true?

Mike: Yes, that's most certainly true.

Psychiatrist: So, to help you notice the difference, I'm going to draw a little movie camera up here above the line [draws a small movie camera at the top right corner of the page] to represent the world that can be seen by others. Below the line is the world inside the skin, where only you can experience it. Again, there's that little circle of "me noticing" both of these types of events.

Mike: Okay, makes sense.

Psychiatrist: We humans can move *away* from things that are not present in the moment and *cannot* be seen by others, such as difficult memories, worries about the future—correct?

Mike: That's certainly true.

Psychiatrist [draws a small movie camera at top left corner of the page]: So this is the bare bones, the basic outline of this point of view, this model, and I'd like to see how it works for you, okay?

Mike: Okay with me. Seems pretty simple, really.

Next, the psychiatrist will guide Mike through an introduction to the ACT Matrix, using five central questions (see Table 4–1).

Psychiatrist: So, Mike, who are some people you care about, people who are important to you?

Mike: Well, Gina [his wife], of course, and my parents.

Psychiatrist: I expect you call them "Mom" and "Dad"? [Writes "Gina," "Mom," and "Dad" in lower-right quadrant]

Mike: Yes, and my brothers, their families, my nieces and nephews.

Psychiatrist: Cool, so, we'll write those in here, and since we're focusing on your nuclear family, can I put you in here as well?

Mike: Well, I don't think I'm doing very well recently, but okay.

Psychiatrist [writes "Myself"]: I think Rex should be in there as well! In quotation marks, so I remember he's a dog. Any other friends of yours or Gina's who are important to you?

Mike: Well, there's Tony and Georgia, whom Gina knows, and some people from the college that I like, Angus and James.

Psychiatrist [writes those down]: And some teacher colleagues?

Mike: Yes, well, some.

Psychiatrist [writes those down]: Excellent. So we have a good range of people who are important to you. Now, what are some things that are important to you in life?

Mike: What do you mean?

Psychiatrist: Well, from our meeting last week, I think learning, and work, and making a living are very important to you?

Mike: Absolutely, but I'm not doing them very much at all!

Psychiatrist: But they are *still* important to you, right? I'll just write those down here: learning, work, and—well, money isn't everything, but we have to pay the bills! Is having fun important to you? Even if you're not in that good of a mood right now?

Mike: Sure, but it's really not happening in my life right now.

Psychiatrist: That's okay, we're just noting in this quadrant who and what you care about in life. I think taking Rex for a walk now and then, getting out in nature?

Mike: Absolutely, and looking after him, which I should be doing more of.

Psychiatrist: So, we'll put caring for others, and nature in there. Is spirituality important to you? Your Catholic faith, and the local congregation?

Mike: Very important, but I'm finding it hard to be with those people just now.

Psychiatrist: I'm a health professional, can I express a bias and put physical and mental health in here as well?

Mike: Sure, but again, I'm not doing very well with those.

Psychiatrist: Great, so we have a range of people and things [explicitly points at each name and valued life interest] that are important to you. Do you find that every single minute of every single day you are able to move toward the people and things [pointing] that are important to you? Or do you find that sometimes stuff shows up and gets in the way of moving toward who and what is important to you?

Mike: For sure, I'm finding it really hard to move toward those things recently.

Psychiatrist: Thank goodness, I'm not the only one who has that problem! Because difficult thoughts and feelings can certainly get in the way of me moving toward people and things I care about sometimes. Now, there are external obstacles [points at the camera in the top left corner], such as distance, time, and money, but I want us to look at the *internal* obstacles that get in the way of you moving toward

who and what is important in your life, such as those difficult thoughts and feelings you mentioned before. Okay?

Mike: Okay, but I'm not quite sure what you mean.

Psychiatrist: I think you mentioned that a lot of anxiety, fear,
and worry show up when you even think about exploring
new work opportunities. Does that stuff get in the way of
you moving toward exploring your career options?

Mike: Absolutely!

Psychiatrist: Awesome, so we just write down here [lower left
quadrant] anxiety, worry, fear. Do you find that frustration
also shows up, and even anger sometimes?

Mike: Certainly, with myself! And sometimes life situations…

Psychiatrist: Excellent, so I'll also write frustration, anger. What
about tiredness?

Mike: Sure thing, and feeling like there's no point in even bothering because I just can't do it.

Psychiatrist: Great, so we'll write in tiredness as something that
gets in the way, and we also have these thoughts of "why
bother" and "I can't do it" that I'm going to write in here.
Can I ask, Mike, who is it that chooses who and what is important [points to lower right quadrant], and who notices
what shows up and gets in the way?

Mike: Well, Gina notices sometimes.

Psychiatrist: Yes, I'm sure that's true, but she can be mistaken
sometimes about your feelings, can't she? Who primarily
chooses who and what is important, and who especially
will *notice* what shows up and gets in the way?

Mike: I suppose you mean me?

Psychiatrist: Absolutely! *You* are the main one choosing [points
to lower right quadrant] and noticing [points to lower left
quadrant]. You are the centerpiece of this point of view,
and we'll keep you there throughout our work [points to
"me noticing" in small circle at center]. Now I'd like to look
at some of the things we can *see* you doing [points to movie
camera at the top left] when you're caught up with or doing things to move away from these difficult thoughts and
feelings that can show up.

Mike: Like when I'm procrastinating all the time, avoiding doing
things?

Psychiatrist: Sure, but what can we *see* you doing when you're
procrastinating and avoiding? For instance, I think you
mentioned you've been sitting on the couch a fair bit,
watching a lot of TV?

Mike: Absolutely, just distracting myself all day long.

Psychiatrist: Great, so I'll write "sitting on the couch, watching a
lot of TV" up here in the top-left quadrant. You mentioned
you used to exercise in the past. Did you ever exercise to
avoid or relieve your emotional distress?

Mike: Yes, in the past.

Psychiatrist: So, we could note "exercised to relieve distress in the past" in here. That's stopped, I presume?

Mike: Well, yes. I did exercise before; I suppose I should exercise at least occasionally, but it was a while ago the last time I did it.

Psychiatrist: That's okay, we'll write it in here anyway. Would you say coming to see me for therapy could also be to help you eliminate or reduce your distress?

Mike: I suppose, but aren't "away" things bad?

Psychiatrist: Not necessarily. We all make away moves from day to day; if we didn't, we'd have been eaten by predators a long time ago and would be stepping into traffic nowadays! [He writes "uses therapy to ease distress" in the top left quadrant.] This is really good stuff, Mike. Now, we've got a nice selection of things you find yourself doing when you get caught up in and try to move away from those difficult thoughts and feelings. I certainly recognize some of those as behaviors that help me move away from unpleasant thoughts or feelings in my own life. Now let's have a look over at this other side [points to camera in the upper right quadrant] to get a sense of some of the things I could see you doing when you're moving *toward* who and what is important to you. For instance, what's a "toward move" I might see you doing with Gina?

Mike: Well, we haven't done many lately.

Psychiatrist: Maybe you did some toward moves in the past, like going out for dinner or taking in a movie?

Mike: Okay, I see, sure—and maybe calling and visiting my parents with Gina?

Psychiatrist: That's exactly it, just simple things we have done, or could do, to move toward who is important to us. What does it look like if you are in a *toward* mode in relation to work at the moment?

Mike: Maybe checking the internet for openings? Doing some work on my resume, mailing it out?

Psychiatrist [writes those in]: Fantastic! How about exercising for fun and health? And perhaps using therapy to perhaps to learn skills to *live* more?

Mike: Okay, and I think I maybe see a little bit of what you're getting at.

Psychiatrist: Now, a final couple of questions to wrap up our discussion of this new point of view. Imagine you could choose between two possible lives: life number one, here on the left [points to entire left side of matrix], in which most of what you do—not all, but most—is about moving away from these uncomfortable thoughts and feelings [points to bottom left], or life number two, here on the right [points to entire right side of matrix], in which what you do is mostly, although not exclusively, about moving toward who or what is important to you [points to bottom right].

> Which of these two lives—the one on the left or the one on the right—would you choose if you were free to choose?
>
> Mike: Well, I'd like to choose the one on the right, but I'm all caught up with this one on the left!
>
> Psychiatrist: Sure, but if you *were* free to choose, which life would you choose?
>
> Mike: Definitely the life on the right.
>
> Psychiatrist: Awesome! That's what I want our work to be all about. Would you be interested in learning skills to help you more easily choose to move toward who and what is important to you [points to the right side of the matrix], even in the presence of this stuff over here [points to the lower-left quadrant]?
>
> Mike: Sure, that would be great to be able to do.
>
> Psychiatrist: Great stuff. By the way, we call this point of view "the matrix," because it's got Keanu Reeves sexy attached to it, and I can guarantee you will never forget the name!
>
> Mike [looks amused]: Gina and I loved that movie.

As the preceding dialogue demonstrates, simply presenting the ACT Matrix point of view and inviting patients to sort their experiences into the matrix can have an immediate positive clinical impact. In addition, approaching the patient's sense of "stuckness" with an attitude of curiosity, openness, and acceptance makes it less stigmatizing for patients to discuss their issues in an open, honest way. Most importantly, patients who, in all likelihood, have come to see the psychiatrist with the goal of getting rid of their unpleasant thoughts, feelings, memories, and urges quickly recognize the futility of following that approach when appraising results within the matrix system (i.e., context sensitivity and workability). Instead, they choose to work on moving more effectively toward who and what is important to them in the realm of public actions (i.e., engagement). In the process of moving toward who and what matters to them, patients must learn skills to more effectively respond to their ongoing private reactions, such as thoughts, feelings, memories, urges, and physical sensations (i.e., openness).

TIPS FOR SUCCESS

The ACT Matrix is a simple, straightforward, interactive method for implementing the CARE approach with patients.

Because the matrix requires ongoing participation by patients, it is an excellent way to motivate them to change their unworkable strategies.

The two basic dimensions of the ACT Matrix are "toward" and "away" moves, which reflects the engagement mechanism of ACT, and mental experiences versus public behaviors, which taps into the openness dimension of ACT.

The "me noticing" reference point reflects being sensitive to context and looking objectively at the workability of toward versus away moves.

Summary

In this chapter, we described the four main components of the CARE interview sequence, which allows the psychiatrist to conduct highly organized, focused, change-oriented, ACT-consistent conversations with patients. The CARE approach identifies specific clinical activities the psychiatrist can engage in to help patients move from a stance of emotional and behavioral avoidance to a stance of experiential openness, self-reflective awareness, and taking perspective of what is and is not working in their lives as well as identify new strategies that will increase their sense of life engagement. This model applies to a multitude of possible practice scenarios, including brief med checks, consultations, and inpatient or outpatient therapy encounters. With repeated practice, the psychiatrist will be able to quickly organize a session and leave it with patients taking ownership of a specific values-based goal. That is a very powerful salsa move indeed!

The Essentials

- Every session, regardless of its purpose or length, is a dance the psychiatrist must organize and take the lead in without stepping on the patient's toes.
- The CARE interview sequence consists of four distinct tasks or clinical activities the psychiatrist should engage in to promote clinical movement:

    Conduct a contextual assessment
    Assess avoidance rules and behaviors
    Reformulate self-instructional rules
    Experiment with new values-based behaviors
- Because clinical change is a qualitative event, every session represents an opportunity for patients to engage in life-altering, transformative change.

- The ACT Matrix approach can be used to develop an interactive, collaboratively completed form of the CARE approach.
- The ACT Matrix often will speed up change by increasing patient motivation and buy-in.

Suggested Readings

Harris R: ACT Made Simple: An Easy to Read Primer on Acceptance and Commitment Therapy. Oakland, CA, New Harbinger, 2009

Luoma J, Hayes S, Walser R: Learning ACT: An Acceptance and Commitment Therapy Skills Training Manual for Therapists, 2nd Edition. Oakland, CA, New Harbinger, 2017

Polk KL, Schoendorff B, Webster M, et al: The Essential Guide to the ACT Matrix: A Step-by-Step Approach to Using the ACT Matrix Model in Clinical Practice. Oakland, CA, New Harbinger, 2016

References

Polk KL, Schoendorff B (eds): The ACT Matrix: A New Approach to Building Psychological Flexibility Across Settings and Populations. Oakland, CA, Context Press/New Harbinger, 2014

Strosahl K, Robinson P, Gustavsson T: Brief Interventions for Radical Change: Principles and Practice of Focused Acceptance and Commitment Therapy. Oakland, CA, New Harbinger, 2012

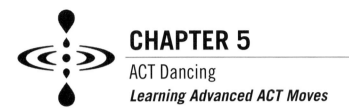

CHAPTER 5

ACT Dancing
Learning Advanced ACT Moves

The moment in between what you once were, and who you are now becoming, is where the dance of life really takes place.

—Barbara De Angelis

Now that you, the psychiatrist, have learned the basic dance steps of the CARE model, it is time to learn some of the more advanced twists and spins available to you in the ACT approach. Recall that in Chapter 2 we described three basic mechanisms that promote psychological resilience: 1) the ability to be self-aware in the context of one's own responding and establish the perspective needed to assess whether those responses are working (context sensitivity/workability); 2) the ability to establish a safe observational distance from distressing, unwanted private experiences to diminish the regulatory influence of unworkable self-instructions triggered by those experiences (openness); and 3) the ability to connect with and articulate personal values and then organize ever-widening patterns of behavior around those values (engagement). As you go through the various components of the CARE interview sequence, seize every opportunity to instigate positive change in one or more of these three core areas. Think of the CARE model as notes of music on the page that set the basic rhythm to be followed and of the clinical interventions you select as the therapeutic conversation unfolds as dance steps to be followed. Any type of dance is difficult to do without a basic rhythm, but once that rhythm is established, you are ready to practice some advanced dance moves.

In this chapter, we revisit the three basic processes that contribute to psychological flexibility and emotional resiliency, with a decidedly clinical focus, to show you several variations of what we call "ACT dancing." First, you must understand the difference between two terms we repeatedly use: therapeutic process and clinical intervention. A *therapeutic process* is an ongoing, dynamic mediator of change that the psychiatrist must continually read and respond to during the clinical interview. As we just described, ACT has three main processes of change, and these can appear and reappear, in and out of sequence, throughout the clinical dialogue. When any one of these core processes is dysfunctional, the patient will be in trouble. When the psychiatrist helps solidify these processes, the patient will be able to respond to life challenges in a more flexible, workable way.

In contrast, a *clinical intervention* is a specific tactic the psychiatrist uses to help "move" a therapeutic process in the right direction. For example, using guided imagery exercises or creating metaphors that help a patient establish an observational distance from an unwanted, distressing emotion are examples of clinical interventions. Such interventions are delivered in the service of teaching the patient how to practice openness in the face of distressing private experiences. Some clinical interventions can actually weaken a core process rather than solidify it. For example, advising a patient that positive coping involves the ability to get rid of, or control, unpleasant emotions would actually undermine the therapeutic process of openness. At the moment of clinical decision making, the psychiatrist must carefully consider the impact a clinical intervention may have on a specific therapeutic process. We call this "ACT dancing" because it involves reading the patient's dance steps as they unfold, determining what therapeutic process is in play, and then matching the clinical intervention to the therapeutic process.

When clinicians get confused about how to apply ACT, or apply it poorly, it is often because they equate clinical interventions with core therapeutic processes. Due to the incredible creativity of ACT therapists over the years, a large and varied set of clinical interventions is available, far too many to describe here. For example, entire books devoted to describing how to deliver ACT-consistent metaphors in clinical practice have been published. The pitfall is that a seemingly ACT-consistent intervention can be delivered in a vacuum if the relevant underlying therapeutic process is not functionally linked to the intervention. So, although many different ACT clinical interventions are available, they all still activate the same three underlying therapeutic processes.

To help avoid any confusion, we organize the major sections of this chapter around the core therapeutic processes of ACT and then demonstrate some typical clinical interventions that can positively affect those processes. First, however, we need to address a defining feature of any successful therapy process: the therapeutic relationship. The ACT approach contains many counterintuitive yet intriguing perspectives on the relationship between the psychiatrist and the patient. Although we do not treat this relationship as a therapeutic process per se, it can be a very powerful vehicle for modeling the three processes that promote psychological resilience. In this sense, the therapeutic relationship is itself a powerful clinical intervention.

The Therapeutic Relationship in ACT

How ACT is practiced within the clinical conversation with the patient flows from the basic assumptions of the model, which were described in Chapter 2. The fundamental processes of human language and the possible traps they include affect us all. Each of us operates in life with the invisible hand of language controlling what we do and how we do it. Moreover, human suffering is ubiquitous, and that understanding ties us to our patients. This recognition of our similarities as human beings generates a stance of equality, compassion, and a genuine desire to help alleviate the patient's suffering.

MODEL HUMILITY

The fact that people with mental problems are trapped in vicious circles of unworkable behavior does not make them stand out as fundamentally different from the rest of us. The mental health clinician or the psychiatrist might even be aware of using the same problematic strategies the patient is using, albeit we hope not to the same extent. In practice, no clear dividing line has been drawn between the dilemmas of daily living we all face and the problems people with mental health problems are facing. This sense of connection and humility brings an aspect of equality into the clinical dialogue.

In a very fundamental way, all people, including patients and psychiatrists, are in the same boat. Recognition of this fact has a therapeutic role in ACT. One way of communicating this to the patient is by using the ACT metaphor described in the following dialogue.

> Sven: Well, you're the expert, I guess…
> Psychiatrist: I would say we're both experts, in our own different ways. There are things I should know, of course, or you wouldn't bother coming to see me. At the same time, you have unique knowledge about the problems you're facing. I figure it's a bit like this: You're climbing your mountain, and in some ways, you're stuck and finding it hard to know how to deal with your situation. I'm across the valley, climbing my mountain, and I know some things about mountain climbing that I hope can be of use to you. At the same time, you're the only one who can climb up your mountain. You are the one noticing how it feels putting your feet where they are right now, and I will have a hard time understanding some parts of your climbing experience, here, perched on my mountain. Some of the barriers you encounter that keep you from climbing in the direction you want to climb will be clearer to you than they are to me. Of course, from where I'm perched I may have an easier time seeing the potential problems you may face. So, I guess we need to share our different points of view. You tell me what it looks like when you are close up, and I'll try to use what I see from here. On and off, I might share something I've learned from climbing my

mountain that may be helpful to you. Naturally, we'll mostly focus on your experience, especially on what happens when you get stuck on your journey.

MODEL OPENNESS

These assumptions also serve as guidelines when something difficult turns up for the psychiatrist during the clinical dialogue; perhaps something a patient says evokes an anxious response, or something happens that is irritating. These will elicit the same core therapeutic processes in the psychiatrist as they do in the patient. Thus, the task of the psychiatrist is to avoid being trapped in these reactions, because that will lead to lecturing or condescending to the patient. In general, remember that patients are doing the best they can with the tools they have at their disposal. The problem is that the tools they have at their disposal do not work, not that something is wrong with them for using those tools.

The skilled ACT psychiatrist will always model openness to whatever experiences show up in the room. This modeling allows patients to see firsthand that they can approach problematic private experiences in a different way. In this case, an overarching value is to serve the patient. Sometimes it might be helpful for the psychiatrist to talk openly about distressing private experiences as they occur in the here and now of the clinical conversation. Sharing such experiences can be a very powerful and immediate way to shape openness in the patient, as the following brief exchange demonstrates.

> Psychiatrist: I notice that I'm also confused right now. It's as if I don't know what to say to help you…[trails off, remains silent for time]. It's okay, though; can we just sit here for a while and be confused together?
> Sven: Okay [long silence]. What should we do now?
> Psychiatrist: I don't know, exactly. What ideas do you have about how to move forward from here?

As this short exchange illustrates, just sitting with a patient, being straightforward, present, and open to what comes next in the conversation can facilitate trust in the therapeutic process and trust in the relationship between the psychiatrist and the patient.

MODEL EQUALITY

The traditional role of the psychiatrist in relation to the patient is one of authority, and this can create an unhealthy power differential in the relationship. Of course, the power of authority is needed in some situations, such as when the patient or other people need to be protected, but the consistent application of authority can negatively influence the therapeutic relationship. The ACT model asks the psychiatrist to move into another position as much as possible—one of authentic equality. This shift entails a radical respect for the patient and genuine humility on the part of the psychiatrist.

MODEL NONJUDGMENTAL CURIOSITY

Another straightforward application of the assumptions of ACT is the way the psychiatrist asks questions and tries to guide the patient in the process and practice of change. The dialogue with the patient should be guided by a stance of *nonjudgmental curiosity.* Curiosity is needed because even though the basic processes entangling the patient are things we have all experienced at one point or another, the specific way an individual person is trapped is unique. Just as no two learning histories are exactly alike, no two depressed patients are identical. Thus, the psychiatrist must "get to know" the patient at a personal level. Acquiring this knowledge involves asking a lot of open-ended questions that signal a genuine interest in what is going on in the patient's life.

The psychiatrist must gather information to help create a snapshot of the patient's life while practicing a stance of nonjudgmental neutrality. The psychiatrist should offer little evaluative commentary or labeling in response when the patient answers a question. Behaviors should not be judged as good or bad or talked about as "signs" of mental illness. Judging the patient is pointless, because whatever experience the patient has is simply the result of a particular learning history. We are all in this mix together, with whatever combination of direct experience and language-based self-narratives comes along. It all fits together once you can fully appreciate the patient's experience. Whatever way the patient is trapped is just another example of the human condition, of trying to live a vital life.

A delicate balance is involved in asking questions and listening to what patients tell you about their experience and history. On one hand, the psychiatrist needs to know enough about the patient to both identify and focus on relevant ACT therapeutic processes as the treatment evolves. On the other hand, not everything that is interesting is helpful in the clinical sense. Taking a nonjudgmental, curious, accepting stance helps the psychiatrist avoid the trap of coming to premature conclusions about the patient that will ultimately lead to ineffective treatment.

TIPS FOR SUCCESS

Therapeutic mechanisms are the underlying processes that directly lead to positive clinical change.

Clinical interventions are the specific strategies or techniques employed to activate a therapeutic mechanism.

ACT has three therapeutic mechanisms of change:

- Being aware of the context of one's own responses and establishing the perspective needed to recognize the unworkability of emotional and behavioral avoidance strategies

- Using self-reflective awareness to establish an observational distance from distressing private experience and the regulatory power of avoidance-based self-instructional rules

- Being willing to engage in values-based approach behaviors in life situations likely to trigger feared or previously avoided inner experiences

The therapeutic relationship is a powerful vehicle for psychiatrists to model the processes that lead to psychological flexibility and emotional resilience.

Psychiatrists should adopt a therapeutic stance of

- Acceptance of patients as "fellow travelers" on the journey of life
- The psychiatrist and patient being equals
- Humility and honesty
- Nonjudgmental curiosity about patients' strategies for dealing with distressing life situations

The Art of ACT Dancing

Although cultivating and nurturing a healthy, horizontal therapeutic relationship is critical, the psychiatrist must also be adept at identifying patient behaviors that reflect the three basic therapeutic processes. As these responses appear during the clinical conversation, the psychiatrist will want to deliver a specific clinical intervention tied to that therapeutic process. In this section, we examine each process using the same case study involving a young, married man with chronic anxiety issues.

Promoting Context Sensitivity and Workability

Mental health conditions typically involve a vicious circle in which the patient, without realizing it, is tricked into following mental rules that promote an enduring pattern of emotional and behavioral avoidance. Her socially conditioned approach is reasonable in its own way but nevertheless functions as a trap that blocks her from moving toward valued life ends. One fundamental task for the psychiatrist is to help the patient develop self-reflective awareness of the contexts in which her problematic behaviors are occurring and then establish the perspective-taking needed to objectively assess both the short- and long-term consequences of avoidance strategies. This is perhaps the hallmark feature of resilient individuals: willingness to try different strategies to see if they work. If a strategy does not work, they try another strategy. Workability is not primarily an intellectual issue; it is not an issue of logical understanding. The mind is good at logic, and patients have many good reasons for doing exactly what they do even though these "reasonable" strategies do not work. They need to make direct experiential contact with the unworkability of their avoidance strategies, to experience workability as a contingency-based form of learning rather than following socially inculcated, arbitrary rules.

To promote this direct contact with the unworkability of avoidance strategies, the psychiatrist may choose to use strategic interviewing to help the patient enter into a stance of *creative hopelessness* (Hayes et al. 2011). Unlike the traditional connotations of the term "hopelessness," when we use this term in ACT, we do not mean that the patient is hopeless. Rather, his continued use of avoidance strategies is destined to fail; as long as the patient continues to use these strategies, remaining stuck and repetitive in the usual ways, he will get the same results as before. Theoretically, this pattern could continue into infinity, and for many patients, this style of responding might have been going on for years or even decades. Once the patient understands the futility of avoidance-based coping, this particular kind of hopelessness prompts him to "give up" on using avoidance. It has not worked, and it will never work. This recognition frees the patient from the need to use the same unworkable strategies over and over again and increases the probability that other strategies will come into play. In a sense, being willing to give up on well-practiced, familiar, and cherished strategies can be a source of great personal creativity.

Getting the patient to talk about her avoidance strategies can be tricky, because she can become preoccupied with trying to control or eliminate the distressing thoughts, feelings, or other private experiences showing up as a result of the clinical conversation itself. On the one hand, the psychiatrist is actively searching for contextual sources that trigger the patient's distressing inner experiences in order to make the issues of workability "come alive" in the session. On the other hand, the psychiatrist must redirect the patient into the present moment and help foster the self-reflective awareness needed to participate in trying acceptance strategies in session. As the following dialogue demonstrates, people with anxiety often need to be redirected to focus on the workability of their coping behaviors rather than on the experience of anxiety in and of itself.

CASE EXAMPLE: PATRICK

Psychiatrist: I'm hearing that you experience a lot of anxiety, and it really gets to you, in many different situations.

Patrick: Yes, I don't know what to do. Often, I feel desperate; it's as if I'll never get rid of this. I have short periods when I feel better, but then it comes back again. It's even getting worse over time. The past few months have been awful; it just gets worse and worse.

Psychiatrist: Can you give me a recent example of when it gets to you?

Patrick: Well, yesterday was really bad. My wife travels a lot as part of her job, and she typically calls me in the morning so I know everything is going well. Yesterday, she didn't call. It really got my anxiety going. I started imagining all kinds of bad things that might have happened. Like, what if she's been involved in a bad car accident? Or that she might be dead. If something happened to her, I don't know what I would do. Then I realize that thinking this way is absurd! I finally got ahold of her about lunchtime; she'd had problems with her cell phone. It was just my anxiety! I don't know what to do.

Psychiatrist: What actually *do* you do?

Patrick: What do you mean? I'm just anxious, I go nuts!

Psychiatrist: Well, I get that it really overwhelms you. What I wonder is this: you've had lots of experiences like this one. Anxiety just hits you, really bad. When it does, what do you try to do? Yesterday, for example. Your wife doesn't call in the morning, and you start to feel anxious. So when this started yesterday, what did you do?

Patrick: I tried to call her, of course. For several hours I tried to contact her. I sent her text messages reminding her to call me. I called the place where she was working, but they didn't know anything and hadn't heard from her either. That set my anxiety off even worse. I called her throughout the whole morning, and then, finally, she picked up during her lunch hour. It's crazy, I get that. Nothing had happened, of course, except that she'd had problems with her phone.

Psychiatrist: So, she doesn't call, you get more and more anxious, and you try to get hold of her in different ways. Let's say that she had answered much earlier than she did, how would that have been?

Patrick: Ahh, then I would've felt much better. That would've calmed me down, of course.

Psychiatrist: Would it be correct to say that the point of trying to get hold of her, calling her and all that, is that it would have calmed you down?

Patrick: Well, yes, I guess. I just can't stand it, you know.

Psychiatrist: Okay. Is this similar to other situations when you get anxious?

Patrick: Yes, it turns up in so many places. Like when I am supposed to take care of my son all by myself. He's 5 years old, you know, and wants to go out to the playground just outside our house and play with my neighbor's kid. Most of the time I try to go out with him so I know what's happening, but sometimes I need to fix something in the house, and he still wants to go outside and play. The place outside is actually pretty safe, and my wife thinks he's old enough to play on his own, but that's another situation when I get really anxious. What if something happened to him? I would never forgive myself if something bad happened.

Psychiatrist: So, what do you do in that situation?

Patrick: If I can't go out with him, you mean? Well, I run back and forth to the window checking all the time, checking to make sure he's safe. It's crazy; I don't get anything else done. I might just as well go out on the playground and sit there.

Psychiatrist: What's the point of running back and forth to the window, checking?

Patrick: To see that he's okay, of course.

Psychiatrist: When you see he's okay, how does that feel?

Patrick: Well, I calm down. For a little while.

Psychiatrist: I think I see a pattern here, and I want to check this out with you to see if it makes sense. First, something makes you anxious, and then you do something meant to calm you down, to get rid of your anxiety. Is that the way it works?

Patrick: Yes, I guess. I haven't thought about it that way, but when you put it that way, yeah, that's what I try to do.

Psychiatrist: How does this approach work? Do you get less anxious?

Patrick: Yes, in the short run. Like, when I see that my boy is safe, I feel less anxious.

Psychiatrist: In the short run it works. At least for a while. But what about in the long run? You mentioned you have to go back to the window to check on him over and over again. So, does this strategy get rid of anxiety in the long run?

Patrick: No, I guess it doesn't, because if it did, I wouldn't have to go back to the window over and over again. It just gives me a little relief, I guess.

Psychiatrist: This seems similar to the approach you take when you get anxious about your wife's safety. You call and call until you get the reassurance you need, but then you have to do the same thing the next day, right?

Patrick: Yes, I guess I'm doing the same thing with her.

Psychiatrist: It's a little like you're walking on this treadmill of reassurance seeking and the treadmill never stops running.

Patrick: Yeah, I just feel worn out and pretty hopeless about ever getting in control of my fears.

Psychiatrist: Maybe this isn't about you *being* hopeless, but the strategy of reassurance seeking is hopeless. As long as you use this approach, your anxiety will probablycontinue to be a big problem. It seems as though you're just buying a temporary reprieve from your anxiety, but it's certain to return in a little while.

Patrick: I think you're right about that, but I don't know what else to do. I feel trapped.

Psychiatrist: Well, it might not be so clear to you at this point what would be an alternative. One thing looks clear to me, though: if you continue doing the very same thing you have done, you will probably get the results you know pretty well by now.

As this dialogue demonstrates, the patient assumes the strategy of "trying to calm myself down" is the natural, normal thing to do. He has probably received similar advice from various friends and family over the years since his anxiety became a "problem." Thus, the strategy itself is seldom questioned, and until it is, Patrick is unlikely to use another strategy. The psychiatrist tries to help the patient contact the unworkability of this approach to dealing with anxiety, hoping that if he makes direct contact with this realization, it will open up the possibility that other strategies will become available to him. The psychiatrist also links different examples of Patrick's avoidance strategy that differ at the topographical level (i.e., checking the window, calling his wife on the phone) but in fact serve the same function (reducing anxiety). Control and avoidance strategies are heavily sanctioned in most human societies, so most patients will have a fairly broad repertoire of functionally similar avoidance strategies.

We can also analyze what has happened in this dialogue from the A-B-C framework. The psychiatrist focused the conversation on the connection between Patrick's avoidance behaviors (B) and the real-world consequences (C) of those behaviors. A connection is also implicitly established between the situations that elicit anxiety-associated avoidance rules (antecedents, A) and the act of engaging in avoidance behaviors (B). Patrick does not get anxious randomly; his anxiety is elicited in specific situations involving possible risk of harm to his loved ones, and his responses are based on his desire to control his emotional reactions in such situations. When helping patients solidify the ability to create perspective on their unworkable patterns of behavior, the psychiatrist will need to help them recognize what they do, what the purpose of their behavior is, when it occurs, and what the short- and long-term results are.

TIPS FOR SUCCESS

Context sensitivity means patients are self-aware of their own responses in specific life contexts and can recognize the situational triggers and short- and long-term consequences of those responses.

Consequences are gauged as negative or positive based on what patients would ideally like to have happen in the given context, often a reflection of their closely held personal beliefs and values.

Workability involves helping patients practice self-reflective awareness and perspective-taking on the actual results of avoidance strategies rather than the results promised by following the mind's avoidance rules.

Workability is not an intellectual issue; it involves helping patients make direct contact with the results of their avoidance so that a new contingency-based rule can be created.

Creative hopelessness involves helping patients realize that using avoidance strategies not only has not worked in the past but also will never work.

When conducting an analysis of patients' avoidance strategies and their workability, remember to look at both the short- and long-term results.

Some avoidance strategies actually work to relieve distress in the short term but guarantee higher levels of distress in the long term.

PROMOTING OPENNESS

As we discussed earlier, the core of the behavioral trap humans easily end up in consists of repeatedly using unworkable avoidance strategies that are closely linked to specific self-instructions. These verbal rules can often be detected by watching what "the mind," or the silent self-instructional dialogue of "the inner advisor" is telling the patient to do in a specific situation. These rules can also be implicit rather than explicit, due to the long and variable learning history that put them in place. Responding in accordance with these mental rules and mandates has a strong habitual quality. The problem is that the patient is *following* these rules, not that she *has* rules. Her inability to create a safe observational distance from these habitual self-instructions allows them to exert their regulatory power on her behavior. When they are overidentified with, avoidance-based self-instructions establish control over dysfunctional behavioral strategies; undoing this chain of control is a major focus in ACT. The ACT therapeutic mechanism of openness involves teaching the patient how to separate herself from her inner experiences so that she is less susceptible to following unworkable self-instructional rules. The success of this new training hinges on the patient's ability to pay attention to what is going on inside and to be in the "here and now," even when being here and now involves making contact with distressing and unwanted inner experiences.

Using the Present Moment

Two basic symbolic contexts determine the quality of the clinical dialogue between the psychiatrist and the patient. The first involves the psychiatrist and the patient interacting in the here and now. Being in the here and now is a critical component of being open to one's private experience. In the here and now, the patient is much less likely to mindlessly follow the avoidance-based self-instructions of the mind. Instead, he will be able to establish an observational distance from those rules and choose what to do based upon his personal values. As we noted in Chapter 2, present-moment awareness (being here, now) is like the windshield wiper on a car. The wiper hinges back and forth and sweeps water off the windshield so the driver can see clearly. In a similar way, present-moment awareness allows the patient to sweep away the life-constricting impact of avoidance-based self-instructions and sweep back into direct contact with a softer, self-compassionate, and values-based experience of self. Indeed, if the ability to be here now is not systematically cultivated by the psychiatrist, then the impact of all three ACT therapeutic processes will be significantly reduced (Strosahl et al. 2015).

The second context that must be incorporated into the clinical dialogue includes all events, situations, or interactions the patient experiences outside of her interaction with the psychiatrist. This includes exchanges about remote to immediate historical events (there/then) and peering into a future that has not yet arrived (now/then). The patient will leave the consultation, med check, or therapy session and enter into this context; the psychiatrist will not have direct access to, or control over, what happens once she leaves. Understanding these two contexts is essential; they create a basic dilemma for the influence the psychiatrist wants to have. The first context is the only one on which the psychiatrist can have any direct influence. The second context, the actual life of the patient, is where she needs change to occur. When talking about the world "out there," the psychiatrist has only the patient's verbal report (and possibly that of significant others) to rely on.

Thus, the challenge is how to use the first context, over which the psychiatrist can exercise considerable control, to influence the patient's behaviors in the second context. To create a meaningful bridge between these two contexts, the psychiatrist must use the present-moment immediacy of the clinical conversation to elicit the unworkable behaviors the patient is using "out there" in the real world and then model and shape the new responses the patient will use instead. Essentially, the clinical dialogue in ACT is designed to promote a kind of exposure-based simulation training, which is why the psychiatrist must focus on creating an accurate snapshot of the patient's life contexts outside the therapy room. The exposure-based simulation must be a reasonably true and accurate reenactment of what the patient actually does "out there" for the new skills learned in the consultation to generalize into similar real-life settings. Talking about unworkable behaviors is not nearly as useful as getting the patient to engage in those behaviors in session. Because ACT conceptualizes most suffering in this context as generated by following avoidance-based self-instructions, the psychiatrist wants to bring the patient into contact with distressing inner experiences that function to trigger avoidance self-instructions and then use the patient's present-moment awareness to create both awareness of, and observational distance from, these self-instructional rules. This requires the psychiatrist to both notice moments of avoidance and take advantage of them in a clinical sense. The psychiatrist must be acutely aware of spontaneous changes in the patient's verbal or nonverbal behaviors that might signal avoidance and be skilled in using verbal instructions that both elicit and amplify present-moment awareness.

 Clinical Tool 20: Phrases Useful for Eliciting and Working With Present-Moment Awareness

---

Patrick: I can see that it doesn't work for me. I get anxious; I get scared something catastrophic might happen. I try to calm myself, I can see that, and it gets me nowhere. If I look back, my problems actually increase. The past few weeks, I've had a hard time going to sleep, too, and then I read this article about how important it is to sleep, about the fact that sleeping disorders can affect the body and cause a lot of problems. What do you think? Can you help me out of this mess? Maybe I should have some other medication?

Psychiatrist: What's happening right now?

Patrick: What do you mean?

Psychiatrist: I get the impression your anxiety level is going up, right now, in the room, as we are talking about this.

Patrick: Yes, I don't know what to do. I can't stand this.

Psychiatrist: Would it be correct to say that right now you're looking for a way to calm yourself down, to lower the anxiety?

Patrick: Well…yes.

Psychiatrist: So we have an example of what you typically do, right here and now? Anxiety shows up, and you do the natural thing: you try to calm yourself down or ask me to reassure you so you can calm yourself down.

Patrick: Yes, this is what typically happens.

Psychiatrist: What does your experience tell you? Does it help?

Patrick: No, it doesn't. It just gets worse. It's almost as though I'm trying to put a fire out by pouring gasoline on it.

Psychiatrist: Can you just notice what the anxiety feels like, maybe by scanning your body or watching what your mind's doing right now?

Patrick: It feels like I have to do something; I can't just sit here and do nothing. I want to move around and unwind. This is an awful feeling. What should I do?

Psychiatrist: That's a good question. I'm not sure I can tell, in any helpful way. Perhaps something like this: What about doing something you typically would not do? Like leaving the fire alone—not trying to put it out, just watching and noticing what goes on.

[Pauses, notices Patrick is holding back and looks confused.] Perhaps something like what you're doing right now?

In this dialogue, the psychiatrist instigates a sufficiently high level of anxiety in Patrick that his normal avoidance strategies are triggered. The psychiatrist keeps him located in the here and now using gentle but specific instructions to "just notice" the private experiences that are showing up. Implicitly, he is being taught, in moment-to-moment fashion, how to accept rather than avoid these experiences. By practicing this ACT dance step, the psychiatrist will become alert to these kinds of instances and can use them to increase the patient's ability to be open to the moment-to-moment flow of distressing, unwanted experiences.

Reformulating Rules

It is worth saying again: avoidance strategies are so pervasive in the general culture that most patients cannot control the urge to use them right in the midst of a psychiatric consultation if appropriate conditions are established by the psychiatrist. Most avoidance behaviors, and the rule-governed mental behaviors that trigger them, are overlearned and habitual in nature. Avoidance moves are more or less a knee-jerk response to the appearance of distressing, unwanted private experiences. Thus, getting patients to exhibit characteristic avoidance behaviors in session is not hard, and from the ACT perspective, this presents the psychiatrist with a golden opportunity to promote powerful, lasting behavior change. To create this outcome, the rules supporting avoidance must be overwritten by superordinate rules that encourage acceptance and approach behaviors. This is perhaps the most daunting aspect of ACT work, because how to accomplish such a transformation is not always obvious. Some general principles have been established that might help guide the psychiatrist in this endeavor, but no hard-and-fast rules exist that will work in every case.

 Clinical Tool 21: Rule Reformulation (Reframing) Worksheet

The need to elicit problematic behaviors in session is not only a prerequisite for rule reformulation that will lead to lasting change but also the main rationale for the use of experiential exercises in ACT. An experiential exercise is a way for the psychiatrist to elicit the patient's problematic behaviors and then model more workable alternative strategies during the interaction. In the dialogue that follows, the psychiatrist deliberately elicits avoidance behaviors in the here and now in order to work with them together with the patient.

Psychiatrist: If we go back to the example of yesterday, when your wife didn't call as you'd expected, what was the first thing you noticed about getting anxious?

Patrick: That creeping feeling in my stomach…

Psychiatrist: Creeping…. So, it doesn't all come at once?

Patrick: No, it starts slow. But when I call to check in and she doesn't answer, it explodes quickly.

Psychiatrist: So, it creeps slowly, and then you call to check; she doesn't answer, and then it explodes?

Patrick: Yes.

Psychiatrist: If we take a closer look at that creeping in your stomach, is there anything more with that creeping?

Patrick: It's strongest in my stomach, but I can feel it all over.

Psychiatrist: That creeping, does it have anything to tell you, does it have a message?

Patrick: Danger, I guess. That something is going on…. I've had this feeling many times, you know. I sort of know where it's going.

Psychiatrist: And it's going toward…?

Patrick: It's getting worse; it's going toward that explosion.

Psychiatrist: We talked earlier about your efforts to calm down. As the creeping starts and you get this message from your stomach, what would you do to calm yourself down?

Patrick: I try to control my breath, to breathe slowly, and I tell myself everything is fine; she'll call later. But it doesn't work, and then it gets worse. I try to call her, she doesn't answer, and then I go nuts.

Psychiatrist: So, that creeping feeling tells you it's going to get worse, you try to calm yourself down, that doesn't work so you take the next step in "calming down" by calling, and then that doesn't work. Then what you called "the explosion" happens?

Patrick: Yes, exactly.

Psychiatrist: Tell me, the explosion, does it contain mental pictures? I remember you said something about seeing your wife in a car accident….

Patrick: Yes, I see all sorts of bad things happening.

Psychiatrist: And yesterday, a car accident?

Patrick: Yes, that's often what comes to mind when I think something has happened to her. She drives a lot.

Psychiatrist: So, you can say this process you go through is a bit like a thriller at a movie theater. First, there's this creeping sense, like the ominous music at the start of the film, as though you know something is on its way. Then, bam! Something happens.

Patrick [laughing a bit]: Yes, I guess.

Psychiatrist: You know, I think it works a bit like a movie, a movie of the mind. It feels so real that you sort of fall into it. That creeping feeling in the stomach, the ominous music, and then…

Patrick: What do you suggest I do, to not fall in?

Psychiatrist: Just watch it, hear the music, let it play. It's a movie of the mind! See what happens if you don't try to turn it off, if you don't leave the theater, and if you don't try to calm your reactions down.

Patrick: Will that stop the explosion from coming?
Psychiatrist: Maybe, maybe not. If it still comes, remain in your seat. It's
     still just a movie of your mind.

In this dialogue, the psychiatrist helps the patient make direct contact with a stance of openness to an unpleasant experience he wants to get rid of. This is done by asking questions about the qualities of the feared experience, which Patrick can only answer by taking an observational distance from the experience. This type of clinical intervention has a twofold purpose. First, the psychiatrist is trying to explore what is actually going on in the patient's here-and-now context, to enrich the conceptualization of how his problem likely plays out in the world "out there." Second, the exposure-based component of this intervention involves creating a new metaphorically delivered rule (i.e., stay in your seat) that makes it increasingly likely he will learn how to make contact with his own experience without the need for avoidance.

This detached, nonjudgmental, nonreactive form of awareness is what we mean by *openness*. From a theoretical perspective, the observational distance that is established ("It is me on one hand and my reactions on the other"; "I am more than the thoughts and feelings I am having right now") decreases the potential behavior-regulating effects of avoidance-based self-instructions while increasing the odds that factors other than the patient's immediate reactions will come to influence his response. Speaking metaphorically about his reactions as "the movie of the mind" is meant to increase the experiential "distance" between whatever shows up in his awareness and his behavioral choices in the moment. After all, ordinary movies appear on a screen, at a distance. The metaphoric talk about the patient's own thoughts and feelings in this way is part of the key strategy for promoting openness: driving a wedge between the human being and the symbolic activity of the mind.

Making Sense of History

The question of what to do about the patient's personal history in the ACT model involves some complex, and seemingly contradictory, perspectives. On the one hand, human cognition involves the ability to link specific historical events together in a sense-making operation we call the "conceptual self," the narrative that people develop to explain their "life history" as it contributes to who they are today. When we ask a person at a social event to "tell me a little bit about yourself," we are eliciting a particular version of the conceptual self-narrative that fits the circumstances in which this request originated. Without this ability to recapitulate and reorganize personal history in highly specific ways, we would not be able to function effectively as members of any social group, much less the complex society in which we live nowadays. The side effect of this unique ability is that avoidance-based self-instructional control can also be carried from distant points of time into the present moment in the form of narratives tied to the conceptual self. The patient can put this sense-making ability in the service of explaining today's issues in terms of sometimes distant historical events. When self-narratives are constructed in this fashion, they can easily come to proactively function as a destructive form of instructional control. In common parlance, patients can apply their self-narratives such that they serve the role of "self-fulfilling prophecy."

A common question raised by patients, especially those who have some previous experience with psychotherapy, is whether it is important to talk about life events that happened many years back, perhaps to childhood. Because of the carrying power of self-narratives, some dominant avoidance strategies probably have been practiced for years. A long learning history is likely behind anything a patient does, but that fact does not necessarily mean that developing "insight" into personal history makes a difference. As we said earlier in this chapter, not everything that is interesting will be helpful, because whatever change the patient makes occurs in the here and now. History is forever gone, and we have no tools to change it. No amount of analysis is going to help the patient escape from his or her historically learned, automatic responses.

Even an event that took place yesterday is, strictly speaking, history. We must rely only on the patient's verbal report to understand what happened yesterday—or 40 years ago, for that matter. So, from a contextual point of view, the only meaningful distinction is between what is occurring in the here and now with the psychiatrist and what the patient experiences outside of the consultation session. As we like to say in ACT, "people vote with their feet." The key to living a vital existence is to be effective in the unfolding context of daily living, with one's historically learned responses carried along. Strictly speaking, personal history does not matter unless vestiges of it show up and function as barriers to effective action in the present moment. Then, personal history becomes very much a target for ACT clinical interventions.

That said, something in the current situation brought the patient to see the psychiatrist, and in that sense, a vestige of the patient's learning history may be blocking her from doing what matters in life. The psychiatrist can bring the tools of functional and contextual interviewing to bear here. The psychiatrist is interested not only in the patient's current life context but also in the trajectory of her problematic avoidance strategies or distressing symptoms that may have been around for years. At the same time, the psychiatrist must remember that the more distant in time a formative life event occurred, the harder it will be for the patient to accurately recollect all of the relevant data. What the psychiatrist collects is a particular kind of self-narrative that the patient uses to both explain and justify her current responses, particularly if those responses are dysfunctional and elicit a need in the patient to explain or justify them. This self-narrative is designed to address the demands of a discussion about the patient's personal problems when these problems are disclosed to another person.

Still, the psychiatrist models curiosity and openness. What happened back then? What was the situation like for the patient? What thoughts, feelings, memories, urges, or sensations does he remember having? What did he do in response? What were the consequences in the short and the long run? These questions can help build a bond between the psychiatrist and the patient and allow him to feel heard and validated. The issue is not whether these accounts are scientifically precise and accurate; most likely they are not. They are functionally important because they contain the self-instructional rules that might be defeating the patient's best interests in the here and now of daily living.

Approaching the patient in a curious and open, nonjudgmental manner is especially salient when she experiences vivid memories of the past, triggered by features of current life situations, as is often seen in patients who are struggling with various forms of posttraumatic stress. These reactions, even though they are situated in historically acquired memories, can still be regarded as something happening in the here and now. This here-and-now experience can trigger habitual dysfunctional responses learned long ago, what we call *embedded self-instructions.* Embedded self-instructions are difficult to access because they reside within the sense-making self-narrative itself, and the patient is often unaware that they are operating in the background. Because they are historically distant, these embedded self-instructions often are located "upstream" in a chain of avoidance rules the patient is following. The degree to which embedded instructions should be targeted or not in the therapeutic dialogue is a pragmatic question. Is it needed for change to occur? Sometimes it is, sometimes not. In the following clinical dialogue with Patrick, the anxious patient described earlier, the psychiatrist suspects that embedded self-instructions may be accelerating both his anxiety level and his corresponding need to avoid anxiety.

> Psychiatrist: If something serious really did happen to your wife, how would that be for you? Of course, most people would find it problematic if something serious happened to their partner, but beyond that, is there some special difficulty for you?
> Patrick: If something bad happened to her, I don't know how I would ever get over it. My life would be ruined, that's for sure. I would never be able to get over losing her.
> Psychiatrist: I'm wondering, when do you first remember feeling like you weren't up to the task of being independent and daring enough to get through a major life setback or loss? Certainly, no one wants to lose a life partner, and that would be hard for anyone to deal with, but in a more general way, do you remember when you first began to question your own daringness and to feel like you couldn't live life on your own terms, even if you had to?

Patrick: The first time? Hmmm [pauses]. I think I must have been in sixth or seventh grade. I had saved up money from mowing lawns to buy a pair of colored sneakers that were a cool thing to have. When I came home with them, my Dad called me a sissy in front of my mom and sister and said maybe I should put a dress on, too. Then he told me to take those "sissy" shoes off and give them to the only real girl in the house, which was of course my sister. He was drunk at the time; he drank all the time. He asked if I wanted to do anything about this—meaning, did I want to fight him. My mom got between us, and he slapped her and stormed out of the house. I guess I never got over how humiliating that was. My dad took what I had earned and treasured and gave it away, and I was too small and afraid to defend myself. I needed my mom to step in and keep me safe, and then she got hurt. I felt so small and like it was my fault. None of this would have happened if I hadn't brought those sneakers home. I can feel it now like it happened yesterday.

Psychiatrist: Wow, that's pretty sad and scary. Not a good thing to go through, and it sounds as though it's left a mark on you. So, another part of this movie thriller is that everything is on the line for you; you have these childhood memories of being unable to defend yourself or to exert your independence, and then somebody else has to protect you and they get hurt, and there you are, meek and alone. Now your wife does the protecting for you, and you are done for if something happens to her. But then when she does protect you, you feel that sense of smallness that your dad gave you. Would you be willing to add this new plot twist to the movie of your mind? And remember, stay in your seat!

The psychiatrist has uncovered embedded self-instructions ("I will never get over losing her; I am incapable of managing life on my own") that need to be contacted directly with a stance of openness. The metaphor-based clinical intervention involving the movie of the mind is flexible enough to incorporate the more chronic and deep-seated embedded self-instructions within the patient's self-story and have the patient relate to them in the same way as immediately accessible ones.

TIPS FOR SUCCESS

Psychiatrists deal with two fundamental contexts: one is the here-and-now immediacy of the clinical conversation; the other is the patient's actual behavior in the real-world context outside of the consultation room.

A key to cultivating openness in patients is to help them get into the present moment so as to bring feared or avoided experiences "into the room."

Various ACT interventions to promote openness are designed to deliberately trigger distressing, unwanted experiences in the here and now.

Openness requires patients to be present, take an observer role on immediate experience, practice nonjudgment, and "lean into" the experience.

Self-instructional rules can be layered as a result of unfolding historically learned responses, such that they exert their influence through a chain of related, more recently learned avoidance rules.

The patient's history is important to the extent that historically acquired behaviors are showing up and interfering with contemporary behaviors.

The conceptual self is a creation of language that attempts to make sense of, and explain, the patient's current level of function or dysfunction using an arbitrary collection of filtered historical events.

Self-narrative components of the conceptual self are constructed largely for the social purposes of explanation and justification, but when practiced repeatedly, they can act as a destructive form of self-instructional control (i.e., "self-fulfilling prophecy").

Promoting Engagement

The third therapeutic process in ACT is to redirect the patient away from living to prevent the occurrence of, or avoiding contact with, distressing, unwanted private experience and toward living according to personal values and life principles. We mentioned previously that the three therapeutic processes occur interchangeably, often in a back-and-forth kind of way, in a typical clinical conversation. Even though the topic of conversation might start with a discussion of the patient's values and what life would be like if the patient were following those values, it can suddenly turn back in the direction of the workability of the patient's avoidance strategies. The therapeutic process of workability reappears in a slightly different form: Once you contact the fact that what you are doing is not getting you where you want to go, the question becomes, "Now, where do you want to go in life?" Indeed, the workability of one's life is directly tied to whether valued life pursuits are being followed. The same conversation can resurface openness in a slightly different form: "Now that you are freed from having to run away from your own experience, what do you want to do with your experience?"

As discussed in Chapter 2, the therapeutic mechanism of life engagement attempts to use the patient's self-instructional rule-following tendency to achieve positive ends. Not only are we under the influence of the direct consequences we have experienced but we also can direct our behavior toward consequences not yet experienced through our ability to simulate the future before we get there and to relate positive consequences to very distant life outcomes. The clinician can help the patient clarify what life pursuits are important and, in the process, construct a new set of self-instructions that will promote a wide-ranging, persistent pattern of approach and engagement rather than avoidance and disengagement. The new self-instructions can be tied to highly specified outcomes in limited situational contexts—what are referred to in ACT as *goals.* Alternatively, they can be more global in nature and refer to a wide array of potential situations unfolding over longer periods of the life span. In ACT, we call this type of self-instruction a *value.* ACT specifically stresses the importance of helping patients connect with their values, because values tend to have strong motivational functions for humans. As the following clinical dialogue with our anxious patient demonstrates, focusing on a more restricted set of values-based goals can be a helpful way to increase the patient's motivation to change.

Psychiatrist: I see how your efforts to control your anxiety, your efforts to "calm yourself down," are both reasonable and problematic.

Patrick: Well, I didn't really see it as problematic before, but rather as the way I had to go. But I can see now that what my anxiety tells me to do is actually very problematic. I just get worse, and I get stuck in the same vicious circle.

Psychiatrist: Let's imagine you got out of this vicious circle, and your life sort of opened up for you. What important things would you shoot for?

Patrick [after a pause]: There are important things in my relationships with both my wife and my son.

Psychiatrist: Like?

Patrick: With my wife, our relationship is getting more and more unbalanced. I'm always relying on her to help me calm down. I'd like to be a more self-reliant partner, and then I could support her in doing the things she needs and wants to do. And I'd like to be more independent at the same time. If I were, I could do more things with my boy. Be more daring, so to speak.

Psychiatrist: Being more daring sounds like a good summary of who you want to be. So, in the moments when "the movie of the mind" tells you to calm down, to feel safe, to hope others can help you, you would actually like to move in another direction, toward being more daring. In your present life situation, what concrete steps could you take to move yourself in that direction?

Patrick: Well, being more independent and more daring in relation to my wife means I wouldn't be calling her just to calm myself down. I'd be more able to deal with not knowing exactly what's going on with her. But what if it gets worse?

Psychiatrist: Yes, we don't know exactly what would happen, do we? But I think it's a good guess that the movie of the mind will fire up and try to get you to do those familiar calming behaviors. What if you just remained in your seat, let the movie unfold on the screen of your mind, and then moved toward what matters to you? Would you be willing to try that strategy when the movie projector turns on?

WILLINGNESS: A PRELUDE TO COMMITTED ACTION

When Patrick actually specifies concrete, values-based actions, the psychiatrist helps him understand that feared and avoided private experiences will very likely show up. In doing so, the psychiatrist is trying to promote the patient's *willingness* level. In ACT, willingness is considered to be a prelude to *committed action*. Most patients, and our anxious patient is no exception, are acutely aware of the dangers posed by entering into previously avoided situations. Willingness is what it says it is: being willing to enter a dangerous situation so a values-based behavioral response, rather than an avoidance strategy, can be implemented. In a very real sense, the first committed action in ACT is being willing to enter into threatening situations in which values-based behavior is possible. Without a willingness to head into dangerous territory, committed action is not possible. In the case of our anxious patient, his anxiety may increase, and the habitual advice from his "inner advisor" to avoid being anxious will undoubtedly show up in awareness. That would lead him to rely on both workability ("What do I want in this situation, and what will work to help me get it?") and openness ("There they are again, the reactions that I typically get. I have them, but I am bigger than my reactions"). Anchoring his awareness in these two processes will increase the likelihood that he will choose more "daring" behaviors in situations that previously have been triggers for unworkable avoidance behaviors.

CONSTRUCTING POWERFUL BEHAVIORAL EXPERIMENTS

Ultimately, the goal of ACT as a behavior therapy is to get the patient to do something different in critical life situations. "Different" means that, instead of using an avoidance strategy, the patient will engage in values-based behavior. This is the "end" that ACT seeks to achieve with every patient, but the means to that end differ with each patient. What different behavior should the patient experiment with? In what situation(s)? Does the patient possess the skills necessary to engage in that behavior?

What is the best strategy for ensuring that something different will in fact happen between this session and the next? Although general guidelines exist for constructing successful behavioral experiments, they must be customized to fit the unique needs of each patient.

✒️ Clinical Tool 22: Guidelines for ACT-Consistent Behavior Experiments

---

A unique feature of the ACT model is the focus on eliciting moment-to-moment contact with positive, imagined consequences of following one's values. In essence, the psychiatrist helps the patient engage his values prior to talking about how he will engage in values-based behaviors in the world "out there."

> Psychiatrist: Let's assume you've taken some of these daring steps and are acting more independently as the partner and father you want to be. What would that look like? If I were a fly on the wall, what would I see you doing?
>
> Patrick: Well, I would take more responsibility for getting things done in our daily life as a family. I postpone so many things right now because I'm afraid they'll give me more anxiety. It would also allow my wife to do some things on her own, like going out with friends on and off. She would really appreciate that! And I 'd also do more things I enjoy, actually. Maybe I'd start kayaking again; I haven't done that for years.... Eventually, I could do that with my son and teach him how to kayak. What a dream come true that would be!
>
> Psychiatrist: Can you just take a moment to imagine yourself doing those things? Letting your wife do something she likes while you go kayaking with your son? Stay with that image for a while!
>
> Patrick: Wow, that would be something.
>
> Psychiatrist: When you first came in here, you just wanted to get rid of your anxiety. That's a reasonable goal, definitely. Anxiety is unpleasant, and it's natural to focus on getting rid of it somehow. But what if our work could be about something bigger, about achieving the things in your life that you really care about and that the anxiety and the movie of the mind have stopped you from? What if you didn't have to get rid of your anxiety to do those things? You could do them even if doing so required you to be willing to let anxiety come along for the ride. It seems your attempts to stop or prevent your anxiety have actually stopped you from living the life you want to live.
>
> Patrick: That puts my anxiety in a very different light, doesn't it?

In this clinical exchange, the psychiatrist focuses on helping Patrick clarify his values regarding his closest relationships and the effect his anxiety and his unwillingness to be anxious have had on that important area of his life context. The psychiatrist then invites the patient to imagine living a life consistent with those values, even though anxiety might show up in the very situations that matter to him the most. Clearly, this type of imaginary "savoring" can instantly produce increased motivation to perform imagined activities. In a basic way, the psychiatrist has helped the patient install a new self-instruction: "Going after what is important to me in my life is more important than controlling my anxiety right now." Once the link is made between pursuing valued life ends and the willingness to have anxiety if it shows up in pursuit of those ends, the same basic strategy can usually be generalized to other areas of life where avoidance behaviors are occurring. With Patrick, for example, the psychiatrist could ask some additional questions about his work situation: Is his mind tricking him there also, in a similar way? Is the fact that he is focusing on "calming himself down" blocking his ability to move forward in his profession? What does he value in connection with his work?

TIPS FOR SUCCESS

At the end of ACT treatment, the psychiatrist will want to capitalize on the patient's capacity to follow rules that encourage exploratory, positively reinforced behaviors.

Engagement involves helping the patient develop new, positively focused forms of self-instructional control.

The new self-instructional rules the patient will follow can be

- Well specified, targeted to limited contexts, and achievable (goals)
- More global in nature and applicable to a wide variety of changing life contexts over a much longer time course (values)

Values tend to have a greater motivational impact in terms of stimulating enduring patterns of behavior change.

Engagement involves implementing values-based approach behaviors and being willing to have any distressing inner experiences that arise.

Using guided imaginal rehearsal exercises that help patients articulate valued actions, and then imagine taking those actions, can have a powerful impact on their motivation to follow through on commitments.

The best values-based actions are those that rapidly generalize to other life areas that matter but in which avoidance behaviors have been occurring.

The Use of Metaphor in ACT

The ACT clinical dialogue requires the psychiatrist to use language to offset and undermine the corrosive effects of language. As we stated earlier, in ACT we are fighting fire with fire. The goal is to not get burned in the process. This is why ACT uses language in some counterintuitive and unconventional ways. In this section, we examine some of the core language conventions that are definitive of the ACT approach.

As we have illustrated in the clinical dialogues, ACT relies heavily on the use of metaphor (Törneke 2017). This reliance serves several important clinical purposes. The first is simply that metaphor is a basic building block of language in general. The question is not whether the psychiatrist should use metaphors but rather how the psychiatrist and patient are *already* using metaphors and how metaphors can be used best to help the patient learn something new. If we look closely into ordinary human dialogue, lots of metaphors exist, some of which have become so conventionalized that we might not even see them as metaphors. You can see this even in the few sentences we have written so far in this section. We said that metaphor is a *basic building block* of language, as though language were a building containing many blocks. We also suggested you *look into* ordinary human dialogue, as though the dialogue were a closed physical space with a peephole or small window through which we could look. Human language is full of what are called *frozen metaphors.* This can be seen in the clinical dialogue earlier in this chapter, when Patrick starts talking about his anxiety as something that starts with a *creeping* sensation in his stomach and ends up as an *explosion* of unmanageable fear responses. The use of metaphor is often more common in a clinical dialogue than in many other types of human dialogue. The emotional problems that bring patients to therapy are often described in metaphorical terms.

A second clinical purpose served by using metaphor is that when unworkable responses (as well as more workable ones) are given a metaphoric name, they will be easier to remember. For example, if the psychiatrist wants a patient to be "on the lookout" (oops, another metaphor!) for a specific unworkable avoidance behavior and try an alternative one instead, creating a metaphorical relationship between the two alternatives can be helpful. When the psychiatrist referred to Patrick's experience of anxiety as akin to seeing a movie thriller at a cinema, a metaphorical relationship was established that included the experience of anxiety itself, the temptation to avoid or escape, and an alternative behavior for the patient to try instead. The anxiety and the central problematic instructions it provides are talked about as "the movie of the mind," and a possible helpful strategy is to "remain in your seat" rather than "try to make the movie go away or try to calm yourself."

As we have mentioned, language-based self-instructions tend to operate silently in the background of awareness. To strengthen the therapeutic process of workability, the patient must learn to recognize and discriminate among a "menu" (hey, another metaphor!) of sometimes competing self-instructional rules. One rule might encourage the patient to accept anxiety without struggle, while the other rule might encourage exactly the opposite response. While asking the patient about different examples of problematic situations, what those experiences are like, and what she tends to do in those situations, the psychiatrist must begin to identify classes of behaviors rather than confine the discussion to one specific behavior that occurs in one specific situation. Because metaphors involve the nonliteral use of language, they can be used to refer to a broad class of behaviors that might look different on the surface but, in fact, share the same functional properties, something that the patient will remember and that can thus be helpful in the continued work for change. In ACT, we encourage you to use metaphors that can be linked to broad classes of behavior exhibited in many different life contexts. This serves the fundamental purpose we mentioned earlier: using moment-to-moment interactions with the patient to influence her behaviors in the world outside the treatment room.

One more clinical purpose is served by using metaphors. Metaphors are a kind of mental shorthand, loaded with meanings and, as we have discussed, with implicit rules. The key problem ACT targets is the patient's habitual reliance on following unworkable rules. Rules or instructions are extremely important for humans, yet they have side effects, and those side effects are what ACT tries to deal with. When a metaphor is used in a helpful way, especially if it describes a class of alternative strategies, the metaphor will eventually function as a new rule. Let's imagine our anxious patient, Patrick, sees the metaphor about *remaining in his seat* when his anxiety increases as a completely new idea. If Patrick then tries to do that in a situation of increased anxiety, he is trying to follow a rule (remain in your seat!). How is that done? He is not literally in a movie theatre, and he is not literally in a seat. The entire self-instruction is metaphorical, not literal. The metaphorical rule establishes a direction, but in other ways it is wide open to interpretation of what "staying in your seat" means. This can then be used clinically to tighten up (oops, another metaphor) the self-instruction as the patient attempts to follow it. In trying to follow the metaphorical rule, the patient must look to the more immediate experience of what he did to "remain in his seat" when anxiety showed up—and to the direct consequences of using that particular version of "remaining in his seat"—to see what actually works. In general, metaphorically established rules will lead to more flexible and adaptable responses compared to literal rules. Metaphorical rules thus allow us to get around the repertoire-narrowing side effects of rule-following.

The use of metaphor is also of special importance in promoting openness. The very essence of openness-based metaphors is to drive a wedge between the human being and the symbolic activity of the mind. Many of the unique language practices distinctive to ACT involve creating the metaphorical difference between the patient and her mind. Typical ACT communications often involve asking the patient to listen to what the mind is advising her to do, within a speaker-listener framework: "Tell me, what does your mind have to say about the subject we're talking about right now?"; "I'm guessing your mind is going to be pretty upset when it finds out you aren't going to follow its advice here!"; "If your mind has its way here, what do you think it will have you do?" Implicit in the speaker-listener metaphor is the ability of the listener to establish an observational distance from the speaker. We do this when we hang up the phone on a telemarketer. The telemarketer is not telling us not to hang up the phone, but we distance ourselves from the emotional pull of what the telemarketer is asking us to do by hanging up the phone. Thus, many if not most patients will have some direct experience with taking an observational distance as well as the consequences of not doing so.

Most people have seen a thriller-type movie. When the patient's immediate reactions are talked about as the *movie of the mind,* metaphorically these reactions are established at a distance. The patient is not establishing an observational distance to avoid the experience in question; rather, he is taking an observational distance to reduce the risk of becoming overidentified with a potentially distressing experience. Such overidentification triggers the unworkable self-instruction to avoid, so—figuratively speaking—watching the "movie of the mind" while "remaining in your seat" allows the patient to have the experience of anxiety at a distance, such that he will not feel compelled to engage in escape and avoidance behaviors. Those temptations may appear in the movie as well, and they can also be seen from an observational distance. Another metaphorical term frequently used to describe this process is *detachment.* The metaphor implies that we first become stuck to something, or tied to it in some way, and then we engage in a strategy that allows us to free ourselves from restraint. We can move as far away from the restraining entity as we please.

One of the most well-known ACT detachment metaphors is the *passengers on the bus* metaphor. Let's see how it can be applied to Patrick.

> Psychiatrist: It's like this: We are like bus drivers in the game of life. We have a route in mind that we want to follow, but on board are lots of passengers—feelings we feel, thoughts we think, and memories we remember. We're driving the bus, and our passengers

have boarded at different times—some of them we know when, but others we have no idea. As a simple example, I grew up in San Francisco, so I have a lot of "passengers" that are memories of San Francisco. They often stand up at the back of the bus, even though I don't live there anymore. Most of these "San Francisco passengers" are fairly neutral; some are pleasant, but some are nasty. Do you have any "San Francisco" passengers on your bus?

Patrick: Yeah. I mean, I'm not from San Francisco, but sure, I have memories from there.

Psychiatrist: Just now, when I mentioned San Francisco, what appeared in your mind?

Patrick: The Golden Gate Bridge, actually.

Psychiatrist: Okay, that's a pretty typical passenger for most people. The pleasant kind, or…?

Patrick: Yeah, I suppose.

Psychiatrist: There are other passengers that aren't so pleasant, aren't there? Like that creeping sensation you've described, and your fear that you will explode with anxiety.

Patrick: Yeah, it really scares me. I just can't stand it.

Psychiatrist: And the advice that you need to "calm down" to get rid of it—it seems to me that *that* passenger is sitting beside the creeping anxiety on your bus.

Patrick: Yes, definitely.

Psychiatrist: I'd like to ask you one thing: Who notices all this? Who can hear what they say, that you have to leave all else to first calm down?

Patrick [A bit confused]: Me, I suppose…?

Psychiatrist: Exactly, and who is driving the bus?

Patrick: That's me, too.

In this interaction, the focus is once more on establishing an observational distance from the patient's symptoms of anxiety and the self-instructions to avoid it. The psychiatrist helps Patrick notice what turns up (the passengers) and also identify who is doing the noticing (himself). As might be obvious, this metaphor, like all good metaphors, has a broad range of applications. It could be used to strengthen any of the three therapeutic processes of ACT. If the psychiatrist wants to use it to strengthen the workability process, the focus of the dialogue could shift to what the patient does when his passengers talk to him and what happens when he follows the passengers' instructions. The metaphor can also easily be used to strengthen engagement by focusing the conversation on the patient's willingness to take his "passengers" with him and see them as part of his "bus service." After all, not every passenger who gets on a city bus is a desirable one. The bus driver learns that part of the job is to allow any and all passengers to board the bus and still continue going in the direction of his own choice. As we show in the next section, this particular metaphor can also be used in a more experiential way, or what in ACT is called a *physical* or *experiential exercise.*

The Use of Experiential Exercises in ACT

As we mentioned earlier, a key ACT principle is that an important part of behavior change happens in the here and now of the clinical dialogue. We do not just want to talk about avoidance, we also want to stimulate it in session and use it to promote change. To instigate avoidance requires that the psychiatrist not be shy about eliciting painful material from the patient. This pain will trigger avoidance behaviors, giving the psychiatrist a chance to have the patient practice the therapeutic processes of context sensitivity/workability, openness, or engagement. In principle, deliberately evoking powerful emotional responses from the patient is similar to exposure therapy, one of the most empirically established interventions in the field of behavior therapy. Take the treatment for spider phobia, for example: the psychiatrist, or any therapist, does not simply make do with talking about how the patient can learn to approach spiders but actually establishes the fear-producing situation using a live spider. This tactic elicits the patient's phobic anxiety response so the therapist can help the patient learn new skills for interacting with this response. The same strategy applies when working with the problem of posttraumatic stress. The psychiatrist attempts to arouse memories that trigger fear responses and avoidance-based self-instructions in the patient. Because the patient is unable to flee the situation, which is what might normally occur in the world outside the consultation room, the patient can learn to relate to the memories—and the fear response they produce—in a different way.

The rationale for using experiential exercises in ACT is slightly different from that for exposure therapy. The clinician wants to initiate clinically relevant responses in the patient so that workability, openness, and engagement responses can be modeled. When comparing the ACT approach with traditional exposure methods, remember to stress that the goal of exposure in ACT is not to reduce or eliminate symptom distress; rather, the goal of ACT-based exposure is to help the patient learn to accept distressing inner experiences for what they are, know that trying to avoid or suppress them does not work, and choose instead to engage in values-based behaviors in those very life situations that matter to the patient but may also be the situations that trigger feared and avoided inner experiences.

ACT experiential exercises (or physical metaphors) also tap into patients' kinesthetic and somatic information processing systems, and for this reason, they avoid many of the pitfalls of using literal language to help patients "process" their feared and avoided inner experiences. For example, many ACT clinicians have a supply of "Chinese finger traps" in their offices. The experience of inserting one's fingers into this device and becoming progressively more alarmed, even panicky, when the expected instruction for how to escape ("To get free, just pull your hands away from each other") does not work, is something the patient will remember long after treatment is finished. In fact, the harder patients try to pull their hands apart, the more firmly bound they become. The only way to get free of the finger trap is to push the fingers together, a completely novel response that runs directly against the primitive urge to escape by pulling away. Thus, something as simple as an oddity sold in a gift shop can function as the perfect physical metaphor for a large number of pivotal ACT concepts. In the clinical dialogue that follows, we show how the psychiatrist can turn the "passengers on the bus" metaphor into an experiential exercise.

> Psychiatrist: Let's stand up, and you can look out that way, as though you are driving your bus in the direction you want to go. Put your hands on the steering wheel, and let's drive. Now, let's say your destination, the route you have in mind, is to be that daring, independent, involved husband and father you described to me earlier. But there are other passengers on your bus that aren't so pleasant, aren't there? Like the creeping anxiety and the fear of the explosion—they're kind of sitting right behind you, right? They don't want you to drive in the direction you want to go; they want you to drive to a place where you are dependent on getting reassurance so you can calm your anxiety. So now, while you drive, I'm going to say the things your creeping sensations and sense of an upcoming explosion of anxiety might say to you.

The psychiatrist and patient begin walking around. The psychiatrist repeats the patient's fear- and anxiety-producing thoughts, including advice to engage calming and reassurance seeking.

> Patrick: This really scares me.
> Psychiatrist: Are you still driving toward your destination? Are they giving you the advice that you need to calm down to get them off your bus, or you can't keep driving? It seems to me that the "calm down" passenger is sitting beside the others, the creeping sensation in your stomach and the image of you exploding with anxiety.
> Patrick: Yes, definitely. They're all there.
> Psychiatrist: I'd like to ask you one thing: Can you hear everything these troublemakers are saying to you and, at the same time, continue to drive your bus to your destination?
> Patrick: I suppose so.

In this brief exchange, the psychiatrist uses the metaphor of "passengers" to communicate an important ACT idea: that the thought of needing to calm down and get rid of the anxiety, the sensation of a creeping feeling in the stomach, or the sense of being about to explode inside are experiences that are separate from the bus driver. They can be present on the bus (a metaphor for the patient's awareness), and the patient can continue to drive onward. The following is another example of an experiential exercise that might be effective with this anxious patient.

Psychiatrist: I have an exercise I sometimes like to use. Would you like to give it a go?

Patrick: Okay.

Psychiatrist [picks up a notepad]: I'm going to write down some of the things that come into your mind in these situations, the things that plague you and that you want to get rid of. That creeping sensation in your stomach, for example [writes it down]. What else?

Patrick: That it gets worse, it feels like the explosion is coming, like I'm going to explode inside. All these thoughts about what might have happened to my wife. And the feeling that I just can't stand this. And now the memory of my dad calling me a sissy, my mother getting hit, and me feeling like I can't defend myself.

Psychiatrist [writes down each item mentioned on the notepad, then holds the notepad directly in front of the patient]: Hold your hand against this notepad, and don't let it get any closer to you!

Patrick [holds his palm up to the paper a little sheepishly]: Okay...

Psychiatrist [presses the notepad from other side]: Resist it! Keep it away from you!

Patrick [presses back with greater force]: Like this?

Psychiatrist: Yes, maybe even harder. [Both apply pressure to their respective sides of the notepad, which hovers back and forth in the space between them.]

Psychiatrist: Okay, well, you certainly did a good job of keeping that notepad from getting too close [lowers the notepad]. For a moment, just zero in on what that felt like! Now, let's try a different way of dealing with these messages and compare this new way with the first way. [The psychiatrist places the notepad in the patient's lap, text side up.] I want you to just read what is on these lines, one at a time, without doing anything to the notepad.

Patrick [after quietly looking down at the words]: Yeah, that certainly was different.

Psychiatrist: In what way?

Patrick: It was easier having it in my lap, of course. In a sense. But it made me feel uncomfortable, too. I could almost sense the creeping feeling.

Psychiatrist: Maybe you can say the two positions are the same and yet different. The same because in both you have contact with the paper and what's written on it.

Patrick: Okay, although resisting it like I did takes more energy. But then it also feels good in a way, too. I am sort of fighting it.

Psychiatrist: If you were to compare how much energy you have to expend to make each of these two strategies work, are they the same or are they different?

Patrick: Resisting it demands all my attention, and my mind's totally set on keeping it away from me. At first, when I got it in my lap and saw what's written on it, I wanted to turn away and resist, but

> then it changed when you told me to just let it be there. It just sits there, you know, and I can let other things in. With the first strategy, I'm totally preoccupied with keeping the pad away from me.
>
> Psychiatrist: What about the experience of just seeing those things that produce anxiety, sadness, and worry written on a piece of paper?
>
> Patrick: It was uncomfortable, at least at first. I can see clearly what's written there, and it just reminds me of all the stuff I can't handle. It's weird, but it was also kind of liberating, seeing it in black and white…. I guess that's when other things start to come in.
>
> Psychiatrist: Which of the positions is most like what you do out in life, do you think?
>
> Patrick: Resisting. It's what I do all the time. It's so obvious to me. That's exactly it. As soon as the creeping feeling starts, that's what I do.
>
> Psychiatrist: And the strategy of letting the paper and what it says just sit in your lap?
>
> Patrick: That is new to me.

Most ACT experiential exercises offer many possible avenues to pursue. In this one, the therapeutic process of openness is the target. The experience of anxiety and what it evokes for this patient are treated as something written on a notepad. This is designed to help him learn to create an observational distance from fear- and anxiety-producing content, thus promoting a stance of openness and the ability to stay in contact with anxiety without using avoidance strategies. Different questions put by the psychiatrist can shift the focus to either of the other two therapeutic processes as well. What are the pros and cons of the different strategies in terms of desired outcome (workability)? In which of the two positions does Patrick have more freedom to act in a values-consistent way in real-life situations (engagement)?

It would also be easy to help the patient use this experience to focus on life "out there." Patrick recognizes that what he does is "resist" the anxiety and the various private experiences that trigger it. What would it mean to leave them "in his lap" in his normal daily life? A possible continuation is to use the exercise as a metaphor for something new that the patient might try between now and the next meeting with the psychiatrist.

> Psychiatrist: If "having it in your lap" could give you greater latitude to act in different situations, and if you could do it at least once this coming week, in what situation would you most want this to happen?
>
> Patrick: This coming weekend, my wife is going out with her sister, and it would be great if I could try this then.
>
> Psychiatrist: Shall we look a little more closely at that situation and see what you can do to allow yourself to just have that creeping feeling sit "in your lap," if it turns up?
>
> Patrick: It would be interesting to see what would happen.

The metaphors that naturally appear during an experiential exercise can be used as a point of reference later in treatment. If the patient returns having gone through a situation that previously produced anxiety, the psychiatrist can ask questions that "rekindle" the metaphor:

- "Would you say that was pushing it away or having it in your lap?"
- "If you want to have that in your lap, how would you go about it?"
- "That sounds like an example of you having it more in your lap. Would you agree?"

TIPS FOR SUCCESS

Using experiential metaphors and exercises is a powerful way to both trigger patients' in-session avoidance behaviors and instigate the three therapeutic processes of ACT.

Experiential exercises tap into information processing systems that are not verbally regulated, thus allowing for different and clinically relevant forms of learning to occur.

Well-constructed experiential exercises refer to multiple core ACT concepts that the psychiatrist can return to and selectively highlight over time.

When an experiential exercise functions well, the lessons learned within that experience can be "repackaged" and applied to new clinical issues that arise.

Summary

In this chapter, we have described some of the advanced steps of ACT dancing so that the psychiatrist can develop and deliver powerful, life-transforming interventions during the clinical conversation. The available ACT literature is replete with amazingly creative and fun-to-use clinical interventions, and we demonstrated some of our favorite ones in this chapter. ACT clinicians frequently comment that helping patients acquire the skills they need to be psychologically resilient is a rewarding and enjoyable enterprise. Helping people does not feel like "work"; rather, it teaches us as clinicians about ourselves as people because the issues with which we help our patients are the same issues we confront in our own lives. The ACT principles so helpful to our patients can also be directly applied to increase our own sense of participation in life.

We hope you can see that many ACT interventions can be delivered very quickly, often within the confines of a 15- to 20-minute medication check or in a single consultation session. Because of the qualitative nature of the core ACT therapeutic mechanisms, it is more important to give patients a well-conceived but small taste of what it feels like to be psychologically resilient. Once this happens, patients will generally become eager to learn more about this approach. They can do this by accessing one of many excellent self-help books on ACT or by coming back to see the psychiatrist for another session or two of ACT dancing!

The Essentials

- The ACT psychiatrist, above all else, models four essential attributes:
  - An open, nonjudgmental, and curious attitude
  - A stance that "we are on the same journey" in life
  - Humility, honesty, and a willingness to be imperfect
  - That the patient and psychiatrist are equals
- The distinction between a therapeutic process and a clinical intervention is critical:
  - A *therapeutic process* is a mechanism that directly mediates positive clinical change.
  - A *clinical intervention* is a specific strategy or tactic the psychiatrist uses to "activate" a therapeutic process.
- In ACT, all clinical interventions touch upon three therapeutic processes: context sensitivity/workability, openness, and engagement.
- Creating sensitivity to life contexts that matter to patients and a willingness to self-reflect on the workability of avoidance behaviors is often the first big "acceptance move" in ACT.
- Promoting openness often requires teaching patients to focus and sustain attention in the moment, thus allowing them to create a safe observational distance from self-instructional rules that show up in awareness.
- Values often function as powerful motivators of life engagement because they refer to a class of behavior that can be applied in many life contexts over time, regardless of short-term negative consequences.

- Physical and language-based metaphors are a core feature of ACT because they work around reductive reasoning and stimulate other forms of information processing.
- Well-constructed ACT metaphors and experiential exercises often simultaneously reference multiple core ACT concepts, such that the metaphor or exercise can be used repeatedly over the course of treatment.

Suggested Readings

Bach P, Moran D, Hayes S: ACT in Practice: Case Conceptualization in Acceptance and Commitment Therapy. Oakland, CA, New Harbinger, 2008

Gorden T, Borushak J: The ACT Approach: A Comprehensive Guide for Acceptance and Commitment Therapy. Eau Claire, WI, PESI, 2017

Stoddard J, Afari N: The Big Book of ACT Metaphors: A Practitioner's Guide to Experiential Exercises and Metaphors in Acceptance and Commitment Therapy. Oakland, CA, New Harbinger, 2014

References

Hayes S, Strosahl K, Wilson K: Acceptance and Commitment Therapy: The Process and Practice of Mindful Change. New York, Guilford, 2011

Strosahl K, Robinson P, Gustavsson T: Inside This Moment: A Clinician's Guide to Promoting Radical Change in Acceptance and Commitment Therapy. Oakland, CA, New Harbinger, 2015

Törneke N: Metaphor in Practice: A Professional's Guide to Using the Science of Language in Psychotherapy. Oakland, CA, New Harbinger, 2017

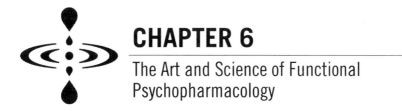

CHAPTER 6

The Art and Science of Functional Psychopharmacology

We cannot direct the wind, but we can adjust our sails.

—Bertha Calloway

Physicians in all practice settings face tremendous pressure to "do something" to help their patients. All too often they face severe systemic barriers to doing so. In low-resource communities in most countries of the Western world, including urban, rural, and frontier settings, psychiatry appointment time is often limited. Because primary care physicians prescribe an enormous amount of psychotropic medications—more, in absolute terms, than do psychiatrists in the United States—patients who are referred to psychiatrists may be especially resistant to first-line therapeutics. With shortages of psychiatrists, tremendous clinical need, and limited access to care resources, a typical initial psychiatric consultation may be very brief, and some patients may wait 3–4 months just to have that initial evaluation.

Given such circumstances, some psychiatrists in these settings feel their practices involve little more than serial prescribing and they have only a limited ability to engage patients fully in discussions about coping strategies other than taking medications. Moreover, patients presenting for psychiatric services typically have significant co-occurring physical, substance, or other mental disorders, making their care very complex. With very little time, increasing new demand for services, limited personnel and system resources, and challenges in managing patients with highly complex health problems, psychiatrists may find it difficult to take a holistic, functionally focused approach to patient care.

As we discussed in Chapter 3, adopting a functional psychiatric approach can nevertheless create additional "leverage" with patients, even when the clinical conversation is short and follow-up visits are few and far between. As several of the case examples in Chapter 1 demonstrated, prescribing a medication is often just the first step in the chain of behavior change.

A critical question naturally arises for psychiatrists who have large numbers of patients requesting or requiring psychotropic medications: "How does this affect my clinical practice when I'm prescribing medication?" In this chapter, we explore how a traditional psychiatric approach to psychopharmacology might be reinvigorated and empowered by augmenting it with a functional contextual approach. To achieve this objective, we must first discuss the history of this approach. Few psychiatrists know about the longstanding link between the fields of behavioral analysis and pharmacology and how instrumental it has been in developing and refining our understanding of the psychological properties of medications and their impact on human behavior. These concepts, in turn, directly inform the practice of functional pharmacology. We delve more deeply into the underlying principles of functional psychopharmacology and demonstrate them in a series of instructional videos and clinical dialogues referenced throughout the chapter. If you, the reader, approach this important feature of psychiatric practice with an open mind and a willingness to try something new, we guarantee you will want to adopt a functional approach in your decision-making process.

The Key Principles of Behavioral Pharmacology

Many of the principles that underpin functional psychopharmacology are derived from a line of scientific research known as *behavioral pharmacology,* which is the behavioral analytic approach to understanding the impact of medications on human behavior. In this section, we outline basic scientific assumptions, theoretical bases, and empirical findings of behavioral pharmacology from its origins in the 1950s to the present day. Behavioral pharmacology is a well-established discipline with strong theoretical foundations and many decades of substantive empirical support. Of late, it is seldom taught in psychiatric residency and fellowship programs, but as you will see, it still has real relevance in contemporary psychiatric practice.

B. F. Skinner had a strong interest in the effects of psychotropic medications on behavior, believing the experimental analysis of the effect of illicit substances and medications on human behavior would unlock the secrets of human genetics and physiology, which he considered to be the real causes of behavior, in combination with environmental influences. Scientific examination of the behavioral effects of psychotropic medications occurred only sporadically up to the mid-1950s, from which time interest skyrocketed, in part galvanized by the introduction of chlorpromazine (Thorazine) into psychiatric practice in the early 1950s. Only 28 studies were published between 1917 and 1954, whereas 274 studies appeared from 1955 to 1963. In 1956, an important conference was sponsored by the National Institute of Mental Health, the National Academy of Sciences, the National Research Council, and the American Psychiatric Association. The conference was called "Techniques for the Study of the Behavioral Effects of Drugs" and was chaired by Skinner and Peter Dews, founder of behavioral pharmacology (Dews 1956). This conference examined the potential utility of using behavioral analytic methods to understand the effects of psychiatric agents, including psychotropic medications, on behavior. Several important principles were established that laid the groundwork for behavioral pharmacology to emerge as a wing of applied behavior analysis. These principles were articulated in the first article published in the flagship journal *Psychopharmacology* by a highly respected contemporary of Skinner, Murry Sidman (1959).

BEHAVIOR IS IMPORTANT IN ITS OWN RIGHT

The functional psychiatric approach informed by behavioral psychopharmacology emphasizes that behavior is a rich and fascinating subject in and of itself and a proper focus of psychiatric interventions. For the practicing psychiatrist with large numbers of patients taking psychotropic medications, the daily lives of our patients—including their thoughts and feelings, and how these activities are affected by medications—are surely of most interest.

EMPHASIZE SINGLE-CASE ANALYSIS

Every human being has a unique learning history, genotypic makeup, and physiological sensitivities that make it difficult to generalize about the likely effects of medications on any particular individual based solely on group-level research data. Each patient will have a personally unique reaction to the introduction of a medication; hence, within-subject study of psychopharmacological agent effects is a more fruitful approach. This means each patient will exhibit a unique pattern of response to medication that can only be measured with reference to that patient's functional objectives in life. These objectives should involve explicit, observable behaviors directly enabled by the introduction of a prescription medication.

USE DIRECT, IDIOGRAPHIC BEHAVIOR MEASURES

Because behavior is of primary interest in its own right, changes in behavior are the best way to determine the "success" of a pharmacological regimen. Procedures (e.g., symptom inventories and checklists) that measure generically chosen behaviors can be problematic because they may or may not predict observable, clinically relevant behaviors for any particular patient. In clinical practice, this means that the most valuable information we have about any medication is what the patient tells us about the experience of improvement (or lack thereof) in being able to move in a chosen and valued direction in life.

ISOLATE AND INFLUENCE FACTORS THAT PRODUCE BEHAVIORAL VARIABILITY

In all cases, functional psychiatrists attempt to promote variability in patients' coping and problem-solving behaviors. When considering the actual effects of medications, the key (and tricky) task is to separate the variability in behavior (including thoughts and feelings) instigated by prescribed psychopharmacological agents from that effected by other sources, such as physical exercise, increased social engagement, and so forth. For a medication to be considered successful, the psychiatrist must be able to conclude that the effects of the prescription medications are what produced the hoped-for change in the patient's functioning. This task requires the psychiatrist to pay close attention to the patient's unfolding exterior and interior life contexts. This will result in a pragmatic, flexible, and personalized medicine approach to prescribing.

TIPS FOR SUCCESS

Behavioral pharmacology is one of the original theoretical traditions of the larger field of pharmacology.

Behavioral pharmacology studies the effects of psychotropic agents on human behavior, with the following guiding principles:

- The behavioral response to medications is an important level of analysis in its own right.
- The effects of medications on human behavior are unique from person to person.
- The most effective level of analysis is repeated measurement of clinically relevant behaviors unique to each patient.

The key outcome of interest is evidence that the agent administered is responsible for increasing both context sensitivity and contingency-based behavior, thus enabling patients to make important life changes that ultimately lead to a natural reduction in symptom distress.

Shared Principles of Psychopharmacology and Behavioral Pharmacology

No clear and absolute distinction can be made between the practices of psychopharmacology and behavioral pharmacology. The term *psychopharmacology* was coined in 1921 to describe a yet-to-be-developed science dealing with the behavioral effects of pharmacological agents (Macht and Mora 1921). Behavior analysis has contributed greatly to the research and principles of behavioral pharmacology, yet any attempt to understand medication effects *also* demands knowledge of the basic principles of pharmacology. These principles arose from the application of scientific methods to the study of psychotropic agents, beginning in the mid-nineteenth century with Bernard in France, Schmiedeberg in Germany, and Abel in the United States (Holmstedt and Liljestrand 1963; Schuster 1962). These researchers and their successors made it clear, for example, that all agents have multiple and dose-dependent actions; these are now basic tenets of behavioral pharmacology. In addition, the concepts of tolerance and physical dependence as well as the receptor model of drug action come from traditional pharmacology. These concepts and findings form an integral part of any adequate knowledge about how psychopharmacological agents affect human behavior (Thompson and Schuster 1968) and must be known by any prescriber of psychiatric medications (Poling and Byrne 2000).

PSYCHOPHARMACOLOGICAL AGENTS VARY IN SPECIFICITY

All psychopharmacological agents vary in the degree to which they selectively target the biological processes hypothesized to produce disease or illness. In the best case, a valid diagnosis leads directly to a limited (or even single) array of medication choices. With respect to this metric, it is safe to say that psychoactive agents are more general, rather than specific, in their effects on behavior. In other words, an important difference exists between the known mechanisms of action of psychotropic agents and those of other well-established medications used to treat common physical health conditions.

Let us consider two hypothetical examples to clarify this important point. In one, after several days with an increasingly sore throat, a woman goes to her primary care physician, who, after conducting a throat culture, determines the woman has a large colony of *Streptococcus pyogenes* bacteria living in her mouth and throat. To treat this condition, the doctor prescribes an antibiotic, amoxicillin, that specifically targets those bacteria by disrupting their cell wall synthesis. The woman's symptoms (complaints of a sore throat) are directly related to the bacteria living in her throat, and the medication prescribed selectively acts on those bacteria via a known mechanism. One week later, the physician can determine the extent to which the prescribed antibiotic has been effective not only by asking the patient how her throat feels but also by conducting a second throat culture. A clear and accessible biological cause (bacteria) of the behavioral symptoms (verbal reports of discomfort) can be identified.

Now consider another scenario. After several weeks of feeling sad and depressed, the same woman begins to feel hopeless and that she will never be socially engaged and happy again. One day, she becomes so distraught that she considers suicide. Troubled by these thoughts, she realizes she needs professional help and visits a psychiatrist. Upon examination, which includes the woman describing her emotional state and her thoughts of suicide, the psychiatrist determines she is experiencing a major depressive episode and prescribes a selective serotonin reuptake inhibitor (SSRI). After 3 weeks, the woman again visits her psychiatrist. She reports she is feeling better and is no longer considering harming herself. In this case, although biochemical *models* of mental illness have been hypothesized, the behavioral symptoms (verbal reports of depression and suicidal ideation) cannot be attributed with certainty to a biological cause, and no practical means are available of ascertaining the effects of the psychopharmacological agent at that precise level of analysis. We cannot administer, for example, a blood test of serotonin deficiency that "proves" the existence of depression and therefore later conclude with any accuracy that the hypothesized toxic biological process has been reversed.

In strep throat, the disease process is fairly precisely understood and consistent across individuals. So, too, is the mechanism through which the medication designed to treat this illness works. Penicillin disrupts cell wall synthesis in gram-negative bacteria, causing the cell walls to leak and the bacteria to die. By killing the bacteria that cause a sore throat, amoxicillin alleviates the symptoms of the disease. The manner in which the bacteria cause symptoms can be described in detail, and the mechanism of therapeutic action is well understood and measurable. Moreover, these processes are generally invariant across individuals with strep throat, and thus, most people with the disorder respond favorably to amoxicillin—in fact, 72% respond within a 7-day period, compared with only 7% who receive a placebo.

In the case of depression, however, the relation between the pharmacological mechanism of action of an SSRI or serotonin-norepinephrine reuptake inhibitor and the symptoms of depression, which themselves vary considerably across individuals, is far more tenuous. Although an antidepressant is known to interfere with the reuptake of serotonin, the manner in which this neurochemical change leads to patient-reported changes in affect and ideation cannot be specified. Put differently, the disease process underlying depression and the manner in which an antidepressant interferes with that process to alleviate symptoms remains a matter of speculation (Krishnan and Nestler 2010). Furthermore, although all antidepressants alleviate symptoms of depression in large group trials, those effects are modest in size and variable across treated individuals. Indeed, it is impossible to predict a priori who will respond favorably to a psychopharmacological agent and who will not.

PSYCHOTROPICS AND PHYSIOLOGICAL DEPENDENCE

Through each period of scientific and technical advance in psychopharmacology, both clinicians and researchers have understandably taken some time to gauge the importance of physiological dependence issues (Lader 1991). Direct-to-consumer advertising since 1985, which accelerated in 1997 when the FDA loosened its rules about listing adverse drug effects, has arguably shaped all of us into a disarming naiveté with regard to the issue of physiological dependence, particularly among the purportedly "nonaddictive" psychotropics (Donohue 2006). Importantly, psychopharmacological principles dating back to the 1950s have emphasized that tolerance and physiological dependence will inevitably occur with *any* psychotropic substance (Poling and Byrne 2000). Increasingly, clinicians and patients have become aware of this fact across the entire range of psychopharmacological agents. Naturally, some medications engender more problematic levels of physiological dependence than others. However, difficulties with withdrawal after prolonged use of any psychotropic compound is to be expected. Our current level of understanding of physiological dependence and psychotropic agent withdrawal syndromes is very limited, and it is difficult to determine how long any particular individual needs to take any particular nonaddictive psychotropic medicine before withdrawal or medication transitions become yet another problem to be managed clinically.

As noted by Witt-Doerring et al. (2018), clinical trials have as yet yielded insufficient information about psychotropic withdrawal or medication transitions. Most clinical trials are not patterned on the lived experiences of patients—a problem of ecological validity and a challenge for clinical practice:

> Medication withdrawal is difficult to assess in the relatively brief 6- to 12-week randomized controlled trials that lead to FDA approvals and marketing. The costs, clinical challenges, and desire to do no more than is needed to show relative safety and efficacy have limited these studies' duration. Such short durations do not typically allow time for participants to develop any level of significant physiological dependence or to produce a difficult or even detectable withdrawal syndrome. These trials, which usually focus on determining efficacy, often have adequate methodology or statistical power to identify and characterize only very common

and relatively severe withdrawal syndromes. Because of these challenges in acquiring the necessary data for educating physicians about any potential withdrawal syndromes, medications come onto the market with many unknowns about their longer-term effects and discontinuation syndromes. Many unidentified problems beyond withdrawal syndromes can take years to become fully appreciated—often requiring an accumulation of published case reports or other observational studies before they become widely known to the medical community. (Witt-Doerring et al. 2018)

As more patients are exposed to longer and longer medication regimens, we no doubt will learn more about the mechanisms underlying problematic physiological dependence in the nonaddictive psychotropic medication classes. The mere existence of physiological dependence necessarily means psychopharmacological agent withdrawal syndromes will become part and parcel of the risk/benefit analysis of any decision to engage in a longer-term medication regimen with a particular patient. This issue cannot be clinically managed simply by acknowledging the risks of longer-term psychopharmacological management. Instead, it argues for prescribing psychiatrists to adopt a significantly new perspective on the use of psychotropic medications, one that is functionally oriented and naturally leads to much more specific, targeted, and time-limited prescribing (Fornaro et al. 2019).

TIPS FOR SUCCESS

Behavioral pharmacology and psychopharmacology share some common principles that provide a basic understanding of how psychiatric medications work.

The effects of drugs occur at multiple levels, including neurological, physiological, psychological, and social.

Pharmacological agent effects at all levels are dose dependent.

Psychopharmacological agent effects vary widely in terms of the specificity of their mechanisms of effect.

In general, psychotropic medications are more general in their mechanisms of action.

Physiological dependence and tolerance are to be expected with *all* psychotropic medications and must be included in any risk/benefit analysis that precedes the prescribing of a medications.

Basic Principles of Functional Psychopharmacology

Before we examine the core features of functional pharmacology, it will be useful to briefly review the main tenets of the functional contextual approach introduced in Chapter 3:

- Human behavior cannot be separated from the context in which it occurs, including both the context external to the acting person (environment) and the private responses of that person (e.g., thoughts, memories, and feelings).
- All behavior is controlled by antecedents (triggering events, including the psychological and physical effects of medications) or consequences (rewards or punishments following a behavior).
- Behavior in turn interacts with and modifies the controlling factors.
- With humans, controlling factors often include behavior-regulatory processes of covert language (the "mind") and self-reflective awareness (the perspective from which the processes of mind are both received and observed).

The prime directive of functional psychopharmacology is to be clear about what functional purpose the medication is serving and to evaluate the effect of the medication based upon that purpose. For example, we know reductions in levels of psychiatric symptoms are only modestly correlated with improvements in functional status (Lin and Yang 2017; McKnight and Kashdan 2009; Vatne and Bjorkly 2008). Feeling less sad, blue, anxious, or fearful is not the same as living a valued, satisfying life. Medications may help lessen feelings of hopelessness or sadness, yet happiness does not automatically fill the void created when hopelessness and sadness disappear. Many times, other equally distressing emotions will fill that void.

To make medications functionally effective, psychiatrists must steer the conversation toward improving patients' participation in, and success with, life contexts that matter to them. As noted in Chapter 3, the functional psychiatrist is not at all averse to prescribing medication, as long as the patient understands that the medication is there primarily to help him achieve meaningful life goals and pursuits. The extent to which a medication is likely to ease or reduce emotional, cognitive, or behavioral barriers to valued action is always the determining factor in the decision to prescribe. Most importantly, the success with which using the medication has helped patients live their lives fully and in a manner congruent with their values should be the central way the medication's effectiveness is assessed. Such an approach is what we mean by "functional psychopharmacology." This stance does not require the psychiatrist to reject the proposition that people have underlying mental disorders. The logic of functional psychiatry, simply stated, is that eliminating or controlling the symptoms of an illness is not the same as improving a patient's sense of health and life vitality. In essence, two objectives are related to the decision to prescribe, not one, and the emphasis in functional psychiatry is firmly on more engagement in "valued living."

ADOPT AND UTILIZE A HOLISTIC VIEW OF MEDICATION EFFECTS

Put succinctly, functional psychopharmacology involves analyzing and assessing the effects of psychotropic medications within the A-B-C framework that is the hallmark of behavior analysis. For example, a psychopharmacological agent can function as an important antecedent, but a human can also interact with that effect in a way that changes the effect. This creates a serious conundrum for strictly biological or neurological accounts of psychopharmacological agent actions and effects on human behavior. The way a human interacts with the experienced effects of a medication can change its effects, including not only its incidental effects but also its main effects. This means symbolic representations of using a medicine can function as powerful antecedents or consequences, regardless of whether the patient is ingesting an active compound or a placebo. Thus, we must both recognize and accept that our patients do not simply *take* medications, they *interact* with them symbolically and socially (Poling and Lesage 1992). This interaction includes the social context in which the medication-taking activity is contemplated and the social cues that are received about the likely effects of taking a prescription medicine. Furthermore, the patient is engaged in producing his own attributions and expectancies about taking the medication (Poling and Lesage 1992). These psychologically mediated interactions can occur in an iterative, progressive fashion; can involve any or all of the interior or exterior contexts surrounding drug-taking behavior; and can result in the same compound producing markedly different effects between patients and, indeed, within the same patient over time. With regard to the effects of psychotropic agents on behavior, this means that private expectancies and beliefs, as well as proximal social cues, have a direct effect upon their functional effects.

The best example of this core tenet of functional pharmacology is the *placebo effect*, arguably one of the most powerful treatments in medicine. When a patient *believes* she is receiving an active agent and expects that chemical substance to produce positive results, the result is often the same as though the patient actually received an active compound (Poling and Lesage 1992). From a behavioral pharmacology perspective, a placebo involves the patient attaching a positive expectancy (antecedent) that creates a powerful, positive drug "effect" (consequence) even though the patient is consuming a pill (a behavior) containing an inert substance. In psychiatric research, the placebo effect is the gold standard against which active medication effects are measured. The problem is, with the massive amount of direct marketing of psychiatric medications, social cues surrounding the act of taking a psychoactive medication are pervasively positive. As a result, the size of the placebo effect associated with all classes of psychiatric medicines has grown closer and closer to the actual effect size of active medication. Indeed, a recent review of the FDA database for antidepressant clinical trials concluded that the placebo response rate in depressed patients has increased 6.2% in the past decade (Khan et al. 2017). This incremental change in placebo effect demonstrates another important principle of behavioral psychopharmacology: cuing activities in the patient's external environment can strongly influence the impact a prescribed medication has on the patient's behavior.

For example, we know the social cues in the immediate environment play an important determining role in a person's response to the ingestion of both alcohol and illicit drugs. An individual who is dependent on alcohol and enters a bar intending to drink is already getting "loaded" before he orders his first beer (Chait and Perry 1992). The substance-using person who expects to get "high" on a drug will report being high even if she has actually consumed a placebo (Chait and Perry 1992). The experience of being intoxicated can be induced simply by creating the expectancy that a placebo beverage contains alcohol (Vuchinich and Sobell 1978). Interestingly, the antecedent functions of alcohol are strengthened by positioning intoxication-consistent social cues in the immediate environment (see Testa et al. 2006 for a review).

FOCUS ON IMPROVING FUNCTIONAL STATUS

From a functional psychopharmacology perspective, psychotropics are unique because they are utilized to deal with problems defined by, measured in terms of, and best understood at the level of overt behavior, *including changes in patient reports of specific inner experiences.* The effects of prescribed medications on the biological processes responsible for any observed changes in behavior are not clearly understood, and their clinical effectiveness cannot be adequately evaluated or understood at this level of analysis. Therefore, from a functional psychiatric perspective, clinical evaluations of psychotropic medications must assess whether medication (the antecedent) significantly improves some targeted aspect(s) of the patient's behavior without producing intolerable or simply unhelpful adverse reactions (side effects) that reduce the emotional valence of the results of the new behavior (consequences).

To determine whether a pharmacological intervention is successful in treating a dysfunctional behavior, three questions must be answered:

1. What were the desired effects of the medication?
2. Were those effects obtained?
3. Did any significant adverse reactions occur?

Although these are easy questions to ask, they are not so easy to answer, and how we psychiatrists (and our patients) understand the role of medications and precisely what questions we ask will *both* profoundly influence the results.

Today, dozens of different psychotropic medications are available. They are prescribed much more broadly and by more diverse clinical providers than in the past. In 1996, psychotropic medications collectively accounted for roughly 10%–15% of all prescriptions written in the United States. By 2013, nearly 17% of U.S. adults reported routinely filling at least one prescription for a psychiatric medication. Primary care physicians are the leading prescribers of psychotropic agents. When psychiatric medications are introduced into a patient's care, whether by a psychiatrist, primary care physician, or another independent practitioner, the goal should be to alter some aspect of the patient's functioning to improve the patient's sense of health and both short- and longer-term vitality. This improvement generally can be achieved by focusing the clinical conversation on the patient's life context and functional integrity within that context.

As we discussed in Chapter 3, the ACT approach regards symptoms of distress as signals of an imbalance in the patient's life context. Once those imbalances have been identified in the psychiatric interview (i.e., the gap between what the patient is seeking and what he is getting from life), medication might play a useful role in alleviating the emotional or cognitive barriers that stand between the patient and more effective living. In practical terms, no compelling reason or particular therapeutic advantage has been found for invoking other explanatory models (i.e., mental illness, correcting a chemical imbalance) to justify using medications or to explain how and why they are helpful. For some psychiatrists, this might constitute a big shift in how the conversation with the patient is oriented and organized. The following case example demonstrates how this functionally focused process of patient education and seeking informed consent might unfold.

CASE EXAMPLE: AMANDA

Amanda is a 28-year-old married primary school teacher seen for long-standing work stress, anxiety, and low mood. She works in a highly demanding private school system and is trying to complete her master's degree in education. She lives with her husband, Tom, who works in a difficult front-line law enforcement job. She has no children. Her main worry is the effect her anxiety will have on her work as a teacher. Her primary care physician prescribed duloxetine after trials with citalopram and venlafaxine proved unhelpful. She had a fairly strong positive response to this medication change but began to experience a resurgence in her symptoms after 3–4 months, suggesting she was beginning to develop a tolerance to the antidepressant (Fava and Offidani 2011). At that point, her doctor decided to refer her for a comprehensive psychiatric workup. Following an initial contextual assessment, the psychiatrist begins a review of Amanda's past psychiatric and medical history and specifically her response to psychotropic medications.

Psychiatrist: I understand from the referral letter that your primary physician has prescribed duloxetine, initially 30 mg and now 60 mg, and this has been for about 3 months?

Amanda: Yes, but like the other ones, it really hasn't been as much help as I'd hoped.

Psychiatrist: Okay, thanks for that overview. Now I'd like to ask a few more specific questions about how you've noticed the duloxetine affecting you. Would that be okay?

Amanda: Sure!

Psychiatrist: What, if anything, have you noticed to have been helpful from the duloxetine?

Amanda: Well, it kind of helped initially, I suppose, to feel a bit less anxious, a bit less sadness, but over a few months it kind of lost that effect.

Psychiatrist: So, you noticed it took the edge off your anxious sensations and low mood and maybe helped you step forward a bit more into life?

Amanda: Yeah, it was certainly better at the beginning, but then we had to bump up the dose after a while, and it didn't seem to work as well. I also had more side effects with the higher dose.

Psychiatrist: About those side effects—what, if anything, have you noticed to be unhelpful about the duloxetine?

Amanda: Well, it certainly numbed out my sex drive. I really don't feel anything much, and things have not been so great with Tom due to that! And feeling kind of numb emotionally. That was kind of what helped in the beginning, but over time it's become more of a hindrance, not feeling pleasure about things that I used to like doing and feeling flat about everything in general in life.

Psychiatrist: Any other adverse effects? Tiredness, stomach problems, troubles with thinking?

Amanda: Not so much, maybe a bit of tiredness ongoing, and going to the bathroom a lot, but that eased off. I noticed that if I miss taking a dose, I feel really fuzzy, nauseated, and weird.

Psychiatrist: Okay, speaking of which, what else do you notice if you miss it accidentally or leave it at home when you go away for the weekend or something?

Amanda: Sure thing. By the early afternoon—and Tom has mentioned this—I feel pretty spaced out, fuzzy headed, and sometimes I get this strong tingling in my neck and head; I will get more irritable and anxious.

Psychiatrist: Sounds difficult. What kind of thoughts go along with those experiences?

Amanda: Well, I worry that it's my anxiety showing up and that I really need the medication.

Psychiatrist: When you start again with the duloxetine, how long does it take for all that to go away?

Amanda: Usually pretty immediately; within half an hour or so of taking the tablet I missed, I feel much better. But sometimes it's taken maybe half the day.

Psychiatrist: If you look at the time course between missing your medication and having these experiences, and then how quickly these experiences ease off after you take the medication again, it would seem pretty clear that this is a physiological dependence on the medication and not so much your anxiety coming back. I don't think your original anxiety symptoms looked like this, did they?

Amanda: No, come to think of it, my symptoms really didn't look like this at all. And I've heard from other folks that withdrawing from antidepressant medications can really be pretty difficult at times. Is that what you're talking about?

Psychiatrist: It's quite possible that's what you were experiencing.

In this brief exchange, the psychiatrist conducts a curious and open-ended inquiry about the patient's previous and ongoing psychiatric medications and goes through a fairly simple and straightforward functional psychopharmacology assessment:

1. What medications are you presently taking, and for how long?
2. What, if anything, have you noticed to be helpful about this medication? Were any other elements in your life changing at the same time?
3. What, if anything, have you noticed to be troublesome about this medication?
4. What do you notice when you forget it for a day or go away for the weekend without it?

Video 21: Medication—Assess Functionally: Benefits, Adverse Effects, Withdrawal Symptoms

---

The psychiatrist must perform a thorough evaluation of the effects, both positive and negative, of each psychotropic medication the patient has taken in the past, as well as those the patient is currently taking. This often provides a useful context for discussing a patient's overall experience with and reactions to the use of medications. The psychiatrist can assume these experiences have shaped the patient's expectancies about the role medications will play in helping improve functional integrity in important life contexts. Some follow-up questioning is often required on the second question, particularly when patients note that certain medications made a significant difference in terms of feeling better. The functional psychiatrist would carefully ask *what else was going on in their lives around that time*. Often, critical, corollary life changes can be entirely overlooked, and improvement can be attributed only to the commencement of medication, when many other critical and sustainable factors—and importantly, ones the patient did for him- or herself—are actually far more responsible for positive mood and life engagement changes!

PICK A LEVEL OF DISCOURSE THAT EMPOWERS THE PATIENT

Another important feature of the initial interview process is to develop an explanatory model for the patient's presenting problems. In the functional contextual approach, the goal is to develop a model of shared understanding that can be used to promote the patient's life goals and best interests over time. Regardless of the psychiatrist's degree of conviction in the construct of "mental disorders" and classification systems such as DSM-5 (American Psychiatric Association 2013), the important question is whether this type of discourse empowers and serves the patient's best interests. Similarly, explanatory "talk" about the mechanisms underlying mental disorders, referencing circuit pathways or chemical imbalances, may be useful to the extent that it empowers the patient to move toward making behavior changes that serve her best interests in life.

 Video 22: Medication—Personalizing Psychiatry: Inquiring, Listening, and Shared Decision Making
Video 23: Medication—Picking a Level of Discourse That Empowers the Patient

---

Patients who believe their problems are the result of a mental illness caused by "chemical imbalances" exhibit more passivity and experience more self-focused stigma (Goldney et al. 2010), may become recipients of more social stigma, and are more likely to view their problems in life as unchanging (Kemp et al. 2014; Pescosolido et al. 2010). Similarly, psychiatrists who see their patient's issues as strictly biological in nature are more pessimistic about the patient's chances of recovery, more likely to rely exclusively on medications, and less likely to combine medications with empirically supported psychotherapies (Lebowitz and Ahn 2014; Pescosolido et al. 2010). Again, we are not taking a position on the scientific validity of any particular theory; we are simply stating that any theory, even if it is scientifically derived and rigorous, may undermine the patient's function if it diminishes or disables his sense of agency or makes it less likely that he will act in ways that serve his best interests.

In the United States, many patients will have been exposed to a heavy dose of direct marketing that explicitly conveys messages about their mental health. Many patients will already be using these concepts to explain their life difficulties and will expect the psychiatrist to remove their "symptoms" so they will no longer have a "mental illness." Psychiatrists inevitably must become involved in this discourse when public and patient attitudes are shaped by such messaging. For the functional psychiatrist, the goal is to help the patient reorient toward more *functionally useful* explanatory models, as demonstrated in the following dialogue with Amanda.

> Amanda: I've been told my anxiety and depression are due to a chemical imbalance in the brain and that this duloxetine helps to correct the imbalance to boost my serotonin. Isn't that right?
>
> Psychiatrist: Well, I'd say the jury is still out on that idea, but it's pretty hard to watch any TV show without hearing that message during drug advertisements. In here, though, the important question is what your life goals are and how we can best get you to live that kind of life. If you believed your anxiety was due to bad genes or chemical imbalances in your brain, how would that affect your sense of having some control over what happens in your life?
>
> Amanda: Well, it would mean someone like you would have to first give me another chemical, like a prescription, to correct that chemical imbalance and so get rid of my anxiety symptoms. Then maybe I could get going in my life.
>
> Psychiatrist: This type of approach makes you wait for your anxiety symptoms to get better before you can get on with your life. Problem is, you've already tried three different medications without much success. You're kind of stuck in limbo waiting for a medication to work. That's why we might want to be aware of the possibility of a chemical imbalance that may or may not be fixed by a medication. Even more important is the possibility that what is going on is more than that, so we don't let our whole game plan be controlled by that possibility.
>
> Amanda: That makes sense; it certainly matches with what I've experienced. When my anxiety comes back even when I'm taking medications, I feel even more frustrated about life. I wonder if I'm going to be plagued with anxiety the rest of my life and if I've got a more severe case of anxiety than almost anyone else! I want it to be something simple—something fixed by a magic medication or whatever—but I know it's more. It's actually quite a relief to have this conversation with you right now.
>
> Psychiatrist: We don't have to conclude that the persistence of your anxiety means your chemicals are out of balance or that you have a severe illness that is worse than other people's. Even in clinical studies, when people have a response to medication therapy, they still exhibit symptoms of anxiety, although typically at lower levels.
>
> Amanda: Wow. I always thought it did, so it's good to hear that having anxiety symptoms is common even when I'm taking medications.
>
> Psychiatrist: What do you know about the longer-term potential adverse effects of these medications? To be honest, we've only become somewhat more aware of them over the years.

Amanda: Well, the paper the pharmacist gave me listed a lot of effects, but when I read it, it was rather scary. And the disclaimers at the end of TV commercials are terrifying!

Psychiatrist: That just tells you that these medications are pretty potent, and we don't want to use them without having very clear and specific goals for them. If the main goal is not to get rid of all your anxiety symptoms, then it could more realistically be to help you function better in the life situations that matter to you.

Amanda: Okay, this is all a bit unsettling for me, but it's good to have this talk. So, we can work together to find medications that are more helpful? To figure out how to manage those side effects?

Psychiatrist: Absolutely. First, we need to get a good sense of what we are trying to achieve with using medications. What are we hoping they will do?

In this exchange, the functional psychiatrist probes Amanda's explanatory system about her ongoing problems with anxiety. The exchange is designed to give the patient a gentle way out of the conceptual trap imposed by excessive allegiance to the mental illness and chemical imbalance messages she has been exposed to in print and on television. The psychiatrist remains neutral about the scientific validity of these theories and instead explores their functional impact on Amanda's sense of agency. The psychiatrist also explores an alternative role that medications might play, specifically, to improve the patient's functional capacities in the context of seeking important life goals.

USE MEDICATIONS TO UNDERMINE AVOIDANCE FUNCTIONS AND STRATEGIES

For our purposes as functional psychiatrists, we must touch upon a basic question: How can we effectively use psychiatric medications to undermine experiential avoidance and perhaps also in other ways help our patients get unstuck? This is a basic fork in the road that determines not only what medications we prescribe but also why we prescribe them. As we have discussed repeatedly, behavioral and emotional avoidance are at the heart of human dysfunction (Kashdan et al. 2006) and are the natural results of our hardwiring and social training. All people, including psychiatrists, engage in avoidance strategies, some more so than others. Overidentifying with socially transmitted rules puts us under a behavior-regulatory system that emphasizes the need to control, eliminate, or suppress distressing, unwanted private experiences. We are all exposed to this ubiquitous form of social conditioning, so it is easy to fall into a pattern of supporting a patient's change agenda of experiential avoidance rather than values-oriented living.

🎥 Video 24: Fostering Emotional Acceptance Rather Than Avoidance

Indeed, one could argue that even the names of our most commonly prescribed classes of psychotropic medications belie a deeply rooted allegiance to the control-and-eliminate social conditioning that leads us all to engage in avoidance behaviors. Medications are called "antidepressant," "antianxiety," or "antipsychotic" medications, as though their defining characteristic is their ability to eliminate depression, anxiety, or psychosis. In modern Western society, many would suggest that we are "anti" anything that does not feel good and apt to quickly generate a "disease" label for it—quickly followed by a treatment that is supposed to eliminate it. The biggest barrier the functional psychiatrist must overcome is the ever-present, socially supported temptation to use medications in a way that might inadvertently reinforce the patient's continued use of emotional and behavioral avoidance strategies.

Part of the short-term appeal of medications is that they can and do suppress unpleasant physical symptoms and distressing inner experiences. Although patients may gain short-term relief from such mental events, the use of emotional and behavioral avoidance can be strongly reinforced. This virtually ensures that the same distressing symptoms will reappear as resulting from the continued use of behavioral and emotional avoidance strategies. The chronic, recurrent nature of many mental disorders may be seen as the result of this "revolving door" pattern of short-term symptom relief at the expense of more sustainable acceptance and values-oriented strategies for living.

The prescribing psychiatrist plays a pivotal role in promoting either a style of living that is organized around the suppression, elimination, or control of painful inner experiences or, alternatively, a style of living that is values-based even if it means experiencing the inevitable pains and misfortunes life has to offer. We believe it is possible to use psychotropic medications in a way that fosters emotional acceptance rather than emotional avoidance in the service of the patient's freely chosen values. The functional, or pragmatic, approach to prescribing is not designed to seek out and destroy all potential sources of human struggle or discomfort. Instead, the psychiatrist targets symptoms in the patient that, if alleviated to a certain extent, would no longer function as major barriers to values-based approach behaviors.

As the following dialogue demonstrates, even the messaging surrounding the prescribing of a psychoactive medication can fundamentally transform the medication's function from reinforcing avoidance to instead promoting an open, accepting, values-based approach to living.

> Psychiatrist: It sounds like your experience with anxiety is that at least some aspects of it are likely going to be a part of your life from here on. Anxiety is a basic human emotion, and most people have anxiety experiences throughout their lives. If we changed focus and concluded that getting rid of all of your anxiety forever is impossible, where would you go next?

Amanda: Well, it's a bit unsettling to hear that from you, because I guess I just assumed that treatment would make anxiety a nonfactor in my life. If that isn't true, and I'm going to have anxiety the rest of my life, then I don't know what to think.

Psychiatrist: Well, what about that? If you have some anxiety the rest of your life? If there is no magic in the medication that makes it all disappear?

Amanda: Well, I guess the goal is how to live with it. It's like my dad used to say—you figure out how it is, and then you get used to it. So, if I have anxiety, I need to get used to it so it doesn't destroy my life.

Psychiatrist: Let's just say that was the goal for you. What parts of your anxiety have the biggest impact on keeping you from living the way you want to live? If we think of anxiety not as one big thing but as a patchwork quilt of uncomfortable thoughts, feelings, and sensations in your body, which pieces are the toughies?

Amanda: When I get really anxious, it's hard for me to think about anything but my anxiety. I can't concentrate on what I'm doing, like a task I need to complete at work. The more anxious I get, the harder it is to refocus. I also feel like I can't relax my muscles, and I can't breathe normally.

Psychiatrist: So how do these experiences get in the way of you living the way you want to live?

Amanda: Well, when it gets really bad, I pull away from people. I pull away from Tom because I feel humiliated that I can't control myself any better. I cancel out on social get-togethers with almost no notice, and then I feel bad about that. I'm sure I've hurt my friends' feelings many times, so I feel bad about that too.

Psychiatrist: Okay. It sounds like when your anxiety gets to a certain level, you get caught up in overfocusing on it—trying to make it go down, I'm guessing—but that just makes it go up even more. Then, you begin to pull away from the people who matter to you, Tom and your various friends that you end up stiffing. I'm guessing that probably makes you even more anxious as new life situations show up. You know—"am I going to get anxious again here, and what if I do"?

Amanda: That's exactly what happens!

Psychiatrist: Any medicine we decide to use should somehow cut into this cycle where you end up losing your focus at work or stiffing the people who matter to you in life. We likely can't eliminate your anxiety altogether, because it's a basic emotion, and you need anxiety to help you in certain situations. If you're walking down a dark alley at night in a part of town you aren't familiar with, I want you to be anxious! I want you to have your senses on full alert and your heart rate up so you can motor out of there if you sense danger. But in certain situations, like some of the ones we were just talking about, we want to dampen your nervous system a little bit so as to take the edge off your anxiety. Then you might be able to practice a different set of responses at a moment in time when you are slightly less anxious. So, if the medication is doing its job, you could refocus on your project at work, you could engage with Tom, you would follow through on your social agreements. If we discover after trying that none of the medications we select is helping you achieve those important life moments, then we won't use medicines. Does that make sense to you?

Amanda: What you're saying is that the medication isn't treating my anxiety problem, it's helping me do the things I want to do in my life, whether or not I have anxiety.

Psychiatrist: Exactly, and the measure of success of any medication we use is whether it helps you do those things.

In this dialogue, the psychiatrist has accomplished two very important objectives in promoting the use of medications in the service of the ACT therapeutic processes of openness and engagement. First is the notion that anxiety is a helpful, basic emotion that all people need in certain contexts. It is not anxiety, per se, that is the "problem," it is anxiety situated in a context, and at certain levels, in which it interferes with the patient's valued life ends. Second, the litmus test of any medication is whether it can alleviate specific symptoms that function as barriers to the patient living a valued life. The medication is not intended to treat all of the anxiety symptoms the patient might experience. Instead, it is targeting the functionally relevant symptoms.

In Chapter 3, we stated a little boldly that the last thing a functional psychiatrist would seek to do is to numb out, eliminate, or unduly regulate a patient's contact with symptoms of distress. These uncomfortable inner experiences are neither random events nor just topographic indicators of an underlying disease state. They are telling the patient something important about imbalances or deficiencies in his current life context. They are important pieces of emotional intelligence that should be responded to rather than treated as problems to be solved. Here we would like to emphasize the terms *numb out, eliminate,* or *unduly regulate.* When the prescriber promotes the value of medications for fostering openness to experience and values-based living, the benefits of medications (i.e., taking the edge off distressing symptoms functioning as barriers to valued living) may well outweigh any adverse side effects, especially in the short run. We must ensure patients are properly informed of the short-, medium-, and longer-term benefits and adverse effects of medications, including the risk of dependence, tolerance, and withdrawal. Most importantly, our patients must be informed about what we do and do not know about how psychiatric medications achieve their positive impacts.

EMULATE MEDICATION EFFECTS VIA PSYCHOLOGICAL MECHANISMS

Humans have the unique ability to induce or augment some of the main effects of medications via strictly psychological processes. This is an important feature of human–medication interactions that the functional psychiatrist will want to use to advantage.

📹 Video 25: Medication—Use Medication Effects to Promote Toward Moves

---

As one example, benzodiazepines work by increasing the efficiency of GABA to decrease the excitability of neurons, which has a calming effect on many activities of the brain. Teaching a patient to deliberately slow down and deepen her respiration rate for 3–5 minutes achieves the same calming effect on the brain. So, for most positive psychoactive medication effects, a corollary end state can be produced via strictly psychological and behavioral mechanisms. The functional psychiatrist is thus in an ideal position to use medication effects as a form of discrimination training designed to help the patient achieve the same basic functional effects using purely psychological or behavioral mechanisms. The following dialogue occurred with Amanda at a follow-up visit 3 weeks after her initial visit, at which a trial of diazepam 2 mg twice daily had been initiated as a short-term intervention.

> Psychiatrist: Since we last met about 3 weeks ago, I'd like to know how you're doing with the life goals we came up with. I think that included being able to refocus at work when anxiety is in the house, engaging with Tom even when you're anxious, and following through on social meetings with your friends. We agreed that you would try this medication on a time-limited basis to see if it helped at all.
>
> Amanda: I think it's helped a lot. I still have anxiety quite often, but it doesn't seem as overwhelming. It's helped for me to focus on just those three specific things we came up with.
>
> Psychiatrist: What do you notice specifically about what the medication does that seems helpful?
>
> Amanda: I don't feel as tight physically, which usually starts to happen for me when I get anxious. It used to feel like my breath went down only as far as my throat, my neck—now it's in my chest. I feel like I can breathe easily and deeply if I need to. That breathing seems to help me get refocused, which is a bit of a surprise. Because I can focus better, I can pay attention to what I want to do at work or at home.
>
> Psychiatrist: Would it be fair to say that when the medication freed you up to try some different responses, you discovered that breathing slowly and deeply helped in and of itself?
>
> Amanda: Yeah, it was sort of a way for me to pull myself together and then focus.
>
> Psychiatrist: A way to divert you away from overfocusing on your anxiety, right? If you're focusing on your breathing and relaxing your muscles, you can't focus on your anxiety. The way this drug works

is it makes it slightly harder for your muscles to get tense, and it blunts the really sharp experience of anxiety. It will slow your respiration rate down slightly. The drug kind of nudges you in the direction of being a little more physically relaxed, of having a slower rate of breathing and being less reactive to anxiety experiences. But it sounds like you took this quite a bit further on your own.

Amanda: I guess once the anxiety didn't totally control my actions, I could try some new things that probably have nothing to do with the pills. I approached Tom and told him I was feeling a bit anxious and wanted to take a walk with him. My friend Sheila and I had agreed to go to a stitch and bitch group after work last Wednesday, and I was about to cancel because I'd had a rough day at work. It wasn't so much about me being anxious, although I was. It was also just work stress. Then I realized I could go anyway and complain about work while I was sewing. You know, both times I ended up feeling a lot better than with just the medication. I know how the medication feels, and this was more than that.

Psychiatrist: Do you think the medication made you do these things? Or did you choose to do these things?

Amanda [laughs]: No, no. I did them.

Psychiatrist: This is important because, as we talked about last time, this particular class of medications can be habit forming, and I want you to take note of the fact that you were acting as your own "chemical" agent here. You don't have to have a pill to help you collect yourself; you can focus on deep breathing and relaxing yourself when you feel tense. You discovered that exercising when you feel anxious actually helps you even more than the antianxiety medication does. You discovered that investing your attention in outward pursuits takes it away from your anxiety, and when your attention is turned away from anxiety, your anxiety won't escalate. So, here we have three specific things that have nothing to do with medications at all but end up dramatically helping you. Practicing deep breathing and consciously relaxing your muscles; exercising, such as taking a fast walk; and creating specific goals that you will put your attention on when you're feeling anxious. Do you think these strategies are things you can practice doing on a regular basis?

Amanda: I guess at one point I thought, "This is a miracle drug," because I'm so used to spiraling out of control when I get anxious, and it didn't happen. And I know these other things really helped too. I just don't want to go back there.

Psychiatrist: And "back there" doesn't mean "I don't want to have anxiety anymore." That's what it used to mean. Now, it means, "I will respond differently to my anxiety if and when it appears. I don't have to overfocus on my anxiety symptoms. I can breathe deeply, relax myself into my anxiety, and refocus on what's important. I don't have to pull back from my husband. I can be with him, talk with him, and be myself with him. I don't have to stiff my friends. I can use my friends to help me stick with my anxieties."

Amanda: I think this is a much better way to go than to be taking pills the rest of my life.

In this brief exchange, the psychiatrist deliberately trains the patient to induce the same psychological effects she experiences with the anti-anxiety agent she is now taking on a short-term basis. Similar conversations can be had about the effects of mood stabilizers, antidepressants, or antipsychotic medications. In all cases, psychotropic medication effects are actually experienced at the psychological level, normally involving decreased symptom acuity and emotional reactivity. This easing of symptom intensity frees up attentional resources in the service of experimenting with new behaviors. Seldom, if ever, do these symptoms completely disappear. For some, the symptoms will be ongoing inhabitants of the patient's perceptual field over the course of a lifetime. Sometimes, symptoms should be "listened to" because they carry important information about the ever-shifting sands of the patient's inner and external contexts. The key goal of discrimination training in ACT is teaching the patient when to listen to symptoms and when to focus one's attention and energies elsewhere.

FOCUS ON TIME-LIMITED MEDICATION TREATMENT

A natural result of following the principles of functional psychopharmacology is that the psychiatrist will tend to use medication in a much more targeted, precise, and time-limited fashion. The goal of prescribing shifts from curing an underlying disease to creating a "learning laboratory" where patients can recruit the resources needed to psychologically mimic active medication effects. This should be good news for most prescribing psychiatrists, given the growing recognition that all classes of psychotropic agents, when taken regularly over longer periods of time, create physiological dependence. Similarly, some emerging anecdotal and research reports suggest that repetitive or long-term use of new-generation psychotropics is associated not only with increased health risks such as diabetes (Salvi et al. 2017) and osteoporosis (Bruyère and Reginster 2015) but also with permanent changes in emotional (El-Mallakh et al. 2011; Price et al. 2009), cognitive (Sayyah et al. 2016), and sexual (Higgins et al. 2010; Lee et al. 2010) functioning.

The seeds of time-limited medication regimens are found in the process of setting functional goals with the patient. The medication does or does not work to help the patient achieve those goals. If the medication does not work, the psychiatrist might try another or, after multiple experiments, conclude that medications are not going to play a role in the patient's treatment. If the medication does work, the process shifts to helping the patient augment or self-induce medication effects via relatively simple psychological or behavioral mechanisms so the drug can be gradually withdrawn. In the brief vignette that follows, the psychiatrist works with Amanda to create a drug discontinuation plan now that she is able to reduce her own anxiety using strictly psychological means.

> Psychiatrist: When we started this experiment with diazepam, our goal wasn't to bring down your anxiety for the sake of reducing or getting rid of it. The outcome we wanted was to allow you to do powerful, positive things in your life: at work as a teacher, at home as a life partner, in your friendship community. Humans have this remarkable ability to do for themselves what medications may do, and sometimes to do them better, longer, and more safely! In your case, you discovered all these wonderful new options you can use to breathe through your anxiety and work with it. That's very cool.
>
> Amanda: I know that most of this is the result of me dealing with my anxiety differently. Yet part of me is anxious about not having access to the medicine. What if I became really anxious and it wasn't available? I know this sounds silly, but it's what I feel.
>
> Psychiatrist: I think anyone in your shoes would have the same nagging fear, so it's not silly at all. Let's view this as another experiment. What would happen if you used your home-grown coping strategies when you get anxious without relying on medication? Perhaps you could leave it at home but still have it available if you're having trouble calming yourself using these natural techniques you've discovered. We'll use the results of the experiment to determine what to do next, whatever those results might be.
>
> Amanda: Are you saying I could start back on the medicine if it turned out I wasn't quite ready to do this on my own?
>
> Psychiatrist: My goal is to help you live the life you want to live. We worked together to identify specific areas of your life anxiety was interfering with and initially used a drug to help you get started pursuing those goals. You've succeeded in many different ways that go way beyond the role medications typically play. We aren't going to go back to where we started. We're going to go forward. If that, or any drug, is needed in the short run, I won't hesitate to use it. The goal will always be the same. You said it yourself: You don't relish the prospect of taking pills for the rest of your life. This is just an experiment to see if you're ready to fly. I think you are.
>
> Amanda: I think I am too.

In this brief exchange, the psychiatrist reframed medication discontinuation as an experiment. A key feature of functional prescribing is that all medication trials are a carefully considered behavior pharmacology "experiment" because every patient inevitably comes with a different physiological, neurochemical, and genetic makeup. Every patient comes equipped with a different learning history and psychological resources and functions in a unique context with chosen life goals that form the basis of our work together. The truth of the matter is that every time we give a patient a medication, it is an educated experiment guided by established behavioral pharmacology principles that require us to carefully monitor the direct and demonstrable effects of the medication on the patient's ability to achieve those life goals. Another feature of this exchange is that the psychiatrist is following the pragmatic truth principle. What is important is what works to help Amanda live—despite her anxiety—the life she wants to live. The psychiatrist is not following a rigid rule about which drugs to prescribe or for how long. The psychiatrist's demonstration of psychological flexibility helps Amanda agree to the experiment and actively recruits her as the *key* participant, carefully noting and reporting on the direct effects of the medication as she experiences them.

TIPS FOR SUCCESS

Functional psychopharmacology involves assessing the effects of medications within the antecedent-behavior-consequence (A-B-C) framework of functional analysis.

Humans interact with medication effects and can mediate them using strictly psychological or behavioral processes.

The focus of functional psychopharmacology is always on improving the functional status and adaptive behaviors of each specific patient, situated within his or her unique life context, rather than on controlling or eliminating distressing symptoms.

Functional psychiatrists use pragmatic, functional, and flexible explanatory models to explain the mechanisms of medication therapy and empower patients.

Functional psychopharmacology also involves describing the use of psychiatric medications to patients in a way that fundamentally reframes and transforms their function from potentially reinforcing further avoidance to strongly promoting the ACT processes of openness to experience and sensitivity to workability in context and life engagement.

A closely related goal of functional prescribing is to heighten patients' awareness of specific psychopharmacological agent effects that are experienced as beneficial, such that ACT discrimination training can be used to help patients induce those effects using psychological or behavioral strategies.

Functional psychopharmacology naturally leads to highly specific, precise, carefully monitored, and in most cases, time-limited medication regimens.

Summary

As psychiatrists, we want to care for our fellow humans, to help our patients overcome or at least cope better with their suffering. As part of our training, we have been encouraged to see patients within the broad context of their biology, psychology, and social settings—to consider their genetic makeup, biological processes, lived histories, and present social contexts. Optimally, we want them to flourish, to be engaged and fully functional in their social contexts. To borrow from Freud and Erikson: to love, work, and play and be healthy! What is the best way to succeed in this mission? We can say with certainty that the latent illness and functional models of psychiatry diverge considerably on this crucial question. The latent-disease-oriented psychiatric approach has typically viewed symptoms not only as signs of underlying mental disorders but also as barriers to effective living in their own right. The natural result of this perspective has been a strong focus on developing medication treatments that can potentially reduce, suppress, or eliminate symptoms, thereby assuring that the underlying disorder has been cured or brought into remission. Although this is in keeping with the generally useful mechanistic orientation of the practice of medicine, using medications in this way may prove more harmful than beneficial in the long run. Medications used for controlling or eliminating symptoms can also inadvertently reinforce patients' use of strategies designed to avoid distressing, unwanted inner experiences. We know that all forms of experiential avoidance, notably emotional and behavior avoidance, have been shown to be the causal mechanism underlying a wide variety of psychopathological conditions. Medications may work in the short run to reduce distressing, unwanted mental experiences, but they also may contribute to the recurrence of symptoms in the long run by reinforcing avoidance-based coping strategies.

Functional psychopharmacology instead focuses on teaching our patients to gently *shift their relationship* to distressing symptoms so these experiences no longer function as barriers to effective living and vitality. Symptoms are viewed as inevitable, natural, health sequelae of living. Furthermore, distressing inner experiences function as feedback loops that can, and should, inform and motivate adaptive change. When symptoms are numbed out to the point that they no longer serve this important purpose, patients fail to make needed adaptations and continue to suffer. Medications are useful to the extent that they can ease the distress associated with specific symptoms so patients have more freedom to make the adaptations needed to live vital, purposeful lives. This approach can fundamentally reframe and transform the function of medications and provide an alternative when the emphasis on symptom suppression is neither effective, sufficient, nor tolerated. If you are intrigued by the possibilities inherent in a functional approach, read on!

The Essentials

- The principles of modern-day functional psychopharmacology are rooted in a much older wing of psychopharmacology known as behavioral pharmacology.
- *Behavioral pharmacology* is the study of the effects of psychopharmacological agents on human behavior, with an emphasis on identifying demonstrable and directly observable causal relationships.
- Research in behavioral pharmacology shows humans do not simply "take" medications or substances, they interact with them on a psychological and social level. These psychological and social processes directly influence the main effects of medications.
- All individuals have a unique response to medications, and the most useful level of analysis is *this* patient, not patients *like this*.
- Functional psychopharmacology holds that focusing too heavily on the use of medications to eliminate or control psychiatric symptoms is highly problematic because it can potentially reinforce emotional and behavioral avoidance behaviors.
- Functional psychopharmacology instead attempts to gently shift the relationship patients have with their distressing inner experiences, cultivating a stance of acceptance and a willingness to have symptoms in the service of living according to freely chosen values.
- Medications are not used primarily for symptom elimination purposes but instead are precisely targeted to remove specific barriers that stand in the way of each patient in his or her quest to live a valued life.
- The three main questions that must be answered to determine whether a psychopharmacological agent is working or not are:

  1. What were the desired effects of the medication?
  2. Were those effects obtained?
  3. Did any significant adverse reactions occur?

Suggested Readings

Andersohn F, Schade R, Suissa S, et al: Long-term use of antidepressants for depressive disorders and the risk of diabetes mellitus. Am J Psychiatry 166:591–598, 2009

Barnard K, Peveler RC, Holt RIG: Antidepressant medication as a risk factor for type 2 diabetes and impaired glucose regulation: systematic review. Diabetes Care 36(10):3337–3345, 2013

Burcu M, Zito JM, Safer DJ, et al: Association of antidepressant medications with incident type 2 diabetes among Medicaid-insured youths. JAMA Pediatr 171(12):1200–1207, 2017

Chouinard C: New classification of selective serotonin reuptake inhibitor withdrawal. Psychother Psychosom 84:63–71, 2015

Clayton AH, Pradko JF, Croft HA, et al: Prevalence of sexual dysfunction among newer antidepressants. J Clin Psychiatry 63(4):357–366, 2002

Davies J, Read J: A systematic review into the incidence, severity and duration of antidepressant withdrawal effects: are guidelines evidence-based? Addict Behav 2018 Epub ahead of print

Fava GA, Gatti A, Belaise C, et al: Withdrawal symptoms after SSRI discontinuation: a systematic review. Psychother Psychosom 84:72–81, 2015

Fava GA, Benasi G, Lucente M, et al: Withdrawal symptoms after serotonin-noradrenaline reuptake inhibitor discontinuation: systematic review. Psychother Psychosom 87(4):195–203, 2018

Haddad P, Anderson IM: Recognising and managing antidepressant discontinuation symptoms. Adv Psychiatr Treat 13:447–457, 2007

Healy D, Le Noury J, Mangin D: Enduring sexual dysfunction after treatment with antidepressants, 5a-reductase inhibitors and isotretinoin: 300 cases. Int J Risk Saf Med 29(3–4):125–134, 2018

Hosenbocus S, Chahal R: SSRIs and SNRIs: a review of the discontinuation syndrome in children and adolescents. J Can Acad Child Adolesc Psychiatry 20(1):60–67, 2011

Kotzalidis GD, Patrizi B, Caltagirone SS, et al: The adult SSRI-SNRI withdrawal syndrome. Clinical Neuropsychiatry 4(2):61–75, 2007

McCracken LM, Vowles KE: Acceptance and commitment therapy and mindfulness for chronic pain: model, process and progress. Am Psychol 69:178–187, 2014

Montejo AL, Llorca G, Izquierdo JA, et al: Incidence of sexual dysfunction associated with antidepressant agents: a prospective multicenter study of 1022 outpatients. Spanish Working Group for the Study of Psychotropic-Related Sexual Dysfunction. J Clin Psychiatry 62(suppl 3):10–21, 2001

Nielsen M, Hansen EH, Gøtzsche PC: What is the difference between dependence and withdrawal reactions? A comparison of benzodiazepines and selective serotonin re-uptake inhibitors. Addiction 107(5):900–908, 2012

Poling A, Lesage M, Methot L: Fundamentals of Behavior Analytic Research. New York, Plenum, 1995

Read J, Gee A, Diggle J, et al: Staying on, and coming off, antidepressants: the experiences of 752 UK adults. Addict Behav 88:82–85, 2019

Rizzoli R, Cooper C, Reginster JY, et al: Antidepressant medications and osteoporosis. Bone 51(3):606–613, 2012

Sansone RA, Sansone LA: SSRIs: bad to the bone? Innov Clin Neurosci 9(7–8):42–47, 2012

Shelton R: The nature of the discontinuation syndrome associated with antidepressant drugs. J Clin Psychiatry 67(suppl 4):3–7, 2006

Viguera AC, Baldessarini RJ, Friedberg J. Discontinuing antidepressant treatment in major depression. Harv Rev Psychiatry 5:293–305, 1998

Villatte JL, Vilardaga R, Villatte M, et al: Acceptance and commitment therapy modules: differential impact on treatment processes and outcomes. Behav Res Ther 77:52–61, 2016

Warner C, Bobo W, Warner C, et al: Antidepressant discontinuation syndrome. Am Fam Physician 74(3)449–456, 2006

Wilson E, Lader M: A review of the management of antidepressant discontinuation symptoms. Ther Adv Psychopharmacol 5(6):357–368, 2015

Wu X, Al-Abedalla K, Rastikerdar E, et al: Selective serotonin reuptake inhibitors and the risk of osseointegrated implant failure: a cohort study. J Dent Res 93(11):1054–1061, 2014

Zwart S, Rovers MM, de Melker RA, et al: Penicillin for acute sore throat: randomised double blind trial of seven days versus three days treatment or placebo in adults. BMJ 320(7228):150–154, 2000

References

American Psychiatric Association: Diagnostic and Statistical Manual of Mental Disorders, 5th Edition. Arlington, VA, American Psychiatric Association, 2013

Bruyère O, Reginster JY: Osteoporosis in patients taking selective serotonin reuptake inhibitors: a focus on fracture outcome. Endocrine 48(1):65–68, 2015 25091520

Chait LD, Perry JL: Factors influencing self-administration of, and subjective response to, placebo marijuana. Behav Pharmacol 3(6):545–552, 1992 11224156

Dews PB (ed): Techniques for the study of behavioral effects of drugs. Ann NY Acad Sci 65(4):247–356, 1956

Donohue J: A history of drug advertising: the evolving roles of consumers and consumer protection. Milbank Q 84(4):659–699, 2006 17096638

El-Mallakh RS, Gao Y, Jeannie Roberts R: Tardive dysphoria: the role of long-term antidepressant use in inducing chronic depression. Med Hypotheses 76(6):769–773, 2011 21459521

Fava G, Offidani E: The mechanisms of tolerance in antidepressant action. Prog Neuropsychopharmacol Biol Psychiatry 35(7):1593–1602, 2011 20728491

Fornaro M, Anastasia A, Novello S, et al: The emergence of loss of efficacy during antidepressant drug treatment for major depressive disorder: an integrative review of evidence, mechanisms, and clinical implications. Pharmacol Res 139:494–502, 2019 30385364

Goldney RD, Eckert KA, Hawthorne G, et al: Changes in the prevalence of major depression in an Australian community sample between 1998 and 2008. Aust NZ J Psychiatry 44(10):901–910, 2010 20932204

Higgins A, Nash M, Lynch AM: Antidepressant-associated sexual dysfunction: impact, effects, and treatment. Drug Health Patient Saf 2:141–150, 2010 21701626

Holmstedt B, Liljestrand G: Readings in Pharmacology. New York, Pergamon, 1963

Kashdan TB, Barrios V, Forsyth JP, et al: Experiential avoidance as a generalized psychological vulnerability: comparisons with coping and emotion regulation strategies. Behav Res Ther 44(9):1301–1320, 2006 16321362

Kemp JJ, Lickel JJ, Deacon BJ: Effects of a chemical imbalance causal explanation on individuals' perceptions of their depressive symptoms. Behav Res Ther 56:47–52, 2014 24657311

Khan A, Fahl Mar K, Faucett J, et al: Has the rising placebo response impacted antidepressant clinical trial outcome? Data from the US Food and Drug Administration 1987–2013. World Psychiatry 16(2):181–192, 2017 28498591

Krishnan V, Nestler EJ: Linking molecules to mood: new insight into the biology of depression. Am J Psychiatry 167(11):1305–1320, 2010 20843874

Lader M: History of benzodiazepine dependence. J Subst Abuse Treat 8(1–2):53–59, 1991 1675692

Lebowitz MS, Ahn WK: Effects of biological explanations for mental disorders on clinicians' empathy. Proc Natl Acad Sci USA 111(50):17786–17790, 2014 25453068

Lee KU, Lee YM, Nam JM, et al: Antidepressant-induced sexual dysfunction among newer antidepressants in a naturalistic setting. Psychiatry Investig 7(1):55–59, 2010 20396434

Lin CH, Yang WC: The relationship between symptom relief and psychosocial functional improvement during acute electroconvulsive therapy for patients with major depressive disorder. Int J Neuropsychopharmacol 20(7):538–545, 2017 28430980

Macht DI, Mora CF: Effects of opium alkaloids on the behavior of rats on the circular maze. J Pharmacol Exp Ther 16:219–235, 1921

McKnight PE, Kashdan TB: The importance of functional impairment to mental health outcomes: a case for reassessing our goals in depression treatment research. Clin Psychol Rev 29(3):243–259, 2009 19269076

Pescosolido BA, Martin JK, Long JS, et al: "A disease like any other"? A decade of change in public reactions to schizophrenia, depression, and alcohol dependence. Am J Psychiatry 167(11):1321–1330, 2010 20843872

Poling A, Byrne T (eds): Introduction to Behavioral Pharmacology. Oakland, CA, Context, 2000

Poling A, Lesage M: Rule-governed behavior and human behavioral pharmacology: a brief commentary on an important topic. Anal Verbal Behav 10:37–44, 1992 22477045

Price J, Cole V, Goodwin GM: Emotional side-effects of selective serotonin reuptake inhibitors: qualitative study. Br J Psychiatry 195(3):211–217, 2009 19721109

Salvi V, Grua I, Cerveri G, et al: The risk of new-onset diabetes in antidepressant users: a systematic review and meta-analysis. PLoS One 12(7):e0182088, 2017 28759599

Sayyah M, Eslami K, AlaiShehni S, et al: Cognitive function before and during treatment with selective serotonin reuptake inhibitors in patients with depression or obsessive-compulsive disorder. Psychiatry J 2016:5480391, 2016 27597949

Schuster L: Readings in Pharmacology. New York, Little, Brown, 1962

Sidman M: Behavioral pharmacology. Psychopharmacology (Berl) 1:1–19, 1959 14446423

Testa M, Fillmore MT, Norris J, et al: Understanding alcohol expectancy effects: revisiting the placebo condition. Alcohol Clin Exp Res 30(2):339–348, 2006 16441283

Thompson T, Schuster CR: Behavioral Pharmacology. Englewood Cliffs, NJ, Prentice-Hall, 1968

Vatne S, Bjorkly S: Empirical evidence for using subjective quality of life as an outcome variable in clinical studies: a meta-analysis of correlates and predictors in persons with a major mental disorder living in the community. Clin Psychol Rev 28(5):869–889, 2008 18280626

Vuchinich RE, Sobell MB: Empirical separation of physiologic and expected effects of alcohol on complex perceptual motor performance. Psychopharmacology (Berl) 60(1):81–85, 1978 104349

Witt-Doerring J, Shorter D, Kosten T: Online communities for drug withdrawal: what can we learn? Psychiatr Times 35(4), 2018. Available at: http://www.psychiatrictimes.com/addiction/online-communities-drug-withdrawal-what-can-we-learn. Accessed May 12, 2018.

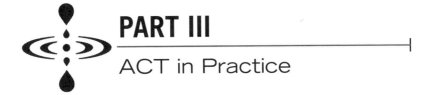

PART III

ACT in Practice

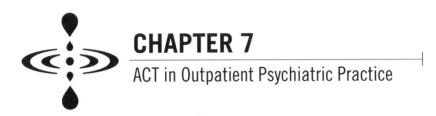

CHAPTER 7

ACT in Outpatient Psychiatric Practice

Right now a moment of time is fleeting by!…
We must become that moment.

—Paul Cezanne

In this chapter, we provide an overview of how to conduct ACT in an outpatient psychiatric setting. The approach described will be of value in a private practice, in a community mental health center, or in a hospital-based outpatient psychiatric clinic. In each of these practice contexts, the structure of treatment might vary from a longer-term, "traditional" approach to brief and time-limited therapy. In some contexts, the sessions might last 1–2 hours, depending on whether the treatment is delivered in an individual or group format. In other contexts, the visit might be part of a 15-minute monthly or bimonthly medication check. Regardless of the practice context, certain basic features of the ACT model will always come into play. The only change is in how compact or extended the delivery of the core therapeutic processes will be.

ACT has been shown to work across a range of outpatient settings, delivery formats, and clinical problems (A-Tjak et al. 2015). The core mechanisms of ACT can be delivered effectively in single-session interventions, brief group formats, half- or full-day workshops, or regular therapy sessions spread across weeks or months. Thus, regardless of the practice setting or timing you may be working in, you can find a way to deliver ACT.

In this chapter, we highlight some key principles that will help guide you in adapting ACT to fit the realities of outpatient practice: maintaining a transdiagnostic focus, relating to psychiatric symptoms in a flexible way, and focusing on improving the patient's functional capacity.

We then demonstrate in clinical dialogues how to activate the three basic therapeutic mechanisms of ACT (i.e., context sensitivity/workability, openness, and engagement) with a representative range of clinical problems frequently seen by the outpatient psychiatrist.

Adapting ACT to Different Practice Contexts: Key Principles

In this section, we examine three core features of the ACT approach that, if followed by the psychiatrist, will greatly increase the likelihood of clinical success across a range of outpatient practice contexts. In essence, these three features reflect the "stance" the psychiatrist will take on the issue of human suffering and psychiatric symptoms and what to do about it (Törneke et al. 2016).

MAINTAIN A TRANSDIAGNOSTIC FOCUS

Providing psychiatric services in an outpatient setting can be challenging in light of the remarkable heterogeneity of the patient population served and often severe constraints on the amount of time available to see patients. Not only do we encounter an extremely wide range of presenting psychiatric problems but also the level of acuity and timing of treatment can vary greatly, from time-limited episodes of treatment to chronic management over months or years. Without the aid of some type of clinical framework that can simplify our approach to this seemingly endless amount of diversity, it would be easy to feel overwhelmed and overmatched.

In ACT, one of our most important advantages is that all psychiatric problems, regardless of their seeming differences, originate in the same underlying processes of context insensitivity/workability and emotional and behavioral avoidance. Diagnostic determinations simply describe the specific topography of a patient's symptom profile and, in that sense, can be integrated as a useful piece of information within the bigger transdiagnostic framework. Genetics, biology, temperament, family environment, prior learning experiences, and cultural practices all influence how individuals experience and express their psychiatric distress. However, our social training and the regulatory processes of the mind's operating system will push people to respond to their symptoms and other sources of life stress in remarkably consistent ways.

ACT is thus not designed as a treatment for a specific "disorder" but as a training of specific behavioral skills or repertoires, all aimed at increasing psychological resilience, that in turn significantly reduce the negative impact of social training and maladaptive "rules" of the mind. Improving psychological flexibility is an important goal for patients with any form of diagnosis because it has been shown to influence the way patients cope with their psychiatric symptoms as well as the environmental stressors that exacerbate those symptoms.

FOCUS ON REAL-WORLD FUNCTIONING

The ACT psychiatrist's stance is that each patient's life context and the self-instructional and avoidance functions situated within that context are unique, and treatment must be customized to promote the patient's successful adaptation. The most important focus of intervention, regardless of the diagnosis attached to the patient's symptom complaints, is to improve the match between the patient's functional capacities and the demands of his life context. At the same time, diagnostic categories often describe the specific components of emotional distress the patient might be avoiding, so including the diagnostic lens from this point of view can be helpful and is in keeping with psychiatric training, because diagnoses are used for so many other reasons and can provide a way to organize psychiatric work. Nevertheless, from an ACT perspective, the focus is on how to help each patient to deal more effectively with the life problems that are generating distressing emotional experiences and, equally important, to deal more effectively with distressing emotional experiences.

The Central Role of Avoidance in Producing Human Dysfunction

As a transdiagnostic, process-based approach to mental and substance use health problems, ACT holds that emotional and behavioral avoidance form a common pathway through which all forms of behavioral dysfunction flow. To demonstrate the parsimony of this approach, we examine how ACT conceptualizes some common mental health conditions seen in daily psychiatric practice.

DEPRESSIVE DISORDERS

Following self-instructions to engage in various forms of emotional and behavioral avoidance is a main determinant of most depressive disorders (Zettle 2007). We suggest that this is the case even though the form of a depressed person's avoided private experiences might be quite different. A person with depression typically struggles with various unpleasant inner experiences such as sadness, interpersonal rejection or loss, unresolved grief, and guilt or lethargy.

In this view, depression itself is not a feeling state or a biological condition; rather, it is thought to be an emotional avoidance strategy designed to eliminate contact (through emotional numbing and anhedonia) with much more intimidating cognitive or emotional experiences the patient wishes to avoid. These aversive underlying experiences trigger verbal self-instructions (explicit or implicit) encouraging passivity, isolation, and withdrawal designed to prevent their continued appearance. Passivity, withdrawal, and self-isolation can be thought of as forms of behavioral avoidance that not only do not prevent the reappearance of underlying symptoms but also function to prevent purposeful action toward valued life domains. Although these strategies may provide a sense of relief in the short run, the aversive emotional feedback loops associated with putting core one's personal values and goals in life on hold will not only continue unabated, they will worsen over time, resulting in a ratcheting up of core symptoms of emotional distress.

PSYCHOSIS

The ACT approach can be applied with more serious mental disorders. In addition to psychopharmacological treatment, ACT has been shown to be effective as a psychotherapeutic approach in the acute (Gaudiano and Herbert 2006; White et al. 2011) and longer-term treatment of psychosis (Bach et al. 2012). In clinical practice, it is useful to analyze how avoidance plays out for individual patients with chronic hallucinations. The perceptual experience of hearing critical or commanding voices or seeing things that other people do not see can be very distressing. It is quite natural for such an individual to begin trying to control or eliminate hallucinations via the same types of avoidance strategies we see in other diagnostic categories.

The patient generates and follows self-instructions to avoid certain situations, be passive, analyze and reanalyze the problem, or postpone important life steps. The goal is controlling the appearance of aversive perceptual experiences such as hallucinations, even if doing so blocks the use of other effective behavioral strategies that would lead to an improved sense of social meaning and integration. The avoidance pattern sets the stage for increased feelings of social distance and alienation, self-stigma, and increased likelihood of aversive perceptual experiences.

PERSONALITY DISORDERS

Let's examine how the ACT framework can be applied to the patient diagnosed with a personality disorder. The ACT approach holds that such a patient engages in behaviors that are

- Pervasive across qualitatively different settings
- Persistent and longstanding
- Resistant to change despite repeated negative consequences
- Not working to promote the patient's best interests in life (Strosahl 2004)

Consider a person with dependent personality disorder in light of these behavioral qualities. Someone who fulfills the criteria for this diagnosis will have difficulty making everyday decisions without reassurance from others; have difficulty expressing disagreement with others, perhaps avoiding initiating projects on his own; and possibly do things that are unpleasant just to obtain the approval of others.

In ACT, these symptoms can be clearly seen as problematic efforts to avoid fears of rejection and abandonment. These aversive experiences can be related verbally both to memories of past experiences of rejection and abandonment and to predictions of a similar catastrophe in the future. This persistent pattern leads to an intense, ongoing sense of vulnerability, fear, and anxiety. The patient's unworkable efforts to control these aversive private experiences share all the features of the vicious circles of avoidance we have already examined.

These behaviors are designed to help the person avoid distressing, unwanted private experiences; her avoidance behaviors produce a sense of relief in the short run because significant others might offer forced reassurances or grudgingly give her yet more emotional support. In the longer run, however, this process erodes the integrity of healthy relationships such that more functional individuals will withdraw emotionally or eventually leave altogether. Those who stay are more likely to exploit her fears to gain emotional control over her. Regardless, each type of outcome "feeds" the patient's need for emotional support and guarantees of safety, but naturally these reassurances do not last. Quite the contrary: in the long run, the sense of uncertainty tends to increase as cues to the possibility the strategy will fail are easily contacted. Inevitably, by following the strategy of avoidance, the patient will fail to consider other potentially available behavioral strategies that could have led to personally valued life ends.

TIPS FOR SUCCESS

The ACT approach is well adapted to, and has been demonstrated to work in, a variety of outpatient psychiatric contexts.

ACT can be applied with equal efficacy in brief and longer-term treatment models and in individual and group therapy formats as well as in half-day and full-day workshops.

The ACT framework provides a parsimonious alternative to having to deliver an ever-growing number of condition-specific evidence-based treatments.

The ACT psychiatrist instead

- Maintains a transdiagnostic approach to treatment using a limited set of therapeutic processes (context sensitivity/workability, openness to inner experiences, and life engagement) to treat all forms of clinically relevant mental and physical health problems
- Focuses on improving patients' functioning in real-world contexts that matter to them
- Recognizes and responds to the central role avoidance plays in producing psychological rigidity and mental suffering

ACT Clinical Interventions: Promoting Context Sensitivity and Workability

Of the three therapeutic mechanisms in ACT, context sensitivity/workability is in many ways the most basic and ubiquitous in the therapeutic conversation. We often say that establishing a clear self-reflective awareness of the unworkable consequences of avoidance strategies is the first big "acceptance move" in ACT. As noted in earlier chapters, context sensitivity requires the patient to get present, adapt a stance of self-reflective awareness, and practice a particular form of perspective-taking that allows the consequences of his actions in the world to be accurately and objectively appraised as to whether they are working to promote his best interests. This form of perspective-taking requires the patient to stand outside of the rules of the mind and appraise things not from the perspective of social training that encourages the control and elimination of distressing, unwanted private experiences but rather from the perspective of what is working and what is not working. *Working* and *not working* are defined exclusively within the framework of the patient's valued life ends, not how he is feeling as those life ends are being pursued. In ordinary language, the psychiatrist is asking: "Given the situation as it is, what do you do and how does that work in terms of your valued outcomes in life?"

In ACT, we assume the patient's avoidance maneuvers, designed to get rid of negative emotions, scary thoughts, bodily sensations, or painful memories, are a central aspect of the present situation. Thus, the therapeutic mechanism of context sensitivity and workability creates an important tension between the temptation to avoid pain and the desire to seek a valued life. Metaphorically speaking, the patient is at a fork in the road of life and must decide to travel in one direction or another. She cannot simultaneously go in both directions. The therapeutic mechanisms of openness and engagement, which we demonstrate later in this chapter, only become relevant when the patient chooses to move toward valued life ends instead of in the direction of avoidance. In this sense, the presence of context sensitivity lessens the likelihood that she will follow unworkable self-instructional rules, thus creating the potential for therapeutic movement to occur.

CASE EXAMPLE: FRANK

Frank, age 52, is a truck driver who lives by himself. For about a year, he has experienced depression. He has been on disability leave from work for almost 5 months and isolates himself in his home. He has tried different antidepressant drugs in adequate dosages and has had modest symptom reduction as a result. He presently uses mirtazapine, 60 mg each night, without serious side effects. He still feels depressed, however, and although mirtazapine has helped with his sleeping problem and improved his mood somewhat, his depression symptoms have not fully remitted. Frank is clear that he really wants to get back to work. He used to be greatly appreciated by both his colleagues and his employer and takes pride in his abilities as a truck driver. He also used to enjoy the friendly social contact with his customers. However, he currently is avoiding all contact with work peers and talks to his employer only by phone and only when he is more or less forced to do so. When asked about his inability to reengage in his work and social behaviors, he repeatedly makes the same statement: "I am too depressed to do anything about all of this."

Psychiatrist: If I get you right, not much has happened since I saw you last time.

Frank: Yeah, I still feel the same, more or less. I sleep better, but I don't do much except make it through the day. I get up in the morning and fix some food. I take a walk with the dog, but that's about it. Then I take my pills at night and hope for at least some good sleep.

Psychiatrist: Have you had any contact with your employer or your co-workers?

Frank: No. I really want to, you know, but I just can't get myself to do it.

Psychiatrist: Okay. It sounds like you've simply parked your truck. It's almost out of gas, and there isn't much run time left in the engine.

Here the psychiatrist is exploring the existing strategy Frank is using, trying to name it metaphorically by talking about "parking." The intention is to involve Frank in a dialogue about the workability of what he is actually doing. This process is a simple way for the psychiatrist to start a functional analysis of Frank's strategies for coping with his depression symptoms: "What are you doing [B, behavior], what are the consequences [C] of doing that, and in what situation [A, antecedent] do you tend to try that strategy?" The psychiatrist is also giving a functionally oriented name to the strategy ("parking your truck"), designed to seek a common terminology that resonates with Frank given his background as a truck driver.

Frank: Yeah, I guess. I need to idle the engine for now, you know. I just
don't have the strength to go on, even though I want to do it.
Psychiatrist: I get it. Parking your truck is sort of the only way to deal
with this situation. I'm sure you hope to go on driving later, but
for now you just need to park.
Frank: Exactly!
Psychiatrist: When do you notice yourself parking? Do you do that
only in relation to your work, or would you say you also park in
other situations?
Frank: With other things, you mean? I'm not sure…
Psychiatrist: I mean, what about contact with your friends, or your
brother and his family? Do you keep driving with them or is some
parking going on there, too?
Frank: I see what you mean. It's pretty much what I do across the board.
Yes, I do seem to be parking a lot, don't I?

Notice a few things in the way the psychiatrist approaches this dialogue. The psychiatrist first develops a new metaphor for Frank's strategy. This new narrative helps Frank contact the connection between what he does and the problematic consequences he experiences. When Frank answers, he seems to understand the metaphor but does not seem to draw a connection between "parking" a lot and the negative consequences he is enduring (e.g., not going back to work; losing his connection with coworkers, friends, and family). These consequences are not protecting Frank from depression, as his avoidance rule promises. They are likely making his depression worsen over time.

Despite this paradoxical result, Frank seems firmly committed to the strategy of parking. Indeed, he specifically defends his strategy ("I need this"). The psychiatrist does not question that at this point. Why? Because Frank needs to make *direct experiential contact* with the relationship between his avoidance strategies and the problematic consequences of using them. By the time Frank comes to see the psychiatrist, many people in his life have already told him he "needs to be active and get out more." If that advice were working, Frank would not be coming in for psychiatric care in the first place. This is a basic ACT position: when patients are engaged in rule-following and do not see the connection between their behaviors and the consequences of those behaviors, the psychiatrist's role is to help them take a closer look at their direct experience and experientially contact those consequences. In the following interaction, the psychiatrist continues to support Frank in recognizing what he does and noticing the results he is getting. If he can notice his strategy of "parking" in other situations as well, it may become easier for him to look closer at his experience of the consequences of those moves.

Psychiatrist: You park a lot, and in some sense, that is the strategy you
need to follow to deal with this depression. How is parking impacting your relationship with your brother and his family?

Frank: Not so well. I haven't seen them for more than a month now. He actually called the other night and asked me over.

Psychiatrist: And?

Frank: No, I didn't go. I was really low and felt I just couldn't make it. I made an excuse that I was feeling like I was getting the flu and said maybe some other time I would come over.

Psychiatrist: So, you parked.

Frank: I do that all the time, I guess.

Psychiatrist: There's something in it for you when you park, I guess, otherwise you wouldn't keep doing it. What do you think parking does for you?

Frank: I just feel too tired. I don't know how to fix it. Just imagine me sitting there, with his kids and all. What would I say? What would they think of me?

Psychiatrist: It sounds like your mind is giving you these bad images of what will happen if you go to your brother's house, and it offers you some advice: "You might just as well park, too many hard corners to take ahead." Then you park.

Frank: Yes, that's how it goes.

Psychiatrist: Although I guess that gives you some rest for the moment, overall, how do you feel parking is working? I mean, for example, when you didn't take your brother up on his invitation, did you end up feeling less depressed?

Frank: No, I felt bad because I basically made up a story. I'm sure he didn't believe it either, but he just said he was sorry I wasn't feeling well and maybe next time. This is why I feel stuck. I can see that this is not really working. Not in the long run.

Notice again that the psychiatrist is not challenging Frank's experience or pushing him to admit that his strategies do not work. Quite the contrary, the psychiatrist is asking Frank to look closer at what he experiences, first by helping him label his strategy and then by looking closer at the connection between what he does and the consequences he is getting. The goal is to increase his ability to step back from rule-following and directly test the workability of his avoidance strategies. This enhanced perspective-taking operation will increase the probability that Frank will start looking for, or at least be receptive to, new strategies.

This dialogue also illustrates how much the three therapeutic mechanisms of ACT play upon each other in a typical clinical interaction. The initial focus of this interaction is on developing context sensitivity and appraising workability, but the other two mechanisms are naturally triggered. The fact that the strategy of "parking" is not working is connected to what is valuable to Frank (i.e., working toward what?). The strategy of avoiding social contact is not workable, given that he values his relationship with his brother and his family. The therapeutic mechanism of engagement could easily be activated by the psychiatrist in this part of the conversation.

Frank also mentions some unpleasant and unwanted private events that seem to trigger avoidance strategies. For example, he complains of feeling tired all the time, with the associated avoidance response being to ramp down his activity level. He was fused with images of what would happen if he indeed did go and visit his brother. These unpleasant private experiences could be targeted using the therapeutic mechanism of openness. Later in this chapter, we demonstrate how focusing the conversation on openness and engagement might look in the ongoing interaction between Frank and the psychiatrist.

CASE EXAMPLE: BEN

Ben, age 45, is divorced and has a 10-year-old daughter who lives with her mother. He sees her on a regular basis. He works as a teacher at a local elementary school. Ben experiences intermittent, intense periods of psychosis. The first episode occurred 25 years ago when he was in college. At that time, he became convinced one of his teachers was giving provocative information about him to the local police, saying he was selling drugs on campus. Knowing he was totally innocent (he never used or sold drugs), he confronted the teacher, who denied knowing anything about Ben or his possible dealings with drugs. His teacher suggested Ben "go see someone who could help him." Ben became more and more upset and finally was hospitalized for a few days. After resting and sleeping well for a few nights, he quickly recovered and was given the diagnosis of "brief psychotic episode."

His hospital attending psychiatrist had prescribed an antipsychotic medication. For some years he took his medication sporadically, usually during times when he felt stressed out and was having trouble sleeping. When he felt fine, he normally stopped taking the medication. He did not like taking the medication because he did not consider himself mentally ill. When he finally decided to stop taking it for good, he had a few periods of time in which he thought people were watching him and relaying information about him to the police. In between these episodes, he did well at his job, although he did not really connect socially with his fellow teachers or school staff. He likes to keep to himself after work. Ben has missed a series of appointments with the psychiatrist that were supposed to occur after his most recent hospitalization. At this time, Ben is searching out a new psychiatrist at a nearby outpatient clinic. He realizes he needs some kind of medical provider, should he need his medication restarted.

Ben: They just misunderstand me, you know. I do get stressed on and off, and if I don't get my sleep, I get into a kind of crisis, but I'm not mentally ill! At the hospital, they just exaggerate everything. And they just focus on medications, just giving me pills.

Psychiatrist: What medicine did they recommend?

Ben: I think it's called Zyprexa, or something like that. I know it starts with a "z."

Psychiatrist: What dosage are you taking?

Ben: Two milligrams.

Psychiatrist: To what extent have you followed their advice?

Ben: Well, I used to take it for a few days in a row, but I got so tired I couldn't do anything.

Psychiatrist: Then what?

Ben: I started taking the pills on and off.

Psychiatrist: What amount? The whole dose, or…?

Ben: Sometimes, sometimes less. It depends on how I'm feeling.

Psychiatrist: What do you think about taking medication? I get that you find it problematic because it makes you too tired. Are there any positive effects at all?

Ben: I don't know. They just keep telling me that "you need it"—for my whole life, I think!

Psychiatrist: What else do you notice when you take the medicine? In addition to getting too tired?

Ben: It does help me get to sleep, and I do need to get decent sleep. Things get pretty hard for me emotionally when I don't sleep well.

Psychiatrist: This crisis you get into on and off, the one you think they exaggerate at the hospital: how much of a problem is this crisis for you when you are in the middle of it?

Ben: Well, it's still a problem, I guess. It causes problems at my work and also in my relationship with my daughter. But that doesn't mean I'm mentally ill the way they say!

The beginning of the "workability and perspective-taking" conversation with Ben is more straightforward and less invasive than was true with Frank. The psychiatrist is trying to build a bond with Ben, given his perceptions of his prior treatment by the staff at the hospital. Even considering this, the psychiatrist follows the basic principles of functional contextual interviewing. The patient's experience is not the problem in and of itself; rather, it is something the psychiatrist will help the patient examine more closely. What is the patient experiencing and doing, and how is that connected to possible problematic consequences?

Psychiatrist: You say they keep telling you that you need this medicine. Did they explain why they think you need it?

Ben: They say I can get psychotic. I'm not really. As I said, I can get into a kind of crisis, but that is not being psychotic.

Psychiatrist: Is that part of the problem with taking the medicine, that it's connected in your mind with being psychotic or mentally ill?

Ben: Yes, I guess it is. Psychiatrists exaggerate everything. What do you think? Am I psychotic?

Psychiatrist: You are definitely not now, as we sit here. When was the last time you had a crisis when you really weren't doing well?

Ben: My last crisis was about a year ago, but it wasn't as bad as some of my earlier ones. I didn't have to go to the hospital or anything, I just took a break from school and slept in and rested at home for a few days.

Psychiatrist: Did you take any meds then?

Ben: Well, I'd forgotten to take it for some time, but then I started to use it again. What do you say, was that a psychosis?

Psychiatrist: What was it like? Earlier you told me that when you get into crisis, you believe other people, like your teacher at college, for example, are giving false information about you to the police.

Ben: Well, that wasn't so bad this time. I get all kinds of thoughts when I get into a crisis, you know. I find it hard to stop thinking about certain ideas I have. They don't always involve other people. Sometimes, I might replay a TV show over and over in my mind and try to see if it has a hidden meaning that other people are missing. You haven't answered my question. Is that psychosis? I don't think so.

Psychiatrist: You're right, I didn't answer your question. For a reason, actually. I get the sense that this kind of debate goes on inside you: is this a crisis or is this a psychosis? That can be kind of a trap. I mean, did you have this debate with your psychiatrist at the hospital? Did it help the two of you develop a good plan to help you function at work and build a life outside of work that you enjoy?

Ben: I guess no, it didn't help. But it's important, right? If I have a psychosis, then I should take the medicine, right?

Psychiatrist: Whether it's helpful or not for you to take the medication is an important question, and that's a different question than whether you have a psychosis or not. Let's say we wouldn't agree on what to call the experiences you're telling me about. You call it a crisis, and I might call it a psychotic episode. It might be something else. Even though we couldn't agree on a name, we could still agree with 100% certainty that you are having these experiences and that they are distressing for you. You told me that in some situations, especially when you're under stress and when you haven't slept well for some days, you begin to believe other people are talking about you, saying things that aren't true. When you act on those beliefs, it causes some additional problems. Could we agree on that?

Ben: Yes, that's happened. I've had that experience. But that doesn't mean I have psychosis.

Psychiatrist: Even if some psychiatrists would call that a psychosis, the word we pick is not important to me. You can call it X if you want. If you want to call it a crisis, I'm okay with that. The important thing for us to agree on, as I see it, is what these experiences are like for you and what you can do to navigate through them so additional bad things don't happen. If it's helpful for you to take some medication when you're in crisis, we can certainly consider that as one part of your coping plan.

In this conversation, context sensitivity/workability is manifesting itself in many different ways. The main emphasis is, of course, on what is working for the patient in the context of his experience (i.e., context sensitivity). The psychiatrist is constantly trying to help Ben attend to his own experience and use that increased awareness in a helpful way. Yet the question of workability is also present for the psychiatrist. What is a helpful way of talking for the psychiatrist? The psychiatrist senses that the term "psychosis" is emotionally loaded for the patient and will likely lead to an unproductive working relationship. This is not a technical argument against calling Ben's condition a "psychosis." That might well be very helpful in certain professional contexts in which Ben's case is being discussed. From a functional psychiatric perspective, however, use of that term is not going to work to help the psychiatrist and patient achieve their mutual objective of sustaining Ben's level of life functioning even in the midst of his periodic crises.

CASE EXAMPLE: JENNY

Jenny, age 42, has a long history of going to psychotherapy. She has seen several therapists through the years and saw her most recent therapist for almost 4 years. That recently ended when the therapist moved to another part of the country. Jenny now comes to see the psychiatrist to establish care. She describes problems in many different aspects of her life. She is married, with no children. She describes her husband as loving and stable and their relationship as "okay," although he does not understand her difficulties as much as she would like. When asked about her difficulties, she describes a chronic, free-floating sense of insecurity, anxiety, dysthymia, and frustration. "I haven't felt good inside for as long as I can remember. Even though I've seen lots of therapists and even psychiatrists like yourself, no one seems to be able to understand what's wrong and actually do something about it." When asked what pharmacological treatment she has tried, she mentions a couple of antidepressants and one mood stabilizer. She is quite clear, however, that she does not want to try any new pharmacological treatment.

Jenny: I've given pills a try, you know, and they don't help me. I used different ones for several years, and I felt a bit better on and off, but it never seemed to last. I stopped taking them a bit more than a year ago, and I don't want to try again. I don't feel any worse now than I did when I was taking the pills. I still feel bad inside almost all the time. I need someone who actually can understand me and get to the core of things. Do you do therapy, or do you know somebody you can recommend?

Psychiatrist: Would it be okay if we talked a bit more about your difficulties and how they impact your everyday life first, and then we can decide together what are the best steps to take next?

Jenny: Sure, if that can help you figure out a way to help me, I'm open to anything.

Psychiatrist: You mentioned feeling low, frustrated, anxious, and insecure about yourself. Does this happen every day, or does it differ from day to day?

Jenny: Well, some. But I never feel okay, really. I look on Facebook, and everyone seems so different from me. They are doing good, having fun. I don't feel like that.

Psychiatrist: What troubles you most, would you say: feeling low? Being frustrated? Being anxious? Or being insecure about yourself?

Jenny: They go together; hard to divide them up, actually.

Psychiatrist: And they trouble you in all areas of your daily life, if I get you right. Is there some area in which they bother you more than in other areas?

Jenny: What do you mean? I told you I never feel okay!

Psychiatrist: I understand. I just mean that for some people their anxiety, for example, becomes worse at work. Even if they're more or less anxious all the time, it's a little better when they're at home. Do you notice any differences like that? That some situations seem to provoke these feelings more than others?

Jenny: I actually have less anxiety at work, although I feel bad there too.

Psychiatrist: What kind of work do you do?

Jenny: I work in an office. It's okay, though people push me a bit too much. They know I have a hard time, but they don't seem to care.

Psychiatrist: How do you feel when that happens?

Jenny: What do you think? I get irritated, frustrated. It's as if nobody really understands.

At this point, the psychiatrist notices two things. First, the psychiatrist has asked questions meant to clarify connections between contextual factors and Jenny's experiences with "feeling bad" but has gotten vague answers in response. The psychiatrist could, of course, go back and try again using other kinds of questions or even have Jenny complete some rating scales. The second notable feature is the way Jenny is struggling to be present in the here and now in her interaction with the psychiatrist. This struggle might actually reveal an important aspect of her longstanding inability to make meaningful changes in her behavior.

Psychiatrist: What's been your experience in your therapies over the years? Have you had the sense your therapists have understood your difficulties?

Jenny: Well, I'm not sure. My last therapist did, to a degree, I guess. But then she moved. I went to her for almost 4 years, and I don't think she really got to the core of my problems.

Psychiatrist: I guess the very fact you've come to see me indicates that you didn't get what you wanted…. Let me ask you another thing about this: here and now, how much do you get the sense that I understand where you're coming from?

Jenny: I don't know. Too early to tell. But I don't give up, you know. There must be some kind of solution for me. Somebody must be able to understand me enough to actually help me.

Psychiatrist: I sense a strength inside you, a determination to live a better life; you don't give up, as you said. Would that be true of you more generally, that you keep pushing, trying to reach things that are important to you?

Jenny: Yes, I don't give up easily. But at the same time, I can't solve my unhappiness with life. Other people can do it, I know, but I need someone to understand and get to the core of this mess. I shouldn't have to feel this way all the time.

Psychiatrist: So, you keep pushing, hoping someone will finally understand you and get to the core of your issues, and will give you the solution…?

Jenny: Yes, what else should I do? Should I give up and resign myself to being unhappy for the rest of my life? Never! I would kill myself instead. I can't stand being this unhappy all of the time. Something has to change.

Psychiatrist: I'm not suggesting you give up your quest to live a good life. As a matter of fact, as I said, I think you're a very determined person. You have the capacity to set your sights on something and keep at it, even though the results might be discouraging. You're a fighter. You don't give up. And then there's this weird thing I've noticed during my career as a psychiatrist: we can easily create problems by using our strengths. In some situations, our strengths actually become our weaknesses, become a part of our problems.

Jenny: I don't get what you mean.

Psychiatrist: It is a bit weird, but not so strange if you think about it. Let's say you are very capable in some way. Like, in your example, you have the capacity to keep pushing, even in a difficult situation. You have a really good tool to use in your life journey. It's an excellent tool, and you know how to use it. In many situations it serves you well. I'm sure your ability to keep going has been helpful to you in many different situations, right?

Jenny: Yeah, I guess.

Psychiatrist: So, this is the downside: You have this excellent tool that's worked well in many other life situations, so you're tempted to try it even in life situations where it doesn't fit. You get into something difficult, and what do you do? You pick up your favorite tool. Quite natural, it's been helpful so many times. But what if there are situations where using this tool will not work? Nothing wrong with the tool; it's a good one. But it doesn't work in all situations. I've seen this so many times, both with patients I've met and in my own life, too. You instinctively pick up your favorite tool, especially when you're in a tricky situation, but the tool doesn't work, and it's hard to accept this is happening, because you're used to it working. So, you keep on using it, even though in this particular situation it simply doesn't work.

Jenny: And you think this is so with me, or what?

Psychiatrist: Yes, I suspect that's what's going on.

Jenny: In what way?

Psychiatrist: Your strength is to be able to keep going, to push on regardless. That's something to cherish. Excellent tool! But I think you're applying it to an area where it might become a trap: hoping someone else will be the solution to the problem of feeling low, being frustrated, anxious, and insecure. Hoping that if you keep trying to find the right person, someone will eventually understand well enough to get to the core of things and solve this problem for you.

Jenny: So, you're saying no one will be able to help me feel better inside and that it's pointless to try to find the therapist who can?

Psychiatrist: Yes, that's what I'm saying.

Jenny: So, there's nothing to be done, I'll be in this situation forever?

Psychiatrist: I understand it could sound like that, but no, that's not what I'm saying. I'm saying that doggedly waiting for someone else to find the solution for you is pointless. Looking at what other people seem to have going in their lives, compared with what you have going, is pointless. You've tried this approach for years, and what does your experience tell you? Have you found that person who has the silver bullet? Not how it looks on Facebook, I mean in real life. How much longer do you want to try this approach, given the results you've been getting? Perhaps you can find another way to use your strength, this excellent tool you have.

Jenny: How can I do that?

Psychiatrist: What if it's like this: There's a new way for you to go, a way to move forward, but to do that you first have to be willing to stop moving in the other direction you've been moving in. Second, this new direction is full of unknowns and uncertainties. It's new territory for you, so you don't know the exact route to take, and neither do I. You'd have to use your dogged determination, that "I'm not a quitter" spirit, to find your way step by step. This would be your show, not someone else's!

Jenny: I don't know.

Psychiatrist: Yes, it's not clear how it will go, exactly. That's okay. You have the ability to persevere. We know that, and we also know that waiting for somebody else to give you the secret to how to live your life's journey has not worked up to now, and it will never work. Yes, there is a way out of this place you are in. Would you be willing to set off on this new journey?

Jenny: This really sounds weird…and I didn't expect it at all.

Psychiatrist: Yes.

Jenny: You're asking a lot.

Psychiatrist. Yes, I know. It's tempting to go on searching for that therapist who will give you the magic solution. You've been down that road many times before. It's easy to go back to familiar strategies that give familiar results. If you try new strategies, you don't know what the results will be, except they will not be the familiar results you've been getting. That's all we can say at this point. The question is whether you're ready to stop doing what hasn't been working and try something different instead.

Jenny: I guess so. Sheesh, what do I have to lose?

In this conversation, the psychiatrist takes direct aim at Jenny's rationale for entering therapy in the first place. Functionally speaking, Jenny has used her past therapies to pursue her agenda of getting rid of "feeling bad" inside. This pattern likely has resulted in all kinds of historical analyses of Jenny's upbringing, critical events in her life, and other "causal" influences that have made her the person she is today. The problem is that none of these things can be changed; only their functions in the present moment can be altered. By turning the conversation toward getting Jenny to "try something different," the psychiatrist is using the workability mechanism to stimulate a change in her approach.

TIPS FOR SUCCESS

Building context sensitivity is a ubiquitous feature of ACT because self-reflective awareness and perspective-taking allow patients to look at the real-world results of following self-instructional rules that encourage avoidance.

Coming into contact with the unworkability of one's own strategies is the first big acceptance move in ACT.

The psychiatrist studiously avoids telling patients that avoidance strategies do not work; instead, the psychiatrist skillfully uses questions that allow patients to discover the real results of avoidance.

The therapeutic process of context sensitivity and workability also plays out in how the psychiatrist approaches a clinical conversation with a patient, such as in choosing words and phrases that do not create defensiveness in the patient.

ACT Clinical Interventions: Promoting Openness

The therapeutic mechanism of openness involves an array of psychological skills that lead to the patient being able to take a detached, nonjudgmental stance in the face of distressing, unwanted thoughts, feelings, urges, memories, sensations, and perceptual experiences. This stance leads to the ability to accept what the patient has previously struggled with and avoided. In this section, we revisit the three patients introduced in the previous section and show via clinical dialogues how the psychiatrist can help patients create a more open, curious, and accepting response to unwanted, distressing private experiences.

OPENNESS AND DEPRESSION: FRANK

Frank has already described some reasons for his self-isolating behavior and social avoidance, what has been metaphorically relabeled as "parking." He is overidentified with "being too tired," which itself functions as a self-instruction to stop doing things. When discussing his reasons for not going to visit his brother and family, he brought up the thought "What would they think of me?" as a barrier to him moving in the valued direction of strengthening his social connections. In the following conversation, the psychiatrist begins to help Frank develop a more open and accepting mental response to these two barriers, such that he can create the needed observational distance from them and escape the influence of the avoidance rules that they trigger.

> Psychiatrist: Did I get it right—when you think about doing things like contacting your colleagues at work or other people you care about, like your brother and his family, the things that tend to stop you are your tiredness on one hand and your fear of them noticing something negative about you on the other?
>
> Frank: Well, that all goes together. I'm sitting here doing nothing, more or less. I can't be the person I want to be. So, if I go to work or go to dinner at my brother's house, they'll see I'm all messed up.
>
> Psychiatrist: So, here you are, in your parking spot. You have an idea of where you want to go, what would be an important direction for you to take, but when you think of actually leaving your parking lot you come up to this stop sign: "Stop, they will see the mess!" So, you stop; you don't pass that sign.
>
> Frank: Yes, something like that.
>
> Psychiatrist: What does it look like, that stop sign?
>
> Frank: Well, it's a scary one for sure. More like a mirror, now that I think about it. I see myself and all the messes I've made in my life.
>
> Psychiatrist: And who is seeing the stop sign mirror?
>
> Frank: I am.
>
> Psychiatrist: Who's driving the car?
>
> Frank: I am. You're suggesting I could just drive by?
>
> Psychiatrist: Have you ever done that, drive on after you've stopped at a stop sign?
>
> Frank: Of course I have. But this is a tough one to drive on from, I guess.
>
> Psychiatrist: So, you notice the stop sign mirror and you stop.

Notice the psychiatrist is not trying to win an argument with Frank about what he should or should not do. The psychiatrist simply reflects Frank's direct experience in a moment-to-moment way so Frank can see what shows up in his awareness, how he reacts to what shows up, and what he does in response to what has shown up. Consistent with the ACT approach, the psychiatrist creates a metaphorical way of talking, a new, shared narrative meant to promote a willingness in Frank to notice his own experience in a way that creates more observational distance, a distinction between the experience he is aware of and himself, the observer. This can be elaborated on further.

> Psychiatrist: This kind of mirror, I wonder…. Have you seen one of those mirrors at a carnival fun house? The kind of mirror that distorts the image of yourself? The mirror we're discussing here is, of course, not a funny one; it's kind of the opposite. But I wonder whether it might be a fun house mirror you're looking at, and to what extent it gives you an accurate view. What do you think?
> Frank: Unfortunately, this one's pretty accurate. At least as it is now.
> Psychiatrist: And even an inaccurate mirror is still a mirror, right? What would happen if you drove by is yet to be seen.

In this brief exchange, the psychiatrist introduces the possibility that Frank's thoughts might not accurately describe how things are. This is done only to support the stance of curiosity and openness, not to discredit and correct Frank's "distorted beliefs." When Frank defends the accuracy of the thoughts contained in the stop sign mirror, the psychiatrist does not push back or challenge him. Instead, the psychiatrist focuses on the distinction between Frank as an acting agent on one hand and what he notices about his own private experiences on the other.

OPENNESS AND PSYCHOSIS: BEN

Ben is not experiencing psychotic symptoms at the time he sees the psychiatrist, but his refusal to use the prescribed medication might be putting him at risk repeated psychotic episodes, which in turn could have negative effects on his life. Having "crises," as Ben calls them, might lead to more hospitalizations and affect his ability to enjoy visits with his daughter and remain on good terms with his ex-wife. The psychiatrist initiates a discussion about the self-instructions Ben might follow that could increase his openness to the perceptual and cognitive experiences that show up when he goes into "crisis." This in turn might help him make effective choices regarding his strategic use of medication.

> Psychiatrist: Your psychiatric providers obviously asked you to take Zyprexa, and sometimes you've taken it, sometimes not. One thing here I think is key. In a sense it's obvious, and at the same time it holds an important truth, I think. Whatever advice you get, you yourself choose what you do. You are the captain of your ship; no one else is going to make that move for you. So, it's one thing to get advice from folks about what you should or shouldn't do. Acting, or not acting, on that advice is another matter.
> Ben: Sure, but I'm not sure what you're getting at.
> Psychiatrist: In the case with the medicine, other people think it would be good for you to take it. But it's true, isn't it, that you also give

yourself advice? If I understand you correctly, you can even hear yourself giving yourself different advice at different times. Like we discussed before, it's a kind of internal debate that goes back and forth for you: Am I psychotic or not? Should I take the medicine or not?

Ben: Yes, the debate is sure going on.

Psychiatrist: This kind of debate goes on within us all, regarding many things. Our minds keep chattering at us about all kinds of things, for example, about the trivial daily choices we make. Pasta or rice for lunch? Watch television tonight or call a friend? What should I do for the upcoming weekend? And so on. This is what it's like to have a mind. Our mind works like a kind of advisor, with the best intentions of guiding us around. At the same time, we can't and don't always have to follow along. Our mind might advise us to do one thing, but what we actually do is another thing. Sometimes we follow our inner advisor, sometimes we don't.

Ben: Okay, I get it. Just to make sure, though. You don't mean voices, right? I've never heard voices. At the hospital they kept asking me about that.

Psychiatrist: No, I don't mean voices, I mean the ordinary chatter of mind we all experience. I do think voices or auditory hallucinations work in a similar way, actually, but that kind of mental chatter is a much more complex experience. I know you haven't had experiences like that. My point now is that we all have an inner advisor constantly telling us to do this or that, reminding us of the consequences for not following along, and so forth. At the same time, we are the ones who listen to the inner advisor, so we are not the same as the inner advisor. Because of that, we're free to move or act independently of that advisor if we choose to. Just because your mental advisor tells you to do something doesn't mean you have to follow along. You still get to choose.

Ben: But what do you do when you can't make up your mind or don't know what advice you should follow?

Psychiatrist: First step, I'd say, is this: Just watch your mental advisor in action! It's doing its thing. Just practicing noticing the activity of your mental advisor can be quite helpful. Reminding yourself that you are more than your mind, you're also the one listening to the mental machinery and you're still the one controlling your arms and your feet. The mind is good as an advisor, but it is not the boss. You are in charge.

Ben: But what should I do, then? I mean, I can't just sit down, listen, and do nothing, can I?

Psychiatrist: You *could* do nothing if doing nothing worked best for you in the situation you're in. You could do nothing when your mental advisor tells you to confront a person whom you think is sharing information about you with the police. Then, in other situations, you must act; in those situations, not acting is acting. For example, not using your medication when you feel at risk is an action, even though it's a nonaction type of action. You can't stop the internal debate about whether you have psychosis and whether you should take medicine. But you can act in a way that promotes your best interests when you feel you're slipping into crisis. Sometimes, you're forced to move your feet in one direction or the other. I'm just saying that if you learn to notice your mind rather than just immediately obeying what it tells you to do, you're in a better position to choose what's actually best for you in the long run.

Ben: Yes, that's what I want to do. I don't want to do things that hurt my own cause in life.

In this conversation, the psychiatrist helps Ben make experiential contact with the distinction between the contents of his mind (the inner advisor) and his sense of self as separate from the mind (the observing self). Creating this observational distance will allow Ben to avoid making impulsive decisions about "what to do" when he is in crisis. If he is in the midst of a psychotic process, his mind will be very busy, full of debates and advice. The best thing for Ben to do in this context is to create observational distance from the chatter of his mind and instead focus on the functional goals that really matter to him.

OPENNESS AND PERSONALITY DISORDER: JENNY

A defining feature of personality disorders is the presence of a narrow behavioral repertoire consisting of rigid overlearned and overpracticed behaviors that affect broad areas of the patient's life. This long-term pattern suggests that these rigid strategies will also show up in a situation such as the clinical interview or consultation. If and when they do, that is a great opportunity for the psychiatrist to intervene to create less behavioral rigidity and a more flexible form of responding. In the conversation that follows, the psychiatrist will try to increase Jenny's ability to take an observational distance from self-instructions that habitually trick her into vicious, self-defeating behavioral circles.

Jenny: So, hoping some therapist will give me the solution or fix my problem is not the way forward, if I get you right. What then?

Psychiatrist: Exactly, that is the key question. It seems to me we don't have an easy, straightforward answer. If hoping for some other person to solve this is not the way to go, we at least know what the answer is not. If another way exists, it has to be different from what you've tried before. We know that, at least.

Jenny: But I need someone to understand!

Psychiatrist: At one level that's very reasonable, isn't it? I mean, that is so human, we all need to have people in our lives who seem to understand us. So, I'm with you on that score. At the same time, you've worked so hard, pushed so far to get a particular kind of understanding, one that will set you free from your suffering. Yet it still seems out of reach.

Jenny: Yes, and at the same time I can do many things. As you said, I have strengths. I know that. But when I feel bad inside, it sort of all falls away. It's like I have no power at all.

Psychiatrist: So, when feeling low, frustrated, anxious, and insecure show up, you can't use your abilities. As you said, the four of them go together, and they seem to be stalking you on a regular basis.

Jenny: Yes, they go together in a long, tough story.

Psychiatrist: If that story were a novel, what would the title be?

Jenny: A novel? How do you mean?

Psychiatrist: I mean, this is a long and tough story about your life journey. All the things you have been through in your life. Your ongoing struggles with wanting to feel satisfied about life and instead feeling low, frustrated, anxious, and insecure about yourself. The story of your endless efforts to find somebody who can understand you and help you solve this puzzle. If this story were a real novel and had a title, what would it be?

Jenny: Somebody should help, or something…

Psychiatrist: Okay, the title would be *Somebody Should Help Jenny!*

Notice how the psychiatrist starts by summarizing the description of Jenny's symptoms with words she has used herself—"feeling low, frustrated, anxious, and insecure"—and incorporating her earlier formulation that "they go together." This is a deliberate strategy aimed at focusing on the part of Jenny's experience (i.e., feelings and embedded self-instructions) thought to have problematic effects on the rest of her behavior. Sensing agreement on this formulation, the psychiatrist can introduce a metaphor (the book and its title) meant to help Jenny create observational distance from her embedded self-instructions. Another term we use in ACT for this complex web of rule-governed self-instructions is the patient's "self-story." Jenny has a dense and well-practiced self-story that has probably been repeatedly reinforced by her previous therapy experiences. The psychiatrist will try to further undermine her literal belief in the contents of her self-story.

Jenny: It really feels like I need that help.

Psychiatrist: Exactly, and I'm sure the book has parts that give good reasons for that. Given what's in there, the title *Somebody Should Help Jenny!* seems right on.

Jenny: But I've been through that, you know. With my therapists, talking about my history over and over, and no one seems to be able to help.

Psychiatrist: In a sense, you cannot "unwrite" this kind of book. I mean, you've had the experiences you've had.

Jenny: So, what then?

Psychiatrist: What if, in a way, the book itself is not the problem? Don't get me wrong, I assume you've been through some really tough things. I get it. But in the here and now, the problem seems to be that the book becomes a script for you to follow, tricking you into doing things that are not really helpful. These books that focus on what has happened in the past, and how the past has shaped us to be who we are, can be interesting to talk about, but they're deceptive. A novel like *Somebody Should Help Jenny!* tends to become predictions about what's going to happen next. Remember, this novel isn't over. The chapters are still being written each and every day.

Jenny: Okay...

Psychiatrist: I mean, what about this story, this experience of yours through the years, your book *Somebody Should Help Jenny!*—wouldn't you say that it tells you what to do, that it recommends you do certain things?

Jenny: Sure, it tells me exactly that, that I need to have somebody help me, somebody to fix this for me.

Psychiatrist: Then you have to put your efforts in that direction, right? You have to use your strength to push for that.

Jenny: Yes.

Psychiatrist: And how has that been working?

Jenny: I get what you're saying. It isn't working at all. But, as I said, what then? What should I be doing instead?

Psychiatrist: Important question. One way to answer would perhaps be this: Is there something outside the main theme of this book, that you will only find happiness if somebody else finds it for you? What if you could find some steps to take that go in a completely different direction, something not dictated by the main message of your story? What if it turned out we're only reading one chapter in your life story? Turns out, we *don't* know the name of the book. We thought we did, but in reality, we're just reading this one chapter in the book called, "Somebody Should Help Jenny." I'm sure some earlier chapters in your life maybe had different titles as well. Maybe coming here today means the "Somebody Should Help Jenny" chapter has ended, and you're beginning to write a new chapter. Maybe this new chapter will have a different title! If you could pick a name for the next chapter, what would you pick?

Jenny: How about, "Jenny Discovers Her Secret Powers" [laughs softly].

Psychiatrist: Now, you get to write that chapter. How cool is that?

Jenny: That would be something.... That would be different. But also scary. I'm not sure what those secret powers would be or how I would find them.

Psychiatrist: That is a beautiful place to start a chapter on discovering secret powers!

In this conversation, the psychiatrist helps extricate Jenny from the behavior-regulating features of her self-story by creating a life course perspective on her travails. The goal is to have her self-story function differently—not as a self-fulfilling prophecy of endless personal failure but as an interesting segment of time in her life journey. The book metaphor itself suggests that each new chapter must be written from the start, and wonderful or terrible things can happen to the main character. The writer is the one who chooses the theme that will carry each chapter. In this way, the psychiatrist uses an ACT perspective-taking intervention to change the function of Jenny's self-story from being disempowered to becoming empowered.

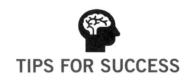

TIPS FOR SUCCESS

The fundamental clinical benefit of practicing openness to inner experiences, whether positive or negative, is that doing so inhibits the regulatory influence of potentially harmful self-instructional rules.

Developing openness basically involves teaching patients to be observers of, rather than participants in, private experiences.

The observer witnesses but remains detached from what is witnessed and therefore does not react to, judge, or evaluate inner experience.

The lack of participation, judgment, and evaluation minimizes the likelihood that avoidance-based self-instructional rules will be triggered or that any self-instructional commands that do show up will be followed, because these too can be witnessed for what they are (products of mind) rather than what they appear to be (mental commands that must be obeyed).

ACT Clinical Interventions: Promoting Engagement

The role of the therapeutic mechanism of engagement is simple in one way and complex in another. In simple terms, life engagement functions as a clear alternative to living a life organized around avoidance behaviors. Once the patient is freed from the necessity of rule-following and avoidance, the natural question is, "What direction will you head in now?" In a more complex sense, engagement is the motivational "fuel" that allows the patient to sustain new values-based ways of living even when the immediate results might be aversive or disappointing. We have repeatedly stressed that the self-instructional rule-following functions embedded in language are essential for effective social organization and cooperation. Rule-following is not the problem; we experience problems when ineffective rules are extended into the wrong areas. The therapeutic mechanism of engagement can be thought of as a process by which new, effective rules are attached to the most meaningful aspects of the patient's life context. In the sections that follow, we examine how engagement tends to unfold in the clinical conversation.

ENGAGEMENT AND DEPRESSION: FRANK

The psychiatrist wants to initiate a conversation with Frank to motivate him to engage in concrete behaviors that will interrupt the vicious depressive spiral he is caught up in. The psychiatrist will talk in ways that help Frank—in the here and now of the clinical conversation—to contact motivating factors or, to use a more specific ACT terminology, to contact his values. Metaphorically speaking, the psychiatrist wants to release a delicious scent into the air, something appealing to the patient, to increase the probability Frank will be motivated to go out and try different things to get more in contact with this wonderful smell.

Psychiatrist: Here you are, at the parking place, seeing that this is not really where you want to be. At the same time, as soon as you even think about driving somewhere you want to go, the stop-sign mirror appears: "What if they see all this mess I've made?"

Frank: Yes, and nothing happens.

Psychiatrist: Let's imagine that somehow you managed to get out on the road again, and the stop sign mirror didn't keep you from going where you want to go. Where would you go? What direction would you head in?

Frank: But that damn sign turns up all the time. It's always there. I just wish it would go away.

Psychiatrist: Ahh, here is the stop sign mirror again. Right here as we are talking about you living your life!

Frank: Okay, yes. It comes easily, doesn't it?

Psychiatrist: It shows up, all right. It seems that if you're going to wait for it to go away, you'll be stuck in this parking lot forever. But let's just imagine! What if you could get out on the road, where would you go?

Frank: Well, it would be nice to see my brother and his family. They are really important to me.

Psychiatrist: Let's imagine you're with them, and you do something together that you like. What would that be?

Frank: Well, just sitting down at their table having dinner with them, talking, feeling that I belong to the family. It's always been such a great thing. Interacting with their kids; I've always been close to them….But what will they say when they see me in this mess? And all the questions they'll ask about how my life is going; how can I explain this mess?

Psychiatrist: Looks like the stop sign mirror just showed up again, right? "What if they see all the mess?" Can you notice that even now, as we talk, you're tempted to put on the brakes, to go back to your parking place?

Frank: Yes, it happens so quickly…

Psychiatrist: I can see how hard this is. A stop sign is a stop sign, right? Feels kind of unnatural to just ignore it and drive through it.

This is once more an example of how the three mechanisms of ACT appear and reappear in the conversation. The psychiatrist is trying to focus on engagement, but as the barriers Frank encounters appear in the here and now, the conversation turns back to workability and openness. At the same time, the psychiatrist begins to use Frank's expressed desire to be a part of his brother's family to move the conversation back to engagement and incorporate openness as a key process component of ongoing engagement.

Psychiatrist: I hear you that your brother's family is really important to you. When you talk about his kids, I also get the feeling that you're important to them and that you being their uncle means a lot to them. Important enough that they'd be concerned about how you're doing and probably would do whatever they could to help. Let's go back and imagine you're at your brother's house spending some quality time with his kids. Can you tell me something about what kind of uncle you want to be?

Frank: Well, a supportive, really "there" uncle. We talk about cars a lot, you know, and we used to build models of special cars. Quite advanced models, actually. The eldest guy, Timothy, is 17, so we've actually started to work together on an old Oldsmobile, a real one I mean. That's stopped now, though.

Psychiatrist: Can you take some time to see yourself back with the kids, doing things like building models, working on the old Oldsmobile? What about closing your eyes, seeing yourself with them? If the stop sign mirror turns up and says you can't drive there, just let it be there and go on interacting with the kids! Can you do that?

Frank [closing his eyes]: Okay. [Silent] Wow, that would be something! Even though it's far from where I am now.

Psychiatrist: I sense the stop sign mirror just showed up, right? At the same time, I wonder a bit more….The relationship with the kids and you being the kind of uncle you want to be is important. Is there not something more here? When you talk about building the models, working on the old car, it sounds to me that there's something there about who you want to be. Something about producing something, being creative. What is that?

Frank: Yes, you're right. I love working with cars and being able to teach those kids how to do their own auto mechanics. That would be great. Not having to worry if your car breaks down. Being able to keep an old car going. Help them have some important skills and save them some money, I think. Helping them out.

Psychiatrist: That's also important in other areas, like at work?

Frank: Yes, definitely. I really like the feeling that I'm helping people out by delivering their goods, putting their deliveries in a place that works for them, seeing their appreciation and excitement when they get new stuff that maybe they've saved up for months to get.

Psychiatrist: So, starting to drive again, even though the stop sign mirror is there, what if that could be about this as well? You want to be creative and feel like you're contributing something positive to people's lives, and this plays out in the relationship with your brother and his family and at work as well. You choose to go out on the road again for the things that really matter to you.

Frank: That would be fantastic, but it sounds so difficult.

Psychiatrist: Yes, difficult things are happening here. The stop sign mirror turns up. What if this is life's challenge to you at this point? Will you stay in this parking place, or will you drive toward the things that matter for you, the things you care about?

Frank: Yes, I want that. Definitely!

Psychiatrist: Then there's the old saying, right? "Even the longest journey starts with a first step." So maybe we can talk about what you can do right now, some action close at hand, that will take you in the direction of creativity and contribution. What would driving in that direction look like, something you could do in the coming week or even today that would tell you were moving in that direction?

In this dialogue, the psychiatrist first establishes an overall valued life direction with Frank and then moves to help him identify the concrete steps he can take that reflect positively on his values. The fact that small, concrete actions in the immediate future can be connected to an overall direction (values) increases the motivating power of those small steps. If Frank, for example, actually contacts his brother and goes to visit him, he not only will have accomplished that but also will contact "being the person he wants to be" in some sense, which probably will increase the reinforcing effect of the consequences following the action.

ENGAGEMENT AND PSYCHOSIS: BEN

If Ben were to take his antipsychotic medication on a more predictable basis, it might prevent him from lapsing into full psychotic episodes and help him avoid the functional consequences such episodes might cause in his life more generally. The dose and rhythm of medication needed to achieve that outcome are still unclear, and discovering them requires Ben's cooperation. Advising him to take the medication would be unwise without first creating a values-based context in which doing so would effectively end up being his decision.

Ben: I like what you said about me being in charge and that I can notice advice, both from others and from myself, and then choose where to go. But I'm still not convinced I should take this medication, and you still haven't told me what you think, what you recommend.

Psychiatrist: I know you'd like to hear what I think, but first I would like to hear what you think. Maybe we could start by talking about the important things in your life and what role medication might play in promoting and protecting those things. What would you say are the important things in your life, the things you would try to stay true to, no matter what?

Ben: Well, that does seem to be off track. Why are you asking that?

Psychiatrist: Because when you're in doubt or don't know what to do, when you get different advice, perhaps even from your own mind, it's often helpful to use these things that really matter to you to guide you.

Ben: I still don't get it....

Psychiatrist: Take this issue about whether to use medication, for example. If you choose to take it, what do you hope it will do for you? In the service of what goals in life would you take it? If you decided *not* to take it, in the service of what goals in life would you make that choice? Will the choice to take or not take the medication potentially have an impact on the things that matter to you in your life right now? If making a certain choice moves you closer to what matters most to you in your life, that would certainly push you in the direction of making that choice.

Ben: Okay, I see what you mean. I must say I've never thought about whether to take the medication or not from that perspective.

Psychiatrist: Okay, so, what are the things you care about, what is ultimately important to you in your life?

Ben: My daughter, of course. Being a good father to Michelle is very important. And my job involves being a teacher and a role model for my students, to give them something that will be valuable to them for the rest of their lives.

Psychiatrist: So, your relationship with your daughter is very important to you, and it sounds like you really like your job and have thoughts about who you want to be as a teacher and in what ways you want to contribute to the growth and development of your students. That is very cool.

Ben: Thanks.

Psychiatrist: These crisis experiences you've had on and off for several years now—when you feel other people are spreading rumors, or you get overwhelmed with all kinds of thoughts, like you said— have these periods of crisis affected your ability to be the father or the teacher you want to be?

Ben: Yes, I guess so. When I go into crisis, I don't go to work. I also cancel out on promises I've made to Michelle. I have really disappointed her quite a few times.

Psychiatrist: Do these results influence your attitude about whether you should take the Zyprexa, or any medication for that matter? The important question now is whether the medication can or cannot help you achieve these important life outcomes you're sharing with me. If the medication can prevent the negative results of disappointing Michelle and missing classroom time with your students, it might make sense to try it. What do you think?

Ben: But I'm still not sure the medication would actually keep me from having a crisis. It does help me sleep, that's clear, but I'm not so sure about whether it keeps me out of crisis.

Psychiatrist: I certainly appreciate that the results are not crystal clear. Would you be interested in pursuing this question a little more systematically?

Ben: What would you recommend?

Psychiatrist: Well, we could start by looking more closely at your experiences with medication over the years to see if there are some patterns we might not see right now. We could experiment with different doses of the medication to find out what is really helpful and what is not.

Ben: Okay, so what would the next steps be?

As this conversation illustrates, turning the clinical conversation in the direction of Ben's values and how those values are being enacted in his life creates enormous behavior-change leverage. It reduces the likelihood of confrontations between the psychiatrist and the patient over issues such as agreeing to take medications in the first place or adhering to medication once it has been prescribed. The thrust of such conversations is not to overpower Ben with the weight of the psychiatrist's authority but to engage him in a cooperative venture designed to improve his sense of life engagement.

ENGAGEMENT AND PERSONALITY DISORDER: JENNY

In her dialogue with the psychiatrist, Jenny seems to see that her strategy of waiting for someone to help her might actually be the problem that has her stuck in life. This is a new and strange insight to her, but it seems to be there, at least to some extent. With the help of the "chapters in a book" metaphor, Jenny also seems to be able to notice her own experience at a certain observational distance, not being as overidentified with her self-narrative as before. The psychiatrist recognizes that developing an alternative strategy for Jenny to follow will be a thorny issue. She has years and years of lived history following her old model of relying on others to make her feel whole inside. A conversation about what really matters to her will be completely new emotional territory.

Psychiatrist: You've felt low, frustrated, anxious, and insecure for as long as you can remember. Of course, many other events in your life probably also produce painful memories, even though we haven't talked much about those things up to now. To make sense of all you've been through, you, like the rest of us, construct a story of your life that acts like kind of a script for you to follow, and you've been following this script courageously and with determination for decades.

Jenny: Yes, I can see I've kind of gotten into this rut of waiting for my issues to go away, but they never do. So what should I do now?

Psychiatrist: What if those negative feelings and your sense of insecurity suddenly and miraculously disappeared? What would you do then in your life? If you were suddenly free to live the life you want to live, what would that look like?

Jenny: I don't know, I would just be happy and free, I guess.

Psychiatrist: If you were happy and free, what would you be doing differently in your life? If I were a fly on the wall, what would I see you doing in your daily life?

Jenny: I don't know. It's hard to even think about that.

In this brief exchange, the psychiatrist is searching for any motivational forces that would help Jenny start experimenting with new approach behaviors, even though none has been identified up to this point in the interaction. How should the psychiatrist respond to patients who respond to the question of what matters to them in life with, "I don't know"? This answer has at least two different possible meanings. One is that "I don't know" really means "I don't want to talk about that because it's too painful." In that case, the psychiatrist should continue trying to elicit value statements in various different ways and eventually talk with the patient about the emotional pain that comes with recognizing one is not living according to personal values. The pain of the "I don't know" response, then, tells us something about what is important to the patient. The psychiatrist has touched upon a raw nerve ending, so to speak.

The second possibility is that "I don't know" is what it says. Perhaps Jenny has created such a pervasive pattern of emotional and behavioral avoidance that it now completely blocks out contact with her underlying life values. We assume that is the case with Jenny. In principle, we then have at least two possible ways to go. One is to go after the pain of living without any sense of a valued life direction. When Jenny is frustrated, for example, she experiences irritation at being blocked in an effort to reach something that is ill defined to her. What is she trying to reach? When she is feeling low, it usually involves a sense of loss or sadness. Sadness implies some kind of loss. What kind of loss is that? There is no frustration if there is nothing important to strive for, and there is no sense of loss if nothing has any importance. Jenny can be asked questions along those lines to see if something of value to her might be lurking in the shadows of her consciousness. The second option is to go back into her historical experience. Has she, somewhere in the past, had a glimpse of something meaningful to her? The psychiatrist pursues that track.

Psychiatrist: I've noticed something many times, when talking with people. Often, a kind of dominant experience—a dominant story—

appears all over the place. Like the experience you've shared with me, of being low, frustrated, anxious, and insecure and pushing for someone else to find a solution. Would it be correct to call that your dominant story?

Jenny: Sure, I can't even look outside it.

Psychiatrist: Then, somewhere in that person's experience is a little short story, almost like a hidden gem. Perhaps just a page or two long. Some life experience that is different in tone but hard to see because it's obscured by the drone of the dominant story. I can't be 100% sure, but I wonder if a story like that lurks around in the shadows of your personal history?

Jenny: I don't know. Not one that just leaps out at me. What if I am that one person who has no hidden gem?

Psychiatrist: As I said, I can't know for 100%. All I can say is that I have yet to meet that person. In my experience, there is always at least a small, perhaps short, alternative experience. A piece of a chapter from another book, so to speak.

Jenny: Now, you mean, or in my past?

Psychiatrist: Could be either or both, I don't know. Would you be willing to look around a little more closely? For example, we talked about your determination and ability to keep going; that you take pride in the fact that you're not a quitter. When you talk about those strengths, I get the feeling that you're proud of them, that they reflect on the better part of you, even with your insecurities. I suspect that you might have learned those things from someone who was a positive influence in your earlier life. Can you put your finger on who influenced you like that?

Jenny: I think it was my school counselor when I was in middle school. He really liked me and believed in me. He had a saying he used all the time: "When the going gets tough, the tough get going." It was a very hard time in my life; he kept me coming to school, and I actually got pretty good grades. He used to tell me I had great things in store for me, that I was very gifted.

Psychiatrist: I think we've found a little gem here, because the look on your face right now as you talk about this is completely different than before.

Jenny [surprised]: Really? I haven't thought about Mr. Evans in years.

As this brief interaction demonstrates, depending upon the patient's life context and personal history, "life engagement" can take on many different appearances. In Jenny's case, simply helping her make contact with a positive, values-based moment in her life journey could change the motivational tone of subsequent clinical conversations. For her, the therapeutic mechanism of engagement might simply result in her experiencing some level of positive self-efficacy. Lack of self-efficacy could severely hinder her ability to sustain new approach-oriented behaviors down the road. So, the psychiatrist slows down the process and tries to help her make contact with a positive, self-referent emotional experience. In contrast, higher-functioning patients, like Frank, respond more immediately to values-based interactions and are ready to begin experimenting with new values-based behaviors.

TIPS FOR SUCCESS

In the delivery of ACT, the therapeutic process of engagement serves three main functions:

- It provides a healthy alternative to avoidance as patients' overarching organizational framework of self-instructional control.
- It provides the "motivational fuel" patients will need to keep moving in the direction of chosen values even when encountering life disappointments or setbacks.
- It provides a new reference point for evaluating the workability of one's behaviors situated in a life context.

Persistent patterns of life engagement result in patients making more contact with, and becoming more responsive to, the impact of positive reinforcements.

Appetitive (values-based) reinforcement results in a higher rate of spontaneous approach behaviors, thus creating an "upward spiral" of positive affect and improved self-efficacy.

Summary

The world of the psychiatrist practicing according to ACT principles is rich with possibilities because of the natural and humane interplay between the processes of context sensitivity/workability, openness, and engagement. The clinical dialogues presented in this chapter show what is possible when patients begin to talk about what is working and not working in their lives and what experiences they are open to having as they pursue the things that really matter to them. In simple terms, the role of the ACT psychiatrist is to help patients stop engaging in strategies that do not work and recalibrate their life compass so that they use strategies based in their personal values. These strategies do not guarantee freedom from personal setbacks or disappointments, but they can promote an ongoing sense of vitality, purpose, and meaning. Clinicians who practice ACT often use terms such as "having fun," "feeling energized," and "personally rewarding" to describe their experience of delivering care within this framework. The principles for adapting ACT to the outpatient psychiatric context and the clinical demonstrations of those principles in action will, we hope, entice you, the psychiatrist, to experiment with ways to incorporate ACT into your outpatient psychiatry practice.

The Essentials

- The ACT framework is a parsimonious, transdiagnostic, pragmatically focused, process-based approach to working with the full range of clinically relevant mental health and substance use problems seen in a typical outpatient psychiatric practice.
- ACT can be delivered in short- or long-term treatment contexts as well as group, classroom, or workshop formats, thus making it an ideal tool for psychiatric practice.
- Most clinically relevant mental health problems, such as depression, psychosis, and personality disorder, arise as a result of the toxic effects of patients habitually and automatically following self-instructional rules that foster emotional and behavioral avoidance.
- Helping patients develop new narratives for their current concerns is a valuable part of conducting ACT.
- When conducting ACT, the psychiatrist must be flexible and allow the therapeutic processes of context sensitivity/workability, openness, and engagement to appear and reappear in the clinical conversation.
- All along, the ultimate focus is on helping patients try out new, more workable values-based behaviors in the world! That is why ACT is a "behavior therapy."

Suggested Readings

Harris R: Getting Unstuck in ACT: A Clinician's Guide to Overcoming Common Obstacles in Acceptance and Commitment Therapy. Oakland, CA, New Harbinger, 2015

Strosahl K, Robinson P, Gustavsson T: Inside this Moment: A Clinician's Guide to Promoting Radical Change in Acceptance and Commitment Therapy. Oakland, CA, New Harbinger, 2015

References

A-Tjak JG, Davis ML, Morina N, et al: A meta-analysis of the efficacy of acceptance and commitment therapy for clinically relevant mental and physical health problems. Psychother Psychosom 84(1):30–36, 2015 25547522

Bach P, Hayes SC, Gallop R: Long-term effects of brief acceptance and commitment therapy for psychosis. Behav Modif 36(2):165–181, 2012 22116935

Gaudiano BA, Herbert JD: Acute treatment of inpatients with psychotic symptoms using acceptance and commitment therapy: pilot results. Behav Res Ther 44(3):415–437, 2006 15893293

Strosahl K: ACT with the multi-problem patient, in A Practical Guide to Acceptance and Commitment Therapy. Edited by Hayes S, Strosahl K. New York, Springer Science and Media, 2004, pp 209–246

Törneke N, Luciano C, Barnes-Holmes Y, et al: RFT for clinical practice: three core strategies in understanding and treating human suffering, in Wiley Handbook of Contextual Behavioral Science. Edited by Zettle RD, Hayes SC, Barnes-Holmes D, et al. Chichester, UK, John Wiley and Sons, 2016, pp 254–272

White R, Gumley A, McTaggart J, et al: A feasibility study of acceptance and commitment therapy for emotional dysfunction following psychosis. Behav Res Ther 49(12):901–907, 2011 21975193

Zettle R: ACT for Depression: A Clinician's Guide to Using Acceptance and Commitment Therapy in Treating Depression. Oakland, CA, New Harbinger, 2007

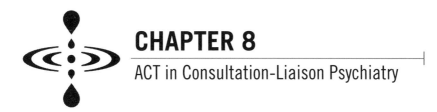

CHAPTER 8
ACT in Consultation-Liaison Psychiatry

A leader is best when people barely know he exists, when
his work is done, his aim fulfilled, they will say: We did
it ourselves.

—Lao Tzu

Consultation-liaison (C-L) psychiatry is an invaluable component
of effective medical and surgical care. Patients with complex physical
and mental health issues do not leave their problems at the hospital's
front door. Mental health concerns interact with and impact the process
and outcomes of physical health care in material ways. Optimal care is
now defined by the collaboration of teams with multidisciplinary exper-
tise to address the complex health needs of patients. C-L psychiatrists
evaluate and suggest best-management strategies for a range of difficult
and bewildering mental health issues that naturally arise in the care of
patients with serious chronic or acute health conditions. They may be
asked for help managing a patient's delirium, mood disorder, anxiety, or
psychosis, not unlike the work psychiatrists already do in more traditional inpatient and outpatient settings. C-L psychiatrists may be called
to assist the clinical care team in assessing whether a patient is suicidal.
Additionally, the C-L psychiatrist is often consulted when a patient dis-
plays difficult or puzzling behaviors that leave members of the team
feeling overwhelmed or fearful, in a state of disagreement, or simply
wanting the patient off their service.

Many psychiatric consultation patients benefit from a straightforward biomedical decision-making approach: Which medication might
be lowering the patient's seizure threshold? What antipsychotics should
be restarted after surgery? At the same time, most if not all patients seen
by a C-L psychiatrist may benefit from a functional psychiatry approach.
Examples include patients who have recently attempted suicide; patients

whose depression makes it hard to engage in treatment; patients whose anxiety is impeding their ability to tolerate badly needed medical procedures; patients displaying "difficult" behaviors that hinder their ability to follow medical recommendations; and substance-using or cognitively impaired patients who may be medically stable but whose challenging behaviors make them difficult to place outside of the hospital. There are many other examples of clinical problems that are hard to tackle without using a more behaviorally focused, functional psychiatry approach.

As consultants, we must realize how challenged and overwhelmed not only the patient but also the treatment team may feel by the time a consult request is made. In a very real sense, both are in need of the guidance of the C-L psychiatrist, and both may require interventions to ensure the best possible medical outcomes. This contextual approach, of course, is the bread and butter of what we have referred to as "functional psychiatry" throughout this book: the behaviors of patients cannot be understood without analyzing the contextual factors involved, including the responses of the hospital staff. These contextual factors not only are environmental but also occur in the realm of private, and often distressing, inner experiences. Similarly, the responses of the clinical team in relationship to the patient cannot be understood without analyzing these same basic contextual forces.

In this chapter, we examine how to apply ACT concepts and strategies across a wide range of patient concerns and with patients showing varying degrees of cognitive and emotional deficits. Illness and hospitalization are usually quite stressful for patients, and those with problem behaviors are frequently stressful for the clinical care team. Therefore, we also focus on decreasing the stress associated with both giving and receiving care, particularly in extended or repeated episodes of care. Working with patients with complex co-occurring physical and mental health issues requires a team-based approach that successfully anticipates and integrates the sometimes competing priorities of the medical unit (i.e., maximizing patient autonomy while addressing hospital safety guidelines). Such an approach is best achieved by creating structured but individualized plans of care. This structure decreases variability in how specific patient issues are addressed by staff; gives them a clear, consistent message about therapeutic expectations; and should decrease the level of emotional reactivity among both patients and staff.

The Benefits of ACT in Consultation-Liaison Psychiatry

Using the ACT framework to add to the existing knowledge base of the C-L psychiatrist can lead to a much more professionally satisfying and organizationally effective form of consulting. Apart from providing effective consulting advice to help with the patient's presenting problem, the ACT approach can be used to foster a deep and beneficial engagement between patients and the members of the clinical care team.

The three therapeutic mechanisms of the ACT model have broad applicability in health care and can be a valuable adjunctive intervention for clinical care team members and patients alike:

1. **Openness:** Approaching unpleasant, distressing events, situations, or interactions with a stance of curiosity, nonjudgment, and acceptance. Being open helps decrease the emotional reactivity associated with labeling and judging patients and their behaviors. Such negativity, when it occurs, only increases the likelihood of patient–staff divisions and confrontations.
2. **Context sensitivity/Workability:** Increasing the ability to be present and to take perspective on the workability of the strategies patients and staff are using. This skill makes it less likely dysfunctional or destructive strategies will continue to be used even when they strategies are clearly not working.
3. **Engagement:** Focusing the energies of patients and staff on developing behavioral options that will lead to positive, health-producing outcomes and a greater sense of vitality, purpose, and meaning. Members of the clinical team are more likely to appreciate how much they share in common with patients in terms of enduring life values. This can promote a more personalized form of medical care in which patients and staff work in a collaborative "win-win" fashion to achieve the best health outcomes possible. Providing care will therefore be more rewarding and values consistent for members of the clinical care team, reducing the risk of professional burnout.

Another distinct advantage of the ACT model is that it can be used to promote brief yet comprehensive and impactful interventions. The C-L psychiatrist often sees a patient only once or twice and must get positive momentum going quickly for both the referred patient and the medical team. The ACT model is quite straightforward, simple, and transparent. The functional contextual perspective inherent in ACT allows the C-L psychiatrist to "hit the ground running" and have intense, direct conversations about things that matter to both the patient and members of the clinical care team. The behavior analytic framework of ACT changes the focus so that consultation requests consisting of imprecise and general questions are replaced by requests for the psychiatrist to assess and make recommendations about how to target specific patient and staff behaviors that are and are not working. The antecedent-behavior-consequence (A-B-C) framework of behavior analysis is generally easily understood by clinical care team members, making it much easier to implement the C-L psychiatrist's recommendations.

TIPS FOR SUCCESS

Medical or surgical care in the hospital and the outcomes of care can be affected by a patient's psychological and behavioral problems that predate, or are exacerbated by, hospital admission.

Functionally based C-L psychiatry, with its emphasis on behavioral analytic methods, is an effective way to focus consultation requests on specific behaviors in specific contexts and to highlight the role played by both patients and members of the treatment team in producing problematic behaviors.

The ACT model allows the consulting psychiatrist to develop brief yet comprehensive and impactful treatment plans that are transparent and easy for members of the clinical care team to implement.

The three therapeutic processes of ACT have broad applicability to the psychological and behavioral issues seen in medical-surgical populations.

Applying ACT to Different Clinical Problems

In this section, we examine several different but "typical" patient problems that lead to a C-L consult request. In some examples, we use clinical dialogues to demonstrate what the C-L psychiatrist might say or do during the patient interview.

THE SUICIDAL PATIENT

Patients at risk for suicide or self-injurious behavior have always been extraordinarily challenging and disruptive to everyday routines on medical-surgical units. The stigma associated with suicidality and the risk of lawsuits in the event of a completed suicide are enough to make most members of a clinical care team feel frightened by the suicidal patient. Avoidance, ambivalence, and anger are natural consequences of their fear, which can damage the therapeutic approach of the team. No-suicide contracts are commonly used on medical-surgical units but have little demonstrated clinical benefit. Such strategies do not "treat" the patient's suicidality. Thus, it is no surprise that such patients are often referred to the C-L psychiatrist, with the hope that the psychiatrist will somehow take care of the problem.

In the ACT framework, suicide is conceptualized as an extreme form of avoidance-based problem solving (Chiles et al. 2018). The "problem" that suicide is designed to solve is "feeling bad inside." Rather than necessarily being a sign of mental illness or an authentic wish to die, suicidal behavior actually serves as a drastic form of emotional avoidance. Destigmatizing suicidal ideation by noting that this has been one of the patient's strategies to avoid painful thoughts, memories, and feelings allows the conversation to proceed to a discussion of the patient's values and aspirations for a meaningful life.

CASE EXAMPLE: JUDY

Judy is a 31-year-old woman expressing suicidal ideation and with a history of self-injurious behavior who is referred for a psychiatric consultation by an emergency department (ED) physician. Judy was brought to the ED by her live-in partner after he discovered that she had been stockpiling pills, apparently to be used to commit suicide. When he confronted her, she told him she "didn't want to go on living like this." Her partner also observed some superficial cuts on her left arm, which Judy admitted she had inflicted on herself earlier that day.

The C-L psychiatrist will first clarify the extent of Judy's suicidal thoughts and behaviors. Drawing on this interaction, the psychiatrist then will try to reframe Judy's suicidal behaviors as a form of problem solving and emotional avoidance behavior, with the hope of engaging her in a context-sensitive assessment of the workability of these actions.

Psychiatrist: You've said that killing yourself seems like the only way out. I'm curious: out of what? What would you be getting out of?

Judy: The terrible way I feel all the time. I'm sick of it.

Psychiatrist: So, killing yourself would be a way to solve this problem you have of feeling terrible inside all the time. Do I have it right?

Judy: Yes, well, I haven't thought about it that way until you mentioned it, but yeah, I guess it would be a way of solving that problem.

Psychiatrist: So suicide is one way of solving the problem of feeling bad inside. Feeling bad inside is pretty common nowadays for a lot of people; would it surprise you to learn that about 25% of all people report having had at least one period in their lives when they seriously contemplated suicide?

Judy: Really? Is it that high? That's hard to believe.

Psychiatrist: So, we can say it's actually pretty common for people to find themselves in the same painful space you find yourself in. When people get into pain they can't tolerate, when they believe they have no way out of the pain, and when they believe the pain will never end, it's pretty natural to start thinking about suicide. I don't think most people want to end up dead; they just don't see any other way to deal with the way they feel.

Judy: That's where I'm at, too.

Psychiatrist: Let's imagine we came up with another way to deal with these painful feelings, and you didn't have to end up dead. What would you be doing in your life that would give you a sense of purpose and meaning? What are the things that matter the most to you in life?

Judy: Well, my children for sure. I'm divorced, and my kids live with their father, but I like seeing them and having fun with them. They love it when I take them to the movies.

Psychiatrist: So being an involved mom and being there for your kids is very, very important to you. You probably want to be there to help them through all of the changes and challenges life can bring.

As the conversation continues to unfold, the psychiatrist could return to the idea that finding other solutions for feeling bad would allow Judy to stick around and pursue her values for parenting and being a life partner. The psychiatrist might conduct a brief five-senses or breath-focused "noticing" exercise with her, stressing that the goal is not to get rid of reactive or judgmental thoughts but to just notice them and not get pushed around by them. The psychiatrist could segue into a discussion of specific small steps Judy could take in the direction of being the kind of mother she wants to be, even while still feeling shaky inside. This type of values-based behavior planning creates a positive framework for living and avoids the coercive features that sometimes arise in no-suicide contracting. As part of the discharge planning in the ED, the psychiatrist might schedule a follow-up consultation to address the possibility of recurrent suicidality by creating a specific relapse prevention action plan for Judy and the ED staff to follow if she presents with suicidality in the future. This patient care approach would also have the salutary result of reassuring the ED staff by giving them a specific, written treatment and management plan to which Judy has already agreed.

SUBSTANCE ABUSE AND ADDICTION

Like suicidal behavior, substance abuse can be viewed as an intricate, habitual form of emotional and behavioral avoidance (Petersen and Zettle 2009; Wilson and Byrd 2004). Beyond their well-documented physiological effects, psychoactive substances of all kinds act extremely quickly to numb out painful private experiences, and in some cases, the substance used replaces emotional pain with an emotional high. Although we focus here on substance addiction proper, in fact, a variety of quick-acting emotional avoidance behaviors can quickly lead to addictive behavior patterns, such as bingeing and purging, sex, self-injury, gambling, and pornography. The problem with all addictive behaviors is basically the same: the quick-acting, positive results of the behavior are eventually undone by its longer-term negative effects. Another important feature of addictive behaviors is the development of psychological dependence crisscrossing with habituation (i.e., tolerance) to the sought-after emotional consequences of engaging in the behavior. In other words, once patients enter an addictive behavior cycle, regardless of what that be-

Table 8–1. Guidelines for ACT-based evaluation and management of substance abuse

1. Fully acknowledge and validate the patient's emotional pain and the extreme difficulty of the patient's current life situation.

2. Establish "context sensitivity" by helping the patient understand that substance addiction represents a collection of specific, unworkable behavioral strategies designed to help him avoid distressing, unwanted private experiences (e.g., thoughts, feelings, memories, urges, bodily sensations).

3. Create direct experiential contact with avoided private experiences so that a stance of "openness" (i.e., emotional acceptance, being nonreactive and nonjudgmental) is cultivated.

4. Engage the patient in a discussion of personal values, with the aim of promoting engagement and creating a positive treatment focus in which abstaining from the addictive substance is an implicit requirement.

5. Schedule regular assessments of how the treatment plan is working for both the patient and the medical team, both while she is in the hospital and after she is discharged.

6. Anticipate that family members or significant others, if they play a functional role in the patient's life, should be involved early on and may play a critical role in ensuring the effectiveness of the plan.

havior is, they have to practice the behavior more and more frequently and at higher "doses" to keep getting the desired effect. Thus, the "real" problem that the C-L psychiatrist must address with both patients and members of the clinical care team is that the main culprit is not the addictive behavior, per se, but the important emotion-regulating function it serves. In a quick C-L consultation visit with a substance-abusing patient, the psychiatrist will want to address each item listed in Table 8–1.

Thus, an ACT-informed plan for treating substance abuse will be more effective if it engages the patient as an active participant in learning new psychological skills for accepting the presence of distressing, unwanted private experiences while shifting the focus to helping the patient pursue valued outcomes in life. In the absence of such a focus, psychopharmacological interventions to address addiction are far less likely to succeed. Almost without exception, the patient will be unable to live a valued life while using substances to numb-out emotionally.

CASE EXAMPLE: TANYA

Tanya is a 45-year-old homeless woman with a 12-year history of drug abuse and addiction. She is divorced from her husband and estranged from her two young adult children. She reports having had a childhood filled with upheavals, abuse, and several losses. Despite this rough start, Tanya married, had two children, and held a job as an office manager for several years. In a way she cannot explain, an opioid prescription for a shoulder injury 7 years ago progressed rapidly from prescription drug abuse to intranasal heroin use and now to intravenous drug abuse. She has been unemployed and living on the street, with acquaintances, or in shelters for the past 5 years. She has no contact with her children and does not seek support from family or friends due to her overwhelming feelings of shame about her current situation. She describes ongoing trauma from the violence she has both witnessed and been subject to while living on the street.

Tanya has already had many contacts with the medical system, although thus far they have not kept her from her steady downhill course. Over the past few years, she has frequently presented to area EDs in an intoxicated state and threatening to kill herself. Afterward, she typically denies suicidal ideation, intent, or urges and requests discharge. Although she has been referred to opiate rehabilitation programs, she has never followed up. She has had repeated bouts of cellulitis at injection sites that were treated at urgent care with oral antibiotics. She apparently stops taking her antibiotics long before the prescription is completed. Last month, Tanya was hospitalized for a more advanced case of cellulitis but left against medical advice before the 7-day course of intravenous antibiotics could be completed. Now she returns to the ED and is hospitalized for the same problem. Obviously, getting her to complete an antibiotic treatment will lessen her overall risk for developing endocarditis, but the members of the clinical care team are concerned she will once again "bolt" from the unit once her acute substance abuse issues have improved.

When the C-L psychiatrist meets Tanya, she is tearful, agitated, and has been verbalizing suicidal ideation to other patients and staff. Staff report that some of her agitation subsided once her acute opiate withdrawal was addressed. Tanya is initially quite difficult to engage, showing limited eye contact and long latencies in her response to questions.

Psychiatrist: This isn't easy. It can be hard and frightening to be inside your skin, because you have a lot of painful stuff in there. It's easy to look for other ways to get away from that stuff. Drugs help numb out the pain, at least for a while. The trouble is, you have to use more and more drugs to stay out of your skin, and pretty soon that's the only thing you have time for. Everything else in life goes by the wayside. You live each day trying to make it from one fix to the next. Nothing else matters, and when you look around, most of the important things in your life are gone.

Tanya [crying softly]: I've been numbed out and lost for years. I've lost everything. I don't want to feel this way. It's too much pain.

Psychiatrist: Can you tell me what life meant to you before the haze of drugs settled over your life? I know you were married, you had some children, and you used to work. Tell me a little about that.

Tanya: My upbringing was a complete mess. I just wanted to have my own family, one that was stable and normal. I wanted to be a good wife to somebody. Then, when I was married and had the kids, I just wanted to be a good wife and mom. But I never felt normal inside. I just couldn't handle it anymore, I guess. I don't know.

Psychiatrist: It sounds like it was very important to you to stop the unhealthy cycle you experienced as a kid. You weren't going to pass that on to your family. Along the way, you somehow got caught up in some of those destructive learning processes you were exposed to as a kid.

Tanya [crying louder]: I didn't want this to happen to me. I'm just so screwed up inside.

Psychiatrist: I understand how painful it is for you to talk about your dreams with me. I appreciate the courage it takes to let yourself think about where you wanted to go in life and where you ended up instead. Would you mind if we try a little experiment to see if it might help you feel a bit more comfortable inside, so we can work together to figure out where to go from here?

Tanya: Nothing will help. It's too late.

Psychiatrist [after remaining silent for a minute]: I understand how stuck you feel and how painful it is to be inside your skin. Would you be willing to try a little exercise that I think might help your mind calm down so you can feel safer when these thoughts and feelings show up?

Tanya: Okay, anything that might help me deal with this. [Psychiatrist walks patient through a five-senses grounding exercise.]

Psychiatrist: What did you notice?

Tanya: It's a little better. [She stops crying and blows her nose.] I feel calmer now, thank you.

Psychiatrist: Notice that I didn't have you try to escape those painful feelings. You just focused your attention in your body. Those thoughts and feelings were still there, but maybe not so in your face as when you try to fight them off or run from them.

Tanya: I'm very good at running, not so good at fighting. I'm not good at being on the streets because of that. I'm scared all the time. I feel like a terrible failure with my kids. I don't know how to cope with being such a bad mom. Everything feels so hopeless.

Psychiatrist: Okay. Is there more?

Tanya: Yes, look at me. How can I see my kids? How can I let my kids see me like this? Heroin helps me feel better. And forget.

Psychiatrist: Maybe a better way to think about it is that heroin helps you run away. When you run, you also run from everything that matters to you. What if you didn't have to run to protect yourself? Maybe learning how to anchor yourself in your body would work better than running away. At least it would give you a chance to turn around and look at the things that matter to you. Even with your sense of failure in your pocket, could you start moving toward those things that matter to you that you told me about?

Tanya: I'd have to get sober and get off the streets. I don't know if I have it in me.

Psychiatrist: I, for one, am absolutely sure you have it in you to get back to living the way you want to live!

As the conversation progressed, Tanya admitted that what she wanted most in the world was to reach out to her children, even if they rejected her at first. She said she was so ashamed of herself that she had not tried to contact them for years. Not surprisingly, she was overidentified with harsh, negative judgments of herself that functioned as self-defeating barriers in situations where she could behave according to her values. The psychiatrist briefly used another openness exercise as a way to begin talking about noticing rather than struggling with or being pushed around by harsh, self-critical thoughts and judgments. The conversation returned repeatedly to how heroin functioned to help Tanya avoid painful inner states and the unworkable results of that avoidance behavior when considering what she wanted to have happen in her life. Tanya and the psychiatrist discussed how practicing being in the present moment—for example, doing a simple 5-minute body scan exercise two or three times a day—could teach her how to ground herself in the here and now so she could just notice painful thoughts, feelings, and memories without trying to control or eliminate them. They discussed how simply allowing her "inner critic" to be present, without needing to judge whether those messages were true or false, might take the edge off the harsh, self-critical self-dialogues that only increased the likelihood she would use heroin. Near the end of this initial conversation, Tanya expressed interest in "getting clean" and finding housing and employment to increase her chances of reuniting with her children.

Because the conversation focused on Tanya's values, she was able to discuss options for care, listen to the recommendations of the clinical care team, and identify barriers to staying in the hospital or following through with a referral for addiction treatment. She participated in brainstorming options to address her concerns about withdrawal symptoms. Tanya decided to accept placement in an inpatient drug rehabilitation program, with a plan to continue the Subutex she had been started on in the hospital. The C-L psychiatrist met briefly each day with Tanya to reinforce the basic messages established in the initial interview and to provide encouragement and emotional support to her for taking the courageous step of committing to getting clean and sober. Tanya finished her course of intravenous antibiotics and transferred to the 4-week residential rehabilitation program, which she completed.

COGNITIVE DECLINE, MEDICAL PROBLEMS, AND DEPRESSION

Feeling "depressed" is a common response in patients with ongoing or worsening medical problems. As mentioned before, the experience of depression can be thought of as a form of avoidance involving emotional numbing and anhedonia. Lots of distressing, unwanted private experiences tend to go hand in hand with chronic medical problems as well as the general physical and cognitive decline associated with aging. Patients may become discouraged about their failure to improve, develop dysphoria when thinking about more health problems coming their way in the future, or respond to minor medical diagnoses with catastrophic interpretations. In other words, they have a lot to avoid. The issue of cognitive decline is also frequently seen in combination with health problems and mood disturbances, particularly among older patients. The C-L psychiatrist is frequently called upon to sort out this maze of overlapping and intertwined problems.

CASE EXAMPLE: ED

Ed is a 73-year-old widower and retired mail carrier. He has hypertension, mild chronic obstructive pulmonary disease, and suspected mild cognitive impairment. Ed was admitted to the hospital with increased shortness of breath after he called an ambulance. His workup revealed pneumonia. He received intravenous antibiotics, and his symptoms quickly improved. Ed's next of kin, a niece who serves as his guardian, reported that he had been refusing to let her visit with him when she dropped off his groceries every Sunday afternoon. She expressed concern about his ability to care for himself independently, noting that he seemed to always be wearing the same clothes and looked unkempt. An occupational therapy evaluation confirmed that Ed had mild cognitive impairment and noted a significant decline in his independent living skills. A plan was developed to discharge him to a step-down facility and then seek long-term placement in an adult family home.

Ed was despondent about this turn of events, however, and refused to engage with physical therapy (PT). He made repeated, concerning comments to nurses and others on his medical team, such as, "I'd rather be dead than live in one of those places." He was vague during questioning about suicidal intent and safety, denying any particular plans but repeatedly saying, "What's the point? What's the point if I can't go home?" When asked if he was safe and would not try to hurt himself in the hospital room, Ed answered, "Who knows?" Because of these safety concerns, a clinical care team member was assigned to provide continuous observation of Ed. Sertraline was started, but no changes were noted in his condition, and the C-L psychiatrist was contacted.

The ages, current life circumstances, and past life experiences of the clinical team members who are caring for Ed may be very different from the life he has lived. For these reasons, individual team members may have a hard time relating to Ed's view of what he wants his life to be about, even at this late stage in his life journey. Talking with him about meaning and purpose and entering into a deeper conversation might help improve Ed's sense of well-being and willingness to engage in treatment.

> On initial assessment, Ed was found to be thin, unkempt, and irritable. He was oriented, was able to comprehend and respond to questions, and cooperated with the psychiatrist during the evaluation. He said he felt angry about being forced to live outside his home, but he also acknowledged that he was uncertain about his ability to return to independent living, and this "cold, hard fact" was making him even more "depressed."

Ed: I don't know what all this nonsense is about me not being able to take of myself. Just because I don't keep my house in tiptop shape and my memory isn't as sharp as it used to be, I don't think that means I have to leave. I've been on my own for years and never had a problem. Now they've decided I need this babysitter invading my privacy [points to staff member engaged in continuous observation].

Psychiatrist: I clearly hear you say that you are able to take care of yourself and support yourself, and that you've done it for years. That is pretty impressive. How long have you lived by yourself?

Ed: My wife died 15 years ago of cancer, and I've been alone since then.

Psychiatrist: That must have been really hard to go through. Watching someone you love go downhill, and there's not much you or anyone else can do about it.

Ed: I still think about her every day. [He pauses.] I think she's in a better place now. Those last weeks were awful to watch. She was such a trooper, right to the very end; she told me that I would be okay and that she would watch over me. We had one hell of a life together.

Psychiatrist: What kinds of things did the two of you enjoy doing together when she was healthy?

Ed: We loved going away camping for the weekend. We had a little camper. We loved being outdoors. She was from far northern Montana and had basically spent her entire childhood hiking, skiing, fishing, camping, you name it. And we were both involved as elders in our church. We helped welcome and initiate people new to our congregation. A lot of them were younger, you know, so they looked up to us. We even started a first-Friday dinner club with some of them. Every month, one of us would put on a dinner, and everyone else was invited to come over. Emily, my wife, was a great cook. She could bake an apple pie to die for.

Psychiatrist: It sounds like you have a lot of time to be by yourself at home. What do you like to do when you're at home?

Ed: Well, I watch a lot of TV. I like the old Westerns. And I have a little garden out back. It isn't much, because I can't bend over and garden for very long before my back hurts. But I enjoy it. I have a glass or two of wine at dinner time to help me relax. If they force me to move to that home for old people, I'm sure they won't let me do those things. There are too many people there, and everyone wants to do something different.

Psychiatrist: You kind of have two sides to you. One is that outdoor person who loves to be on his own, or sort of on his own, with his better half. As you are getting older, you really enjoy getting outdoors in your garden. The other side of you is a guy who likes to kick back and have fun doing things by himself or with other people. I'm curious—most of the things you said that you do now are things you do by yourself. Do you ever get out and have social activities? Like going to church or maybe seeing some of your old friends?

Ed: Not really. I'd like to get out more, but it's hard to do it by myself. I doubt I'd even be safe camping or traveling by myself now. But I think I could spend more time with people. Listen, when you get older, you'll understand why it's harder to do things. No one's around to get me going, so it's harder to do things like getting out of the house.

Psychiatrist: Yes, that's a huge barrier to getting yourself going. I'm not sure I'd be able to cope with always having to get myself in gear. My husband does such a good job of that! So, even if living around other people has some drawbacks, one upside is that it wouldn't always be up to you to get yourself going. Another is that you might like being around people more, because that was important to you in the past, and it sounds like that's kind of gone away in your life.

Ed: You might be right about that part. But that doesn't mean I can't live by myself!

Psychiatrist: Maybe moving doesn't have to be about "I can't live by myself." You could be plenty capable of living by yourself but choose to move anyway because your new digs have real benefits, like we've been talking about. It might be less work and less of a drain on you than living alone and having to always clean up, do dishes, wash clothes, vacuum floors, or clean the bathroom. And you'll be seeing people. That might be more like your old life. Of course, you'll always miss some things about living in your own house, no doubt about it.

Ed: I appreciate you talking with me about this. My niece won't even answer my phone calls anymore, and she's the one calling all the shots. I've been to quite a few adult family homes, and a lot of times they have backyard gardens, they have multiple TVs, they allow folks to drink wine.

Armed with information from this conversation, the C-L psychiatrist spoke with Ed's case manager, who knew of several adult family homes where the owners would gladly let Ed help with the gardening, give him access to his own television so that he could watch his Westerns, and let him enjoy a glass of wine a few times a week if he did not pose a fall risk. The psychiatrist met with Ed again to review his options. Ed's case manager provided information and went over various placement options with Ed and his niece. With his niece in agreement, Ed acknowledged that it might be nice to spend more time with people, as long as he could also garden and watch the television shows he preferred. Ed's affect improved markedly after the initial conversation with the C-L psychiatrist. He began participating in PT because he was now looking forward to leaving the hospital. He ceased making vague comments about wanting to die. The C-L psychiatrist instructed the medical team to focus conversations on the exciting prospect of Ed being able to garden and watch his favorite Westerns. The result was that staff reported having far more pleasant interactions with Ed during his last few days in the hospital.

ANXIETY AND INTOLERANCE OF MEDICAL PROCEDURES

Patients with various types of anxiety frequently have difficulty tolerating certain medical tests or interventions. The constraints placed upon their ability to escape or avoid an anxiety-producing medical test or procedure triggers their fight or flight system, which creates intense anxiety and fearfulness. Often, traumatized patients will stop participating in medical treatment, even though it may be essential to maintaining their health and well-being.

As demonstrated in the following case example, the ACT approach to anxiety stresses that overidentification with the "threat messages" of the mind triggers rule-following designed to help the patient eliminate, suppress, or control the resulting fear response. This avoidance maneuver backfires, resulting in a ratcheting up of the fear response, which eventually escalates into full-blown panic. Thus, teaching the patient to be willing to have that anxiety and its physical symptoms without trying to control those symptoms will short-circuit this upward spiraling process.

CASE EXAMPLE: ALICE

Alice is a 51-year-old woman who originally presented to the hospital with increasing shortness of breath and lung pathology leading to a several-week course of ventilation. She has a remote history of alcohol dependence that has been in remission for 24 years. She had damaged her lungs through exposure to toxic fumes while cleaning a shed she was planning to use as a greenhouse. While Alice was on a ventilator, she initially experienced several life-threatening events due to poor pulmonary function. After 10 weeks, however, she was able to be weaned off the ventilator and onto peripheral oxygen. Her pulmonary specialist thought she had made a remarkable recovery given her initial presentation, although she was left with chronic lung impairment requiring external oxygen for even moderate physical exertion. The plan was for Alice to work with PT so she could regain adequate strength to be transferred to a skilled nursing facility. Flu season was approaching, so her clinical care team was hoping Alice could leave the hospital before she would be exposed to this heightened risk for respiratory infection.

Although Alice agreed to receive PT, she reported shortness of breath ("oxygen hunger") with even minimal exertion and would quickly refuse further participation. She said, "I just can't! I'm so short of breath, I'm going to ruin my lungs." In reality, prior stress tests had shown that her oxygen saturation was normal during prolonged exertion. As an initial intervention, an electronic readout was placed so Alice could see that her oxygen saturations remained in the high 90s, even during more physically taxing forms of PT. Unfortunately, this strategy was not successful in increasing her engagement. Additionally, even when she was not exerting herself, she continued to report experiencing shortness of breath, leading her to reach for nasal oxygen despite showing good oxygen saturation on pulse oximetry. She reported feeling oxygen hunger in each of these circumstances, with increased heart and respiratory rates, and having the recurrent thought, "I'm not going to get enough air, and I'll suffocate and die."

After a few days on the unit, Alice's anxiety complaints worsened, and she refused to work with any unfamiliar PT staff. She reported that just seeing an unknown clinical care team member would trigger panic symptoms. At this point, the C-L psychiatrist was asked to help with her anxiety so she could increase her participation in PT. Benzodiazepines were contraindicated, given her underlying illness and past history of alcohol dependency. During an initial brief triage assessment, the psychiatrist determined that Alice might have mixed depression-anxiety and prescribed a serotonin-norepinephrine reuptake inhibitor, knowing it was not likely to be effective in addressing her symptoms in the short term. Later that day, the psychiatrist administered a contextual interview to see what gave meaning to Alice's life.

Psychiatrist: I understand you're facing a really tough situation here. When you've gone through the type of medical crises you've been through, it's natural to feel somewhat traumatized—it's tough to feel so nervous and vulnerable.

Alice: Yeah, these past several months have been the worst of my life, and that's saying something.

Psychiatrist: Let's see if we can do something about that. Tell me a little bit about your life before this all happened. What was life like before all of these medical problems showed up?

Alice: Well, I had a pretty good life. I really liked my job. I worked as a manager at a title company. We were making good money. My husband and I were getting along really well. Our daughters were doing great in school and socially, too. Then the bottom fell out.

Psychiatrist: That's when you accidentally injured your lungs, right?

Alice: Yeah, it was a total fluke. I had no idea something like that could happen to me. I've always been a go-getter; I was in really good physical condition. I loved outdoor activities like hiking, cross-country skiing….In fact, I was planning a hike down the Appalachian trail with my two daughters. They're twins, you know, and sometimes twins don't get along, or they get jealous and compete with each other. But my daughters are like two peas in a pod; they love each other to death and are such nice people. I love spending time with them. It's a real disappointment that I can't go with them. They probably will never go if I don't go, so I feel like it's my fault the trip's going to fall through for everyone.

Psychiatrist: So, a really huge change in your life. Probably more financial pressure now that you're off work, and going from a healthy, physically active person, and what sounds like a very involved mother and life partner, to being physically compromised and in some ways dependent on others. Seems like you have lost a lot. You must be feeling pretty sad about the big changes here, and I would guess anxious about what the future holds?

Alice: This is very difficult for me to accept. You're right; I worry about what's going to happen to my health. I don't know if you've ever had trouble breathing, but it's about the worst thing imaginable. I get anxious just thinking about what that feels like, not being able to get enough air.

Psychiatrist: Did you ever have issues with anxiety or things like that when you were younger? Something that might have gone away for a long time but got triggered when you injured your lungs?

Alice: I've always been a worrier and pretty high strung. I react strongly to things—I think I tend to overreact to things that worry me. Way back when, I started drinking because it helped me relax. I had to stop drinking because it was getting out of hand, so I just had to learn how to calm myself down when I would start worrying or begin overreacting.

Psychiatrist: Interesting. What did you discover worked to help you calm down when you would worry or start overreacting?

Alice: Well, if I let myself get into worrying, I can't get myself out of it, so I just have to say "no" to getting into it. Just move off in a different direction. Put my attention on something else.

Psychiatrist: Let me see if I'm hearing you right. You learned way back when that you get to choose whether you're going to worry or not. It's not like you can keep those worrisome thoughts and images from appearing, but you can choose whether to join them. If you join them, you'll get carried away by them. If you don't join them and put your attention somewhere else instead, they don't disappear, but they also don't hook you. You can keep functioning and doing what's important. Do I have it right?

Alice: Well, you put it a lot more clearly than what I actually think I'm doing at the time, but yeah, that sounds like what I do. Although I don't always do it—sometimes I can get lost in my worries.

Psychiatrist: What about now, like this situation you're in? No doubt, you have a lot to worry about, a lot to be anxious about. It's not as though you can choose not to have anxious and worrisome thoughts around, because your life situation is really challenging. To add insult to injury, you're mainly anxious about being short of breath due to your injury and what that might mean for your future lifestyle. The problem is, anxiety itself often creates shortness of breath. That's a core symptom of anxiety. So, when you're feeling short of breath, it could be because of your lungs, but it also could be the result of you joining in with your anxiety.

Alice: I hadn't really connected my earlier phase in life to this phase, but I see what you're saying. I do pay super-close attention to the oxygen meter when I'm in PT. Maybe I'm so keyed up that I overreact to changes in the readout. They told me they were putting the meter in there to help me feel less anxious about my oxygen readings, but it's actually making me more anxious! It might be better to do the PT exercises without looking at the meter.

Psychiatrist: Even without a meter, you might still get to a point in your training where you feel a little short of breath, and those very basic memories of being out of breath are sure to show up. You can count on it. But you still have the same choice on the table: to join your anxiety or finish your rehab so you can get on with life. Maybe before you start a PT session, you could take a moment to gather your wits about you and remind yourself that you are able to choose. You can choose to let anxiety and worry hang out while you work to restore your physical health as best you can, so you can participate in all the things that matter to you in your life.

Alice: That makes sense to me. As I said, I tend to overreact to certain things, and anxiety is one of those things. This would give me a different way to go.

Based upon this conversation, the C-L psychiatrist recommended the clinical care team include the following verbal cueing to Alice prior to having her engage in a PT session: "We're going to give you a moment to get yourself mentally prepared for PT." The physical therapist was asked to stop the PT exercise when Alice's respiration rate exceeded a certain level, to help Alice engage in 1–2 minutes of belly breathing until her respiration rate returned to an acceptable level, and to then resume the PT intervention. Subsequent feedback from the clinical care team indicated that Alice was far less anxious and avoidant during PT, and she seemed far more engaged in her rehabilitation.

Alice's tendency to respond with anxiety and avoidance when approached by PT staff whom she did not know was slowing down her progress, and staff rotations made it impossible to avoid this scenario because it was impossible to provide her with the same PT specialist every day. The C-L psychiatrist recommended that PT staff who did not know Alice use the following script when starting a PT session with her: "Yes, it's a little nerve wracking to work with someone you've never worked with before, let's just give it a try"; "Yeah, it's hard to do this, but let's keep your eye on the prize, which is to go home and be with your family"; and "Let's just see how far we get today." Feedback from the PT staff indicated that this way of accepting the newness of the situation and re-orienting Alice to her underlying goals was very helpful. As a result of these ACT-based interventions, Alice increased her level of engagement in PT and ancillary treatments and was discharged to a skilled nursing facility after 10 days.

CHALLENGING PATIENTS

Patients who feel overwhelmed by their life difficulties often have trouble being in the hospital. They may seek discharge before they have been stabilized, risking poorer health outcomes and, paradoxically, requiring more frequent care and higher overall health care costs. These patients often encounter an institutional system of behavioral control that exacerbates their anxieties and makes their behavior even more unpredictable. Such patients may resort to angry outbursts and threats of self-harm or simply refuse to cooperate with treatment providers. These behaviors are not typically well received by members of the clinical care team, who expect patients to be grateful and obedient. Team members might feel threatened and overwhelmed by difficult patient behaviors. They may apply pejorative labels to describe these behaviors, which only serve to alert other team members to expect more of the same from the patient. As the next case demonstrates, the C-L psychiatrist often is called in with the explicit purpose of getting the patient to comply with the social norms and routines of the clinical care team.

CASE EXAMPLE: NED

Ned is a 19-year-old patient admitted to a surgery unit to receive intravenous antibiotics for an infected hand wound that was healing poorly after a compound fracture. When a staff member came to check his vital signs, Ned was lying in a fetal position on the bed, so his nurse was called in for a more comprehensive assessment. The nurse was solicitous and attempted to draw Ned into a meaningful interaction, particularly given previous notations in his chart about depression and self-injurious behavior. Ned remained irritable and would not talk with his nurse or any member of the team. Because of his uncommunicative and unconventional presentation, he was thought to be at risk for potential self-harm. He was put on continuous observation until he could be seen by the C-L psychiatrist. Multiple staff members approached the psychiatrist to warn her that Ned was "difficult," "uncooperative," "manipulative," and "attention seeking." The psychiatrist, using a functional approach, wished to engage Ned and then focus on understanding his current sources of stress within his life context.

Psychiatrist: Ned, I know you came in because of that nasty infection on your hand. That must hurt something awful. Are you okay?

Ned [long pause; looks up at the ceiling]: Yeah, I'm okay. I just want to get out of here.

Psychiatrist: That's what we want, too. We want to help get your hand treated—the infection and the bone repair—so you can go home and go back to work, I'm guessing. What happened last night when you came in? Sounds like you were pretty upset. Maybe freaked out a little. The nurses said you wouldn't talk to anybody about what was going on.

Ned: I was sort of panicking. My hand really hurt bad. I didn't know what they were going to do to help it. I can't afford to pay for any of this, so what's going to happen when I get the bill? Every day that I'm here I'm not at work and I don't get paid. Then, they put this guy in my room—I guess because they didn't trust me—but he was just getting in my face, and that made it even worse. I couldn't calm down. When I get stressed out like that, I freeze up inside. I find it really hard to talk. I suppose I could've said something to my nurse, but like I said, I just tend to freeze.

Psychiatrist: So, lots of things were going on inside that made coming here tough. Then, you feel like people are getting in your face and don't trust you. Not a good formula, for sure. It sounds like you do better when you're stressed or feeling pressured if people give you some space. How does being by yourself help?

Ned: It lets me just sit, close my eyes, and take a few deep breaths. Because when I get stressed, I start remembering things that happened in my family, like my dad being drunk and driving on the wrong side of the road at night and beating us—like, coming after me with a fire poker. Things I don't like to remember because they really upset me. Like my dad hitting my mom in the face, and all this blood coming out of her nose as she fell to the ground, crying for help. I still have those memories like it was yesterday.

Psychiatrist: Wow, that must have been just a horrible, horrible thing to go through. I'm so sorry you had to go through that. So, what seems to help when you get stressed is you kind of ground yourself by sitting with your eyes closed and breathing slowly. You sort of become an observer of what's going on in your body and mind, if you know what I mean. You're probably aware that you're stressed, but you don't make it worse.

Ned: When it's getting really bad, that's when I've hurt myself in the past. I don't like doing that. Just sitting and chilling myself out works better, but I have to have my space.

Psychiatrist: How can we make sure you have your space? How can you let the nurse know that now is a time for you to be alone? We'll have to figure something out, some type of signal you can give, or something like that. You're going to be here for a few days, so let's figure out how to make communication work between you and the nursing staff.

Ned: Well, since I kind of freeze up when someone comes to change my bandages or check my IV [intravenous line], maybe they could just come in 5 minutes or so earlier and tell me what's going to happen next. That would give me time to prepare myself. Watching them replace my bandages or change my IV is stressful. It still hurts a lot.

Psychiatrist: Let me check with the nurses and see if that might work for them. I know they want this to go better for you, so maybe this will do the trick.

Based on this conversation, the C-L psychiatrist concluded that Ned had undergone significant trauma earlier in his life and that many of his re-actions were self-protective rather than designed to thwart the efforts of the clinical care team. When team members were reminded that self-protective, hypervigilant responses are typical of patients with trauma histories, they became more understanding and sympathetic. When the advance notice plan developed with Ned was shared with the team, their appraisal went from viewing Ned as "difficult" to having compas-sion for him and being willing to work with his requests. Giving Ned "space" and asking permission to come into his room were written into the care plan. He was able to stay on the unit for the full course of his antibiotics, underwent reparative surgery, and left fully healed and able to return to work. At discharge, he went to several team members and personally thanked them for being so kind and helpful.

ACT Interventions Delivered by the Medical Team

The C-L psychiatrist is frequently consulted for help with managing pa-tients who have major neurocognitive illnesses when agitation or other forms of behavioral dysregulation interfere with medical care. The same issues come into play once the patient living with dementia is medically stable and the task turns to finding a suitable residential placement. Of-ten, the failure to behaviorally analyze problematic behaviors while the patient is on the medical unit results in protracted inpatient stays. With-out a plan of intervention with demonstrated effectiveness to accom-pany the patient to the new setting, many facilities will simply refuse the placement.

One major feature of C-L psychiatry is that the clinical care team is often the main "customer" of the psychiatrist's recommendations. In general, although interacting with a C-L psychiatrist may have some benefit for patients, the real benefits come when a functional psychiatric approach is applied to understanding the entire context of the treatment milieu. Even patients with severe cognitive impairments engage in be-haviors that serve specific functions. Furthermore, medications may have a positive impact but can lead to oversedation or other problematic side effects. The inability to communicate one's needs or to self-regulate one's emotional experiences can lead to even more agitated behaviors. Therefore, the ACT strategy of carefully investigating the antecedents and consequences of problematic behaviors will lead to a more precise plan of intervention. Very often, making subtle adjustments in the envi-ronment can decrease the likelihood of problematic behaviors. Table 8–2 lists a few examples of common environmental adjustments that are the result of following a contextually focused intervention approach.

Table 8–2. Functional interventions delivered by members of the treatment team

1. Monitor and adjust the level of sensory inputs: light versus dark, quiet versus loud, warm versus cold, even the texture or temperature of food.
2. Alert patients before beginning care and give them time to respond before initiating care.
3. Realize that response times among the medically ill are frequently slowed, so allow for longer periods while awaiting a response.
4. Determine whether the patient prefers to be talked to while receiving care. If so, what name does she like to go by? Does she like to talk about certain topics?
5. Consider and adjust intensity of touch: Some patients respond best to vigorous tactile input. However, unless the patient's preferences are known, start with gentle touch and watch for a response.
6. If the patient is agitated, pause for a few seconds, reassure him using his first name, and slowly restate any instructions.
7. Emphasize consistency and predictability in the patient's daily routine to increase the sense of safety and decrease arousal associated with unpredictable events.
8. Gather information from staff and family to allow ongoing monitoring of which interventions do and do not work to reduce problematic behaviors.
9. Ensure that all staff are responding in essentially the same way to the same problematic behavior. This is best achieved by creating a clear, behaviorally focused treatment plan.

CASE EXAMPLE: HERB

Herb is a 73-year-old divorced male with significantly impaired cognition as well as impairment of motor coordination, including speech. He can be calm and cooperative but then have episodes of yelling and becoming physically agitated every few days. A single such episode seems to trigger several similar episodes. Herb was always calm when seen by the C-L psychiatrist, but due to his cognitive and expressive deficits he was unable to explain why he was getting agitated in other settings and circumstances. No residential or nursing home facility would accept him because of his intermittent agitation, yet he did not meet criteria for inpatient geriatric psychiatry. Various standing and as-needed medications were tried (olanzapine, quetiapine, valproate) to control his agitation, but they produced mainly sedation after the fact and did not seem to prevent the episodic problems with agitation and verbal outbursts. Indeed, some were concerned the medications were increasing the likelihood of later episodes because their sedative effects made it even more difficult for Herb to make himself understood. To better understand various staff viewpoints on what was working and not working, the C-L psychiatrist arranged a meeting with three front-line nursing staff.

Psychiatrist: I hear Herb is having some difficulties. Please help me understand what you're seeing and why you think it happens.

Team member 1: He starts shouting. I ask him why he's shouting. He says he's not shouting, that his butt hurts. I ask him to stop shouting, and he shouts more.

Psychiatrist: Okay, so he's trying to communicate about something?

Team member 1: Yes, but it's hard to understand him when he yells.

Psychiatrist: What helps him calm down?

Team member 1: Nothing, he just likes to yell. I don't think anything helps.

Psychiatrist: Has anyone found something that does help?

Team member 2: When he's yelling, if I speak slower or ask him to spell the word he said that I didn't understand, that works better.

Psychiatrist: So, speaking slower, asking him to spell words. Good. Anything else?

Team member 3: I think he's frustrated. I try to slow down and look at his face when he's talking. He sees I'm trying to listen. When I'm more rushed, he gets more upset.

Psychiatrist: Speaking slower, asking him to spell words, looking at his face when he's talking, trying to slow down your pace. Anything else?

Team members [nodding in agreement]: No.

Psychiatrist: Can you put this in his plan of care so everyone who is taking care of him can see it? Do you see any barriers to trying this out over the next couple of days? It really helps if the charting records the number of times he resorts to yelling during any particular shift, so we can see if what we are trying is working or not. I'll drop by tomorrow to see how it's working.

This case example illustrates how the C-L psychiatrist helps the patient not through direct intervention but rather by developing a behavioral intervention plan that will be applied by the clinical care team. Steps to help the team include providing clear, specific documentation of the plan in the patient's medical record; conducting brief, regular reviews of the plan with staff during team meetings; and ensuring all members of the clinical care team are actually adhering to the plan.

DOCUMENT THE PLAN

Documentation is the primary tool for analyzing problematic behaviors and helping the staff and C-L psychiatrist work as a team to test interventions designed to decrease those behaviors. This requires all team members to enter information in the electronic health record in such a way that the A-B-Cs detailed in the intervention plan can be followed over time. Often, members of the team will benefit from clear guidance about what should be documented. Make sure an up-to-date treatment plan is being reviewed regularly and together with the full clinical care team. To be readily used by the team, keep the plan brief, no more than one or two pages in length. Have one place where the guidance plan can always be found in the electronic health record, and have a laminated copy in the patient's room.

EVALUATE THE PLAN DURING TEAM MEETINGS

Team meetings that are focused constructively on new approaches to the patient's care are invaluable. If possible, prior to a clinical care team meeting, collect data from front-line staff about the patient's problematic behaviors and what seems to have worked best so far to help the patient. For example, "What seemed to set him off? What was tried to settle him down? What worked and what didn't work?" Continue shaping the plan based on feedback from staff who are having an "easier" time with the patient. Set the expectation that the plan will be revised and adapted based on what is learned from the intervention protocol. Reinforce the notion that effective problem solving requires a team approach, with every member of the team playing an important role. Emphasize that no "one size fits all" approach exists for dealing with problematic behaviors; each patient has a unique learning history, temperament, and response pattern.

ENSURE THE PLAN IS BEING FOLLOWED

The clinical care team and, when necessary, the hospital administration must be willing to commit the resources needed to ensure ongoing adherence and fidelity with the care plan. The team may find it helpful to designate a point person in charge of reviewing the documentation of interventions and their effects as well as staff adherence to the intervention. When problematic behaviors do reappear, team debriefings should involve a full A-B-C analysis of these behaviors to identify unrecognized antecedents and ineffective staff responses that potentially are reinforcing them. The C-L psychiatrist should conduct regular staff reviews of the behavioral plan (including developing specific scripting if needed), highlighting wins and brainstorming breakdowns. As team members learn these new techniques and approaches, validate their occasional frustration with learning new skills and share techniques designed to keep them from overreacting to temporary setbacks (i.e., grounding exercises, compassion, and self-compassion experiential exercises). At all times, the C-L psychiatrist should model a patient, nonjudgmental, curious, and open demeanor and encourage all staff to take a creative, experimental approach to addressing problematic behaviors.

TIPS FOR SUCCESS

Development of medical problems that lead to hospitalization can itself be a major cause of stress, demoralization, anxiety, and hopelessness. The C-L psychiatrist helps unit staff balance the goals of patient autonomy with the need for unit routines and patient safety.

Frequently, the C-L psychiatrist will "give voice" to patient concerns that have not been well understood by medical staff so patients begin to feel heard and that their emotional concerns are being addressed.

The perspective of functional psychiatry is that *all* behavior serves a function, even among patients diagnosed with severe cognitive or emotional deficits and even when their behaviors seem to make "no sense."

Many types of medical procedures, tests, and treatments can create distressing and unwanted private experiences that can lead to emotional and behavioral avoidance by the patient.

Often, the clinical care team is the main customer of the consultation process because the treatment plan will be implemented by the team rather than by the consulting psychiatrist.

In the functional approach, the goal of the consulting psychiatrist is always to

- Develop a specific, behaviorally focused intervention plan
- Document the plan in the patient's medical record in simple, direct terms
- Create a method for measuring progress and making changes to the plan
- Ensure all involved medical team members are aware of the behavioral intervention plan and following it

Summary

This chapter provides several examples of how ACT principles and practices may be integrated into the care of complex medical and surgical patients seen by the C-L psychiatrist. Demonstrating a stance of openness, curiosity, and nonjudgment about the strategies patients are using to make their lives work naturally leads to increased patient engagement with the psychiatrist and a willingness to try different strategies. Helping patients identify the things that really matter to them in life allows medical issues to be situated within that context, rather than simply experiencing medical problems without a useful point of reference to help guide the patient's coping responses. The value of being healthy is directly tied to the things a person would do in her life if her health permitted her to do it.

These three core processes of ACT (context sensitivity/workability, openness, and engagement) are straightforward and feasible and are typically well received by the clinical care team. When applied with consistency and fidelity, these powerful therapeutic mechanisms produce positive changes not only in the life-coping skills of patients but also in how those patients interface with the health care team, both now and in the future. The C-L psychiatrist must appreciate how challenged and overwhelmed team members may feel. The ACT approach emphasizes an empathic, perspective-taking stance that results in compassion for both the patients and the professionals who care for them. On both sides of this relationship, the ACT psychiatrist tries to create increased emotional processing capabilities and a sense of personal resilience. If we do this well, the lives of patients and all of their clinical care providers will become much richer and more rewarding.

The Essentials

- The functional psychiatry approach is "tailor made" for application with medical-surgical populations because the hospital milieu is a powerful behavior-influencing context.
- The functional psychiatric consultant uses behavior analytic methods to determine the antecedents and consequences of problematic patient behaviors and then works with the patient and staff to alter those factors.
- The toxic effects of rule-following and avoidance are nearly universal in medical-surgical patients because changes in health status can trigger unpleasant, unwanted inner experiences, resulting in unworkable patterns of avoidance being injected into medical care. This, in turn, affects acute medical outcomes and increases longer-term health risks.
- The ACT therapeutic processes of context sensitivity/workability, openness, and engagement are directly applicable to the wide range of psychiatric, medical, and cognitive issues typically seen in a medical population.

- An ACT-based consultation frequently results in very brief, comprehensive, and effective interventions for patients on medical-surgical units.
- Often, the behavior of clinical care team members is directly linked to problematic patient behaviors, and thus the behavior intervention plan will necessarily involve changing specific staff responses.
- ACT-consistent treatment plans are generally easily understood and agreed to by members of the clinical care team.

Suggested Reading

Losada A, Márquez-González M, Romero-Moreno R, et al: Cognitive-behavioral therapy (CBT) versus acceptance and commitment therapy (ACT) for dementia family caregivers with significant depressive symptoms: results of a randomized clinical trial. J Consult Clin Psychol 83(4):760–772, 2015

References

Chiles J, Strosahl K, Roberts L: Clinical Manual for the Assessment and Treatment of Suicidal Patients, 2nd Edition. Washington, DC, American Psychiatric Association Publishing, 2018

Petersen C, Zettle R: Treating inpatients with comorbid depression and alcohol use disorder: a comparison of acceptance and commitment therapy versus treatment as usual. Psychol Rec 59(4):521–536, 2009

Wilson KG, Byrd MR: ACT for substance abuse and dependence, in A Practical Guide to Acceptance and Commitment Therapy. Edited by Hayes SC, Strosahl KD. New York, Springer, 2004, pp 153–184

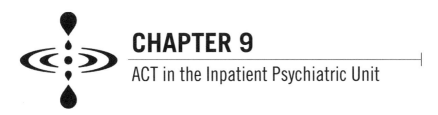

CHAPTER 9

ACT in the Inpatient Psychiatric Unit

We must accept finite disappointment but never lose infinite hope.

—Martin Luther King Jr.

Over the past several decades, a trend in public financing for mental health services has been to systematically shift the available resources toward medication-based treatments and away from psychotherapeutic services. The tide may be turning, however, because increasing research evidence supports the clinical and financial benefits of integrating empirically supported psychotherapeutic approaches with existing biological interventions, particularly in the care of patients with severe and complex illness who are hospitalized on psychiatric units.

In this chapter, we show how ACT can be implemented within a typical psychiatric inpatient unit. To start, we examine growing research evidence suggesting that ACT enhances the clinical impact of traditional inpatient treatment. Effecting change at the institutional level can be a complicated and sometimes discouraging undertaking, however, so we examine some of the system-level challenges the psychiatrist is likely to face when attempting to help a more "traditional" psychiatric unit transition to the ACT model of care. Assuming the interested and committed psychiatrist stays the course and is able to create a new ACT-centered program for the inpatient unit staff to implement, many important questions will remain to be answered regarding how to structure such a unit-based program from top to bottom. To give you a practical sense of what such an ACT-based program looks like in action, we spend considerable time describing the components of an inpatient ACT treatment program that can be delivered in a brief 5- to 7-day hospital stay.

Evidence for ACT as a Clinically Effective Inpatient Treatment

A small but rapidly evolving empirical literature suggests that ACT protocols have beneficial effects on clinical service utilization and overall health outcomes in psychiatric inpatient settings. ACT implemented on inpatient units can reduce readmission rates, for example, and has led to documented improvements in patient wellness ratings (Gaudiano et al. 2017; Thekiso et al. 2015). Studies have been published on the efficacy of ACT for inpatients diagnosed with any form of psychosis compared with treatment as usual (TAU). These studies have consistently shown that a brief, three- or four-session ACT protocol reduces the 1-year readmission rate to 20%, compared with 40% among patients with psychosis receiving inpatient TAU. The purported mechanism of change is that ACT reduces the believability of psychotic symptoms, and this change is strongly associated with a decrease in distress related to psychotic experiences (Bach and Hayes 2002; Gaudiano and Herbert 2006; Gaudiano et al. 2013). A subsequent follow-up analysis of these studies demonstrated that the benefits persisted in the ACT group at 4 months (Gaudiano et al. 2013) and 1 year after the index discharge (Bach et al. 2012). A recent study conducted in Sweden (Tyrberg et al. 2017b) found a significantly higher risk for hospitalization in the TAU group after controlling for age, gender, and pretreatment values-based living scores. A trend was also reported in the ACT-treated group toward an increased values-based living score. However, the numbers included were smaller than those included in previous studies, and the average number of ACT treatment sessions was only two, due to the short inpatient stay model employed on this psychiatric unit. These differences may explain the slightly less favorable results in the Swedish study when compared with the U.S. studies cited earlier.

A meta-analysis of 14 studies examining a variety of mindfulness-based treatment approaches (including ACT) for psychosis reported a moderate effect size across all interventions (Khoury et al. 2013). Although each was different in form, their underlying similarity was the focus on changing the patient's relationship to psychotic symptoms rather than helping the patient control or eliminate them.

The transdiagnostic framework of ACT, with its focus on core therapeutic mechanisms such as context sensitivity/workability and openness, makes it an ideal approach for patients with co-occurring mental and substance use disorders. Indeed, a growing body of research points to the benefits of incorporating the ACT approach in inpatient treatment programs targeting dual-diagnosed patients (Petersen and Zettle 2009; Thekiso et al. 2015). Both of these studies used the same conceptual argument: that emotional and behavioral avoidance underpin substance use disorder and function as a core psychopathological process in affective and anxiety disorders. Petersen and Zettle (2009) demonstrated that dual-diagnosed patients assigned to an ACT treatment program met discharge criteria earlier and required less time in individual therapy than patients assigned to TAU, which was based on a 12-step recovery model. Interestingly, no differences were observed on posttreatment depression scores between the two groups. Still, a difference was found in self-reported levels of experiential avoidance, with the TAU group reporting significantly higher levels. Reductions in experiential avoidance may explain the more rapid positive impact of ACT on addictive behaviors. The authors also demonstrated that the ACT program resulted in savings of approximately $12,000 per patient treated when compared with the cost of the TAU program (Petersen and Zettle 2009).

Thekiso et al. (2015) found that dual-diagnosed patients treated with an ACT protocol reported significantly higher cumulative abstinence duration scores, significantly lower depression and anxiety scores, and significantly lower binge drinking scores at 3 months after inpatient treatment compared with a matched group of dual-diagnosed patients who received only TAU. The clinical benefits of the ACT treatment were sustained over a 6-month follow-up period.

Ducasse et al. (2014) studied the impact of an add-on ACT program for high-risk patients with recurrent suicidal ideation and serious psychiatric disorders such as bipolar disorder, addictions, or borderline personality disorder. No suicide attempts were reported during the 3-month follow-up period, and dosages of benzodiazepine medication were reduced for 65% of the patients. Participants in the ACT program demonstrated strong reductions in experiential avoidance and an increased likelihood of engaging in values-based behaviors. The researchers concluded that an increased acceptance of internal experiences and a focus on values may have mediated the decrease in suicidal ideation and suicidal attempts. Although this study was conducted in an outpatient clinic setting, it is relevant to our discussion because of the prevalence of suicidal ideation, suicide attempts, and completed suicides on psychiatric units and the well-documented increased risk of suicide during the month following discharge from hospital.

The Challenges and Rewards of Creating an ACT Treatment Milieu

Even with a substantial evidence base arguing for it, establishing an ACT inpatient program is a challenging endeavor for many reasons. To begin with, inpatients comprise the more severely ill of those with mental health problems, often presenting with multiple health problems and with a high incidence of cognitive impairments, at least in the acute phase. For example, initially necessary sedative medications can render administration of psychological interventions more difficult. Inpatient stays tend to be brief and orientated toward crisis management. Even within specialized units for affective disorders, personality disorders, eating disorders, or psychosis, heterogeneity and comorbidity tend to be the rule. Patients tend to have multiple symptoms spanning different diagnoses, making the use of more manualized interventions problematic. Involuntary admissions can decrease patient buy-in and create barriers to psychotherapeutic interventions.

Being actively involved in the delivery of ACT may clash with the psychiatrist's concept of his or her own role on the psychiatric treatment team. A recent editorial in the *British Journal of Psychiatry* (Prosser et al. 2016) highlighted these two divergent views: one favored a more inclusive approach to psychiatric treatment, whereas the other advocated for a more reductionist stance limited to traditional psychiatric assessment and biological interventions. Indeed, balancing between a psychotherapeutic holistic model that encourages patients to accept the presence of symptoms and instead put their focus on what gives their lives value and a more reductionistic model focused on eliminating or lessening those same symptoms can be a difficult task.

Institutional challenges can also include inadequate or inconsistent staffing practices, ambivalent management torn between financial pragmatism and clinical realism, and an excessive focus on what are essentially custodial roles of inpatient staff. Additionally, psychiatrists faced with heavy clinical and administrative workloads, in which responsibilities for conducting assessments and managing medications are not optional, may find themselves pressed to find time for psychotherapeutic interventions. Psychiatrists adopting an integrative approach may find themselves operating with little support from peers, indifference from management, and pressure from patients and families who expect the psychiatrist to find the right medication to control the patient's aberrant or abnormal behaviors.

Given these difficulties, why bother? Rewards include increased patient satisfaction, improved therapeutic alliance, less use of medication, reduced rehospitalization rates, and decreased risk of professional burnout in both the psychiatrist and other staff exposed to ACT interventions. Additionally, increasing evidence from the neurosciences favors an integrative approach to patient care if the goal is to increase quality of life and decrease disability and readmissions. Integrating ACT into an inpatient setting is also in harmony with the shift in mental health policy toward a more holistic recovery model defined as "a deeply personal, unique process of changing one's attitudes, values, feelings, goals, skills, and/or roles" (Leamy et al. 2011, p. 445). Like ACT, the recovery model does not focus on symptom resolution but instead tries to build resilience and hope and to increase the likelihood that people with mental illness can lead meaningful lives even in the presence of treatment-refractory symptoms. Like ACT, the recovery approach views life as a process, not as a single destination (Jacob 2015).

TIPS FOR SUCCESS

ACT has been shown to be an effective intervention for hospitalized patients with psychotic symptoms, resulting in much lower rehospitalization rates compared with traditional inpatient treatment.

ACT is consistent with recovery-based approaches to serious, persistent mental health problems because it emphasizes learning to live with, rather than trying to get rid of, residual symptoms of mental distress.

Some of the bigger challenges to converting a unit to the ACT approach involve the psychiatrist becoming stretched too thin due to a multitude of competing job duties and responsibilities, lack of buy-in and support from hospital administrators, and resistance among unit staff to taking on a "therapeutic" as opposed to a "custodial" role with patients.

Benefits of creating a unit-wide ACT protocol include more productive and satisfying therapeutic relationships with patients, more consistency in the therapeutic interventions delivered to patients, and an increase in job satisfaction among unit floor staff as well as members of the clinical care team.

A Brief-Stay Inpatient ACT Protocol

We now describe a protocol for delivering a consistent, high-quality ACT-based approach on the inpatient unit from admission to discharge. We hope to provide a basic template of how to implement this approach in terms of diagnosis, medication use, and the roles of various unit staff in delivering ACT during individual, group, and unit meetings. Although ACT can be used in many ways during inpatient care, we examine how to implement it on an open or locked unit with a 5- to 7-day average length of stay. Inpatient programs with longer anticipated lengths of stay can simply expand on the protocol presented here, for example, by adding in more ACT group sessions. Our other major assumption is that the inpatient population is transdiagnostic, reflecting the clinical heterogeneity encountered on most inpatient units. ACT-informed inpatient protocols have been used in diagnosis-specific units, such as those that only treat patients with affective disorders or borderline personality disorder, so be aware that the principles, treatment formats, and intervention strategies we describe could be applied with equal benefit to more homogeneous inpatient populations. The full ACT protocol is shown in Table 9–1.

The ACT approach is based on helping people lead full and valued lives in the presence of distressing, unwanted thoughts, feelings, urges, memories, or sensations by being aware and accepting of their experiences and focusing on actions that reflect their core values and life purposes. This contrasts with the focus of a traditional inpatient unit on symptom reduction through biological interventions. This approach is based on the premise that once symptoms are controlled, the patient will again function as before. Symptom reduction is also typically the expectation of patients, family members, and significant others. However, recent studies have shown that symptom reduction via purely biological interventions is usually partial and only modestly correlated with improvements in the patient's levels of functioning. For example, a 2-year follow-up study has shown full symptom remission in 97% of first-episode manic patients with psychotic symptoms, but only 37% showed full functional recovery (Tohen et al. 2000).

The growing recognition that symptom status and functional status may be two relatively independent domains has led to an increased emphasis on inpatient interventions that improve functional outcomes. The ACT approach supports these goals because symptoms are not viewed as signs of a latent underlying illness but rather as "environmental inputs" that signal the presence of functional deficits in certain core areas of the patient's life context. Unless the responsible functional deficit is targeted and changed, the patient will continue to experience a high level of functional impairment even after biological treatments have been applied. Although some symptoms may be controlled through biological intervention, the underlying functional mechanisms that are producing symptoms in the first place have not been altered. In some cases, symptom intensity is such a problem in and of itself that, if left untreated, it would serve as a major barrier to any attempts by the patient to improve functioning in a particular life area. Therefore, an ACT-based approach supports the use of appropriate medication interventions by helping the patient and the clinical care team construct a personally meaningful framework to help her assess, in a more targeted, strategic way, the pros and cons of consistently taking medications. This personalized approach increases the likelihood of medication adherence when psychological interventions alone will not suffice, such as when the patient has a severe depressive illness with melancholic features or a severe psychotic illness with formal thought disorder. Appropriate, precisely targeted medication interventions can be used in combination with ACT interventions designed to promote an increased willingness to engage in values-based committed actions, both on and off the inpatient unit.

Table 9–1. A 1-week protocol for inpatient ACT treatment

Clinical activity	ACT process	By whom
Day 1		
Initial admission interviews	Assessment of fusion, avoidance, and psychological flexibility	Psychiatrist and nursing staff
	Functional analysis of behavior leading to admission	
Multidisciplinary treatment planning	Relative strengths of workability, openness, and engagement	Psychiatrist, psychologist, nursing staff
Diagnosis	Functional impact of medication for this patient	
Treatment plan:	Functional impact of diagnosis	
Core process targets		
Medication		
Group activities		Psychologist, nurse, social worker
Individual treatment session	Introduction to ACT	Psychologist, unit therapist
	Functional analysis and workability of behavior; present-moment noticing	
	Values clarification	
General unit activities	Mindful movements/breathing practices	Nursing staff, auxiliary staff
Day 2		
FACT group	Session 1: Functional analysis, workability, noticing, values	Psychologist, psychiatrist

Table 9–1.   A 1-week protocol for inpatient ACT treatment *(continued)*

	Clinical activity	ACT process	By whom
Day 2 *(continued)*	Individual treatment sessions	Functional analysis and workability of behavior, present-moment noticing, function of medication, diagnosis, values clarification	Psychologist, unit therapist
	Individual/Group	Values, communication skills/problem resolution	Nursing staff
	Treatment adherence group	Functional approach to understanding how medications work; discussion about avoidance of or nonadherence to medications in the context of personal values and important life pursuits	Psychiatrist, nursing staff
	General unit activity	Mindful movements/relaxation	Nursing staff, auxiliary staff
Day 3	Unit meeting with all patients	ACT-related themes organized using the matrix method	Team volunteers, psychiatrist, nursing staff, psychologist
	Individual treatment session	Workability of avoidance behaviors, noticing, developing openness, and shifting focus from avoidance to values-based behavior patterns	Psychologist, staff therapist
	FACT group	Session 2: Noticing, learning about values, engagement	Psychiatrist, psychologist
	General unit activity	Mindful movement/breathing practices	Nursing staff, auxiliary staff

Table 9–1. A 1-week protocol for inpatient ACT treatment *(continued)*

	Clinical activity	ACT process	By whom
Day 4	Initial treatment plan review with patient	Functional analysis of avoidance behaviors observed on unit (e.g., staying in bed, not answering phone, missing group or ward sessions, requesting as-needed medications, verbalizing suicidal ideation, self-injurious behavior, fixating on "causes" of suffering, adamant that avoidance behaviors actually work); patient experience with ACT processes so far (individual therapy, FACT group, mindful movements and breathing exercises)	Psychiatrist, nursing staff, psychologist, social worker
	FACT group individual interviews	Session 3: Noticing, openness, perspective-taking, engagement	Psychiatrist, psychologist
	Self-stigma group	Noticing internal experiences of shame, self-stigmatizing thoughts; learning to see labels as labels, being open and self-compassionate, willing to "live and learn" based on personal beliefs and values	Nursing staff, psychologist
	General unit activity (end of day)	Mindful movements/breathing practices	Nursing staff, auxiliary staff
Day 5	Multidisciplinary team meeting	Treatment progress review:	Psychiatrist, psychologist, nursing staff, social worker
		ACT processes the patient seems to "get" and "not get"	
		Future directions for outpatient individual or group ACT	

Table 9–1. A 1-week protocol for inpatient ACT treatment (*continued*)

Clinical activity	ACT process	By whom
Day 5 (*continued*)	Treatment progress review (*continued*):	
	Decision about readiness for discharge or to prolong hospital stay	
FACT group	Session 4: Compassion, willingness, and committed action	Psychiatrist, psychologist
Discharge orders for next day		Psychiatrist
General unit activity	Mindful movements/breathing practices	Nursing staff, auxiliary staff
Day 6–7 Individual interviews	Accepting internal experiences, focusing on workability of actions using values as a yardstick	Nursing staff, psychologist
Individual treatment sessions	Reinforce values-based action developed in FACT group; troubleshoot barriers to follow through, function of medication	Psychologist, psychiatrist
Discharge		

Note. FACT=Focused Acceptance and Commitment Therapy.

Asking the patient to engage in values-based actions in the presence of painful, sometimes crippling symptoms is a delicate task. From the onset, orient the inpatient stay toward enabling him to see himself as a whole person rather than as a collection of symptoms with an associated label given to him by a member of the clinical care team.

Focusing on the actual behavior and how it accords with the patient's values can be helpful. One patient with bipolar disorder and borderline personality disorder recounted how she had everything she wanted and could not understand why she cut herself, had bulimic crises and recurrent suicidal ideation, and spent her days in bed. Acknowledging her good fortune and then homing in on the workability of her avoidance behaviors in light of her stated values gave her food for thought and opened the door to decreasing her requests for as-needed medication while demonstrating an increased willingness to accept her feelings and negative thoughts. Suicidal ideation and the urge to abandon all activities resurfaced just before her discharge in response to serious relationship problems. The psychiatrist and unit staff helped her focus on values and sought to normalize her emotions given the painful context in which she found herself, and this enabled her to leave the hospital on the planned discharge date.

The Importance of an ACT-Consistent Admission Interview

An ACT-based approach is integrated in the initial admission interview to whatever extent is possible given the circumstances and constraints placed on the attending psychiatrist. If necessary, the data collection process can be continued over the next few days in subsequent interviews as time allows and by collecting collateral information from family or close friends. The ACT approach can be quite easily folded into the formal psychiatric interview. In addition to the standard practices of assessing suicidal risk and dangerousness, formulating a differential diagnosis to guide treatment strategies, and conducting a full developmental and longitudinal personal, physical, social, and family history, the psychiatrist can begin looking for the core toxic processes that drive the patient's problematic and unworkable behaviors. The initial interview can help the psychiatrist quickly identify processes of emotional and behavior avoidance, context insensitivity, rule-following, problems with self-reflective awareness and perspective-taking, and the degree to which the patient is living according to stated values and life principles.

Often, the psychiatrist will develop an initial impression of how a newly admitted inpatient interprets, responds to, and interacts with his symptoms. The functional analysis of the "problem" behavior(s) begins with the initial interview and enables the psychiatrist to develop insight into the function of a behavior that may have worked at one stage of the person's life but now has becomes a source of suffering and a barrier to living a meaningful life. Inpatient stays are short, so training the patient to notice his behavior—the function and workability of that behavior over his life span and in the present moment—will help him become more psychologically flexible after leaving the hospital.

CASE EXAMPLE: PAT

Pat is a 46-year-old man admitted with severe chronic depression, suicidal ideation, and a diagnosis of bipolar disorder. He had been treated for years with three different mood stabilizers, including two atypical antipsychotics and an antidepressant. He is very invested in his work, and in his spare time erratically practices sports. He does not feel a sense of pleasure when engaged in any of his leisure activities. All of his activities are results and performance oriented, and this has always been the case. He dates this behavior back to his childhood, when, due to intellectual precocity, he skipped a grade in elementary school. He believed that to be accepted by his older classmates, he had to prove himself both academically and athletically equal to them. The function of a results- and performance-based approach was perhaps adaptive in that situation. When he continued to rigidly apply it throughout his adult life, however, it became a source of mental and physical exhaustion that was no longer working for him or his family.

Psychiatrist: You said your motto in life is to come in first place and always be the best. How does that feel inside? What does it do to your sense of calm?

Pat: It's like a burden inside I can never get rid of. I can't ever let up. I have to keep driving myself to the point of exhaustion.

Psychiatrist: I guess, as you said, you learned this way of doing things a long time ago, back in grade school when you had to prove yourself to your classmates. Would you say that way of doing business is still very active in your life?

Pat: I guess so. I never questioned it until I just couldn't keep it up anymore. But what other way is there? I don't know any other way; this is who I am. Am I just going to be depressed the rest of my life?

Psychiatrist: I think it's a positive sign you're able to step back and look at your life strategy and whether it's working for you. That's sometimes an important first step in making any change at all.

As this brief dialogue demonstrates, introducing core ACT concepts during the admission interview provides a wealth of clinically useful information about the patient that can be used in subsequent treatment while she is on the unit: sources of rigidity in her behavioral repertoire, present-moment awareness and perspective-taking abilities (context sensitivity), and the presence of values and values-based behaviors that might be targeted in treatment. Just helping the patient see how she responds in certain life situations is often the first step toward making a change, because those life situations tend to come up again and again. If the patient knows what does not work in those situations, she can begin to experiment with strategies that might work better.

To this end, the initial interview focuses on cultivating awareness and helping create a clear connection between the antecedents and consequences of problem behaviors. Emphasis is placed on the workability of avoidance strategies designed to control or eliminate distressing private experiences. The cost of unworkable avoidance strategies is often seen in deficits in key life domains such as work, intimate relationships, relationships with children, and friendships or in how leisure and "me time" is experienced. To ground the admission interview process, we recommend the psychiatrist use the ACT-consistent questions described in Table 9–2 as a guideline for the type of patient information that will yield the most powerful treatment plan (Strosahl et al. 2012). These questions can be integrated quite easily and naturally into a psychiatric interview, even when time is significantly constrained.

Depending on the context, more than one initial interview with the patient may be necessary after admission. The psychiatrist, nurse, psychologist, or therapist might each have a chance to interview the patient. This is a golden opportunity for each of them to use a common language grounded in ACT principles. Similar questions are expressed in a different manner throughout each interview, with the objective of developing the patient's capacity for self-observation, perspective-taking, and workability assessment. Table 9–2 provides examples of ACT-consistent assessment questions that can be woven into the initial and subsequent interviews. The functional analysis of behavior is an ongoing process throughout the inpatient stay. The "magic wand" question opens up a vista for the patient that extends beyond the constraints of his current symptom struggles and helps redirect the conversation toward his closely held values and potential life goals after discharge.

Although the unit treatment program is based on an ACT protocol, each patient's care plan needs to be highly personalized. Inpatient units comprise a population of severely mentally ill patients, and we need to be aware of our own urges to fix things too quickly. Some patients have been stuck for years, have built their lives on a scaffolding of avoidance and rule-following, and are overidentified with the belief they are sick, weak, or defective. They have lived their lives relying on very high doses of various medications that allow them to stay away from their chronic feelings of emptiness, pain, and despair. Significant others are often integrated into this scaffolding, which leads to an extreme dependence on family members that may feed into those family members' own needs. The treatment team must tread carefully and remain flexible in how they apply the ACT model in each particular case. Staff can easily become

Table 9–2. Guidelines for an ACT-consistent initial admission interview

Relevant ACT interview targets	ACT-relevant questions
Focus on the patient's use of avoidance strategies and their consequences	How would you know you were doing better? What would "better" look like?
	What have you tried to "get better"?
	How has that worked in the short term? In the long term?
	What are the consequences or costs of using these strategies?
	What are you missing out on in life that is important to you?
Conduct a functional analysis of behavioral strategies to date and their workability	When did you first begin to use that behavior?
	Where does it come from?
	Where did you learn it?
	What purpose did it serve in other settings?
	Did it work in those settings?
	How is it working now?
	Does it work in every domain?
	Are there areas where it works and areas where it doesn't work?
Assess ability to establish awareness of and discriminate among inner experiences	What feelings are showing up now as we talk about this?
	Where in your body do you notice them?
	What thoughts, feelings, memories, or urges show up at the same time?
	What's happening in your body now as these other things show up?
Examine connection to personal values and current life goals	The "magic wand" question: If I had a magic wand and could take away your [problem], what would you be doing in your life that you are not doing now? Why would that be important to you?

Table 9–2. Guidelines for an ACT-consistent initial admission interview *(continued)*

Relevant ACT interview targets	ACT-relevant questions
Assess self-reflective awareness and perspective-taking abilities	What feeling(s) show up in that situation?
	When that feeling shows up, what do you do next?
	When you buy into those feelings, what happens inside? What do you do next?
	Does it help you feel better?
	What purpose does "feeling better" serve for you?
	In the long run, what happens to those feelings?

overidentified with their own rules—for example, that it is wrong to prescribe extra medication no matter what the patient is going through. Alternatively, staff may experience a sense of disappointment when a distressed patient resorts to requesting additional medication, because they believe it functions as an avoidance strategy.

CASE EXAMPLE: SAM

At nursing rounds, staff reported that Sam, who had been on leave from the unit, had experienced a difficult weekend at home with his family. Sam requested several additional doses of his benzodiazepines when he returned to the unit, which led the nursing staff to believe he was regressing and might need a reassessment. The psychiatrist briefly met with Sam to assess the situation further.

Psychiatrist: How did your weekend go? I heard from the staff that you had some difficulties.

Sam: Very difficult; I was very anxious all day yesterday.

Psychiatrist: On Saturday, what did you do? And how did it go?

Sam: I spent Saturday with my wife and daughter.

Psychiatrist: That sounds like fun. What did you guys do together?

Sam: We had lunch together and then went for a long walk along the sea. Then I realized I had to return here.

Psychiatrist: How did you feel when that thought showed up?

Sam: I was happy to see my wife and daughter and to spend time with them, so I was okay for a while.

Psychiatrist: Yesterday, the day before you had to come back here, how did that go?

Sam: I was okay until the afternoon. Then I was alone, bored, didn't know what to do, and began to feel agitated.

Psychiatrist: What did you notice inside when you got agitated?

Sam: I just kept feeling more upset and agitated. It increased as if I was going to explode.

Psychiatrist: Where did you notice the agitation in your body?

Sam: It was mainly in my head, and a feeling of tension.

Psychiatrist: Where else in your body did you notice your tension and agitation?

Sam: My chest—a feeling of heaviness, pain.

Psychiatrist: What did you want to do when those feelings and sensations showed up?

Sam: I banged my head against the wall.

Psychiatrist: What did you notice show up after you banged your head against the wall?

Sam: I told the nurses what I'd done, because I knew they would give me more pills for my anxiety. They gave me medication and told me to talk to you about it today.

Psychiatrist: What purpose did banging your head against the wall serve?

Sam: As I said, I knew if I told the nurses what I did, they'd give me medication and I'd feel better.

Psychiatrist: What would've happened if you'd stayed with that feeling of being anxious and agitated at the thought of leaving your wife and daughter and coming back here?

Sam: I don't know. I was enraged at the idea of having to come back. I didn't want to come back, but I knew my wife would tell me not to come home if I wasn't going to finish my treatment. That's what she did before to get me in here. Just sitting on those feelings, I don't know what would've happened. It was unbearable.

Psychiatrist: So, you got anxious, then bored and anxious inside, and then you got really mad about having to be here. Do any of those feelings seem way out of whack, given your current situation of being in here?

Sam: No, I guess they don't, but I wasn't aware that I had so many reactions.

This interview was conducted during a general unit meeting where 12 other patients were also interviewed over the course of 2 hours. It illustrates the fact that a busy psychiatrist can effectively integrate ACT into a brief interview such as this, designed to help patients recognize and better respond to challenging internal experiences. This exchange enabled Sam to notice and name the emotion of anger, of which he had been unaware until then, and opened up the possibility for him to work on this in individual sessions. Since his admission, Sam's high-dose medication regimen had been slowly and cautiously decreased. In this treatment context, the psychiatrist could help Sam identify and accept more and more of his avoided internal experiences. A balancing act of gradually titrating his medication downward and increasing his ability to accept painful internal experiences was in motion. It was important to respect his rhythm and to accept that sometimes the balancing act would tilt more in one direction than the other. The psychiatrist needed to be flexible enough not to get lost in a tug of war between using medications and promoting emotional acceptance.

In the ACT protocol, we have to respect the patient's readiness to engage in the treatment process, consider the resources and limitations of the unit context, and ensure the safety of unit staff and other patients. The first priority is to make sure that formulating and communicating a diagnosis to the patient can be achieved in an ACT-consistent way. Bearing all of this in mind, and if the patient's mental state permits, she can be integrated into the ACT protocol. This protocol functions at several levels including individual ACT, group, and general unit sessions.

MANAGING THE FUNCTIONS OF DIAGNOSIS

The psychiatrist must be clear about the function of diagnosis and how it can help the patient. Diagnoses within a hospital setting serve administrative, statistical, quality management, and clinical purposes. The function of a diagnosis for a patient may depend on how it is presented; if done flatly and categorically, it may induce feelings of despair, helplessness, and pessimism about the future and promote self-stigmatizing thoughts and behaviors. Placing the diagnosis within the patient's unfolding life context may help diminish any sense of being to blame and responsible for his life problems. Placed in context, the disappointing results the patient is getting in life are not his fault, given the lifelong learning experiences he has had. If only his life had been different, then maybe....This is the rub that leads to sadness, grieving, and ultimately, one hopes, acceptance.

Be sure to emphasize that the patient is not the same as her diagnosis. Many patients take their diagnoses literally and begin to identify with them. Statements such as, "I'm bipolar," "I'm depressed," or "I have schizophrenia" all suggest that the sum of the patient's identity is captured by the diagnostic label(s) attached by a mental health professional. When explaining a diagnosis to a patient, emphasize that everyone has many different roles to occupy in life and help her clarify the roles important to her. This also opens up a space in which to discuss values and committed actions as well as the function of medication, which presumably could be used to improve the patient's ability to function in one or more important life roles.

Sometimes, delivering a diagnosis may be unhelpful. In this case, it may be more workable to focus on the three ACT therapeutic processes and simply not discuss the diagnosis. An example might be an individual diagnosed with schizoid personality disorder. Given the avoidant, concrete cognitive processing tendencies of patients with this disorder, focusing on the diagnosis itself likely will be perceived as unhelpful and stigmatizing. Here, an ACT explanation focusing on the important role avoidance, passivity, and withdrawal play to protect us from uncertainty, criticism, or judgment by others may make far more sense to the patient. This would open the door to another conversation about the consequences of avoidance in terms of its pivotal role in obstructing his values and important life aspirations.

IMPLEMENTING A FUNCTIONAL PSYCHOPHARMACOLOGY APPROACH

Agreeing to take a medication and taking it as prescribed can be seen in many circumstances as a committed action by the patient in the service of her core life values. For example, taking a medication may reduce or remove emotional barriers that currently block the patient from returning to work or being the type of parent or spouse that she would like to be. Viewed in this way, taking medication can be seen as a freely chosen action in the service of her values as opposed to something ordered and coercively imposed by the psychiatrist. The "free choice" model of prescribing allows for more open and honest conversation about the obstacles to taking medication. This includes such topics as fear about being controlled by medication, fears about potential side effects, and the risk of physical or psychological dependence. The type of discussion will depend on the context, but the aim is to enable the patient to see the positive function of medication in the short and the long term and how using the medication supports her pursuit of valued life ends.

CASE EXAMPLE: CANDICE

Candice is a 55-year-old woman with bipolar disorder who has experienced several manic relapses with psychotic symptoms. She has experienced repeated hospitalizations, nearly all of them after stopping her lithium treatment, which usually happens when her symptoms are under control and she feels that she is "normal" again.

Candice: I stop taking lithium when I feel well. It's like a test to see how I will be when I stop my medication.

Psychiatrist: What typically happens when you stop lithium? You've tried this quite a few times in the past.

Candice: Nothing really changes for a while.

Psychiatrist: Then what happens?

Candice: I start to feel very happy, enthusiastic. I can do loads of things; I become very active and productive.

Psychiatrist: Do you notice that change every time you stop lithium? That nothing changes for a while and then you start to get really happy, enthusiastic, active, and productive?

Candice: Yes, I feel very good. I'm not so sure lithium is good for me. I like being that way, you know; I like feeling confident, witty, and able to talk to everyone. I have a lot of great ideas and do things I wouldn't normally do.

Psychiatrist: How do your family and other people around you react?

Candice: Sometimes I can be very irritable and impatient toward others, and that sometimes causes me problems. I won't listen to anyone.

Psychiatrist: What else have you noticed happens after a while?

Candice: The way I act changes. I get weird. I start to do and say strange things.

Psychiatrist: So, you do and say strange things. What are the consequences of these changes in your behavior? What happens next?

Candice: Well, it embarrasses my family. Once I remember my sons wouldn't talk to me for several weeks, they were so angry and disappointed about my behavior in public.

Psychiatrist: Anything else in the way of disappointing results?

Candice: The last time I was in the hospital, my son came to see me, and he began to scold me and lecture me like a parent would to a child. I felt terrible. I thought, "I'm the mother, and he's treating me as if I were a child." He was talking down to me! It really hit me here [points to her heart]. I really felt our roles had been reversed. I don't want that to happen again.

Psychiatrist: Sounds like that was an eye opener for you, and very painful at that. So, every time you stop lithium, first you notice a period of time when you feel joyful, active, and productive, which you like, and you also notice that you become more irritable, impatient, and unreasonable and that this has negative effects on your relationship with your sons, is that correct?

Candice: Yes, I don't want that to happen again. I don't want that feeling of being treated like a child by my own children.

Psychiatrist: How do you think you can protect yourself from having that happen again, where your roles get reversed? It sounds like you want to be in the mother role here, that being their mother is really important to you. What do you think would help you succeed in your quest to be their mother again?

Candice: I suppose taking the lithium and not stopping it even if I'm tempted to do so.

Psychiatrist: Would you be willing to continue taking your lithium, even if you don't like to take medication and even though you know you'll probably feel good to start with—really good, in fact? Would you still choose to stay on your lithium in order to continue having the relationship that you would like to have with your sons?

Candice: Yes, it would be worthwhile for me to make that choice when I look at it that way.

In this dialogue, the psychiatrist initiated a values-based discussion with the patient about her reluctance to continue taking medication in spite of its beneficial effects on her ability to function in important areas of her life. Although the psychiatrist was able to secure a commitment from the patient, her choice to be adherent needs to be reinforced by other members of the unit staff in subsequent treatment sessions.

An ACT-based intervention may also be needed when concern arises that medication use is potentially functioning as an avoidance strategy for the patient. Consistently taking medication to avoid severe anxiety, boredom, or a sense of emptiness, or when it helps him "check out" of the urge to act in an impulsive, self-destructive way, may actually promote the use of avoidance strategies. In one context, taking medication may be in the service of values during a transitional period in which the patient abandons self-harming behaviors while developing and working on acceptance and a new behavioral repertoire. In another context, however, it may constitute a form of avoidance in which fear of a more restrictive staff response (e.g., seclusion, restraints, continuous observation) to impulsive, self-defeating behaviors is likely. This may lead him to resort to higher doses of medication to avoid those anticipated aversive consequences.

CASE EXAMPLE: MARY

Mary is a 42-year-old woman with bipolar disorder and borderline personality disorder admitted for a depressed state with mixed features. She has previously been noted to have a poor response to treatment and has tended to request benzodiazepines at high levels when she becomes agitated and suicidal. She has been on a high dose of an atypical antipsychotic for several months, and she is very attached to using this medication now that she has learned she will no longer get any benzodiazepines.

Mary: I feel okay in the morning; it's the afternoons and evenings that are terrible. I feel very sad, anxious, and would like to go to sleep and never wake up. I go to bed between 7 P.M. and 8 P.M. and just try to sleep as long as I can. I do this at home as well; I practically never see my husband. It's been like this for a long time.

Psychiatrist: What do you notice in the afternoons?

Mary: The mornings are fine; I'm busy. It starts in the early afternoon, when it's quieter. I begin to feel anxious and empty inside. Sometimes, if I take enough medication, it helps get rid of those feelings. That's why I don't want you to even think about stopping my meds. Because if I stop the medications, I know those things will start again.

Psychiatrist: What do you do when anxiety and feeling empty inside show up?

Mary: Usually, I eat and make myself vomit, but I don't do that here. Or I cut myself. I do it on my waist so no one can see it. But I won't try to cut myself here. I just go to bed.

Psychiatrist: What do you notice when you eat and vomit or when you cut yourself?

Mary: It relieves me. I feel better.

Psychiatrist: So, you notice relief from that anxiety and sense of emptiness inside. How long do you stay relieved?

Mary: Oh, it works for a long time, for several hours, at least until the next day. It helps me.

Psychiatrist: And then?

Mary: It starts up again, and I end up doing them again.

Psychiatrist: You say it helps you. In what way do you experience it helping?

Mary: When I feel the physical pain, I forget the rest. It also makes me feel alive when I cut myself. I see the blood, and that's reassuring. I sometimes add alcohol to clean the wound. It really hurts, and that makes me feel even better.

Psychiatrist: If I've got it right, the number one strategy you use when anxiety and a sense of emptiness shows up is to do whatever you can to get rid of them. That might be by eating and vomiting, cutting yourself, or taking medication. When you're here, you don't try vomiting or cutting; you just sleep a lot.

Mary: Yeah, that's right. Because there's no way I can handle those feelings. It just feels like I'm about to explode inside.

This brief exchange illustrates how stuck this patient is in her use of emotional and behavioral avoidance strategies. During the interview, she seems strongly resistant to any notion of accepting her anxiety or sense of boredom and emptiness. She also has difficulty describing her emotions, which is not unusual for this type of patient. The psychiatrist will focus on improving her present-moment awareness and developing openness to her difficult inner experiences. However, engaging this patient will be difficult, given her fear her medications might be changed if she gets better. Mary's use of medication functions as an avoidance behavior because it decreases her awareness of her anxiety and boredom and helps control her urges to eat and vomit or to cut herself. After the first ACT session, Mary's attitude changed; she expressed an interest in finding other ways she could handle anxiety and emptiness other than through quick-acting, but ultimately ineffective, avoidance behaviors.

THE ROLE OF INDIVIDUAL ACT SESSIONS

The topics covered in individual ACT therapy sessions will vary depending on the team member's role on the team. Individual interviews with the psychiatrist are more likely to focus on diagnosis, symptoms, and treatment strategies, because these are subjects frequently raised by patients in interviews. Individual sessions with other members of the psychiatric treatment team can help create a more intensive, in-depth ACT approach. Attending psychiatrists rarely have the time needed to be the primary therapist for a patient. Thus, other members of the team must be familiar with ACT and able to deliver the same ACT-consistent messages to the patient. Individual sessions can focus on normalizing distressing, unwanted private experiences; raising the patient's level of awareness of the short- and long-term workability of avoidance behaviors; and using experiential exercises to increase openness, present-moment awareness, perspective-taking, and connection with personal values.

The content of sessions between a patient and different clinical care team professionals will overlap considerably. This type of redundancy is actually helpful because it leads to a consistent, unit-wide focus on the workability of avoidance behaviors, cultivates openness as an alternative to avoidance, and promotes positive conversations about the patient's aspirations in life. Many hospitalized patients feel life has all but passed them by, and the positive, optimistic tone of ACT is captivating and motivating at the same time. Simple mindfulness exercises can also be practiced during the individual sessions. Staff nursing interventions, which may be brief depending on the time available, can focus on validating the patient's distress in response to unwanted private experiences while encouraging present-moment awareness so difficult experiences can be named and accepted for what they are, not what they appear to be. The conversation can evolve toward encouraging a willingness to have such distressing experiences while at the same time focusing on values-based actions the patient can take, both on the ward and after leaving the hospital. Nurses often play a key role in the administration of medications, particularly as-needed requests, and thus are in an ideal position to address the function of medication-seeking behavior and to reframe it within an avoidance-oriented versus values-based framework. The urgency of such requests is no longer the determining factor in whether the request is granted, which is a godsend for any member of the ward staff who is feeling pressured to prescribe medications that may help alleviate immediate distress but will also reinforce avoidance tendencies in the long run.

Patients frequently talk about their symptoms during interviews with other clinical care team members (e.g., nurse, psychologist, social worker, therapist) and demand relief or try to elicit explanations from others for why they feel the way they feel. Often, the harsh, self-critical, and highly evaluative stance patients take toward their own symptoms and inner experiences can elevate a bad moment into a psychiatric crisis.

CASE EXAMPLE: LAURA

Laura is a severely depressed young woman diagnosed with bipolar disorder. She is currently undergoing electroconvulsive therapy (ECT) because all other treatment options have failed, but her response to ECT has been slow. She has been severely depressed for more than 10 months and has very high anxiety levels. This high level of distress is difficult for Laura and her family to bear, and also for staff, whom she frequently solicits to provide emotional reassurance or additional short-term anxiety medications.

Laura: I can't take this any longer. I'm not able to do anything; it's terrible. I look at others on the unit and see all they do. I'm incapable of doing anything. I feel worthless, useless.

Psychiatrist: Your mind is busy comparing yourself with others on the unit and then tells you how useless you are. How does comparing yourself to others help you?

Laura: I know it doesn't help me. It makes me worse, but I can't help it.

Psychiatrist: Your mind constantly compares you with others in a negative way, and you notice that instead of helping you, it makes you feel worse.

Laura: It makes me want to hide away, stay in bed all day. I don't see any change. I'm fed up; I make my family suffer; everyone suffers. I'd like to go to sleep and never wake up. I'm frightened I'll never get better. If I could, I would take medication or cut myself and end my life, but I can't do that here.

Psychiatrist: This is the first time I've ever heard you talk about ending your life. I can understand you have a feeling of despair, but what purpose would ending your life serve? What problem in your life would be solved by killing yourself?

Laura: Well, I wouldn't have to suffer anymore. I would be dead.

Psychiatrist: So, one way to solve this problem of feeling bad inside all the time would be to kill yourself, right?

Laura: Yeah, it would be over.

Psychiatrist: Very over! And you might miss out on an opportunity to feel better without having to do yourself in.

Laura: What do you mean, miss out? Is there something I'm missing out on?

Psychiatrist: You've been like this before, and what happened?

Laura: I got better, at least for a while. I could do things that made me feel like a person.

Psychiatrist: Yes, from your experience you know your moods can change, and you go on to do a lot of things. You even found work. You helped your family; you looked after your grandparents and helped at the food bank. Sometimes you even helped too much.

Laura: Well, those times are gone now. Back in the black hole of my life again.

Psychiatrist: For all of us, change is always happening, and sometimes in the wrong direction. But that will change, too. What would it be like for your family if you ended your life?

Laura: I don't know. They'd be very sad, I guess.

Psychiatrist: Maybe there's another solution, and that is to put a little less trust in what your inner critic tells you. The critic is telling you you're incapable of doing anything, but let's look at your actual experience. We know that not too long ago you were capable of doing a lot of things, good things, and people- and caring-oriented things. Maybe even right now, your inner critic has it wrong. What's been happening in the past day or two here? What did you do this morning?

Laura: I got up, had a shower, went out for a smoke, and then went to activities.

Psychiatrist: Yes, and I noticed you participated really well in the activities. The staff even wrote that you seemed to be enjoying yourself.

Laura: I did, but it didn't last, and I feel really oppressed again.

Psychiatrist: Did the inner critic show up and tell you everything that's wrong with you?

Laura: Well, sort of. I mean, I'm in a psychiatric unit, so I can't be that worthwhile inside.

Psychiatrist: So, your mind is telling you you're useless and can't do anything, and your experience shows you're doing more and even contributing to group activities on the unit. I also noticed that your facial expression is more relaxed than last week and less submerged by anxiety.

Laura: My mind's telling me do this, do that. I don't know what to do, and I don't do anything with my day. I try to pause, do the "stop" like you showed me, but it's very difficult. I try to let the thoughts go by, but there are so many that I feel completely paralyzed—

Psychiatrist: Really, the task is not to get rid of the inner critic—we all have one, and we all get raked over the coals by that critical voice inside. More, it's about learning to let the critic chatter away while focusing on what's important to you, like all of those activities you did for your family, friends, relatives, and people in need.

This conversation illustrates Laura's lack of observational distance with regard to her negative, judgmental internal dialogue and the psychiatrist's efforts to get her to create a productive distinction between her actual experience and what her mind tells her. In this case, the same interview will be repeated on several occasions, albeit in a slightly different manner, in order to cultivate noticing and the consequences on her behavior and mood of overidentifying with her critical mind.

THE ROLE OF GROUP THERAPY SESSIONS

Group therapy activities may include closed groups, stand-alone group sessions that are ideal for 5- to 7-day inpatient stays, or open-ended ACT psychoeducation sessions. Group therapy or psychoeducational class sessions can focus on a single ACT process (i.e., openness) or may combine all the ACT therapeutic processes into a single session. Groups may address specific dimensions of psychopathology, such as psychosis, or be more general, as in a Focused ACT (FACT; Strosahl et al. 2012) group. A FACT group consisting of four sessions fits nicely into a ward context because it ensures most patients will be exposed to all parts of the therapeutic model before they are discharged. An outline of the session-by-session content and treatment objectives of a FACT group is presented in Table 9–3.

FACT group sessions generally last between 60 and 75 minutes and allow a maximum of four to six patients. There are numerous reasons for this. Patients who may not have had any prior experience in groups are

Table 9–3. Session-by-session agendas for an inpatient FACT group

Session #1	Objectives
Group introductions and rules	Participants introduce themselves; leaders go over group rules.
Brief lecture	An introduction to ACT
Opening metaphor	"You are at a crossroad and have to make a choice between taking one of two roads. One is a smooth, well-maintained road leading to nowhere. The second is a rocky, pothole-riddled, briar-covered road that leads to all that is important in one's life." [Patients are asked to choose which road they would take.]
	Which road have you been traveling on?
Exercise	The FACT focus questions are then posed within this metaphor:
	1. What road have you been trying to go down?
	2. What have you tried (to make that road work for you)?
	3. How have your strategies worked up to now?
	4. What have these strategies cost you in terms of your life's vitality and meaning?
Introduction to the "life path"	Patients are asked to position themselves in the direction in which they are traveling (i.e., toward a life of struggle for control or a meaningful, valued life)
	What would a meaningful life actually look like?
	What would you be doing?
The "180° turnaround" metaphor	Illustrates the dangers of trying to change too much, too fast; the help and motivation required to change; and the need to slow down and observe. Patients are asked to walk rapidly in a straight line and, on a signal, to do an abrupt 180° turn. This rapid change of direction creates imbalance and confusion (some turn 360°). It shows the difficulty of changing without stopping, observing, and choosing one's direction.
Homework	Mindfulness exercises to practice on the ward (e.g., body scan, breathing control, thought watching)

Table 9–3. Session-by-session agendas for an inpatient FACT
group *(continued)*

Session #1 *(continued)*	Objectives
Assessment	Bullseye values exercise is given to each participant to complete and rate before leaving session.
Evaluation of group by the participants	
Session 2	**Objectives**
Intention-setting exercise	What if a miracle happened and you could learn anything today?
Homework review	How often did you practice the mindfulness exercises? What did you learn about your mind?
Opening mindfulness exercise	"Raisin" exercise and debriefing. The raisin exercise is a mindfulness exercise that involves exploring a raisin with the five senses as though it were an unknown entity. The exercise illustrates our tendency to function on automatic pilot and to allow our thoughts and experiences to intervene between us and our experience.
Learning about private events	Three circles of emotions, thoughts, and behavior and their interconnections
Learning about values	A life direction freely chosen, not goals, not feeling dependent, not always pleasant
Group roleplay	"Passengers on the bus" metaphor with debriefing
Mindfulness practice	Brief body scan if sufficient time
Homework	Patients describe values-based actions to implement before the next session.
Assessment	Re-rate values-behavior consistency on Bullseye exercise.
Evaluation of group by the participants	
Session 3	**Objectives**
Intention-setting exercise	What do you want to get out of today's class and what are you prepared to do to get it?
Homework review	Values-based action assignment from Session 2

Table 9–3. Session-by-session agendas for an inpatient FACT group *(continued)*

Session 3 *(continued)*	Objectives
Openness	Being present, nonjudgmental, nonreactive; avoiding the temptation to run, hide, or escape. Openness is not wanting to have something painful or distressing; it is being willing to accept it is there.
Openness exercise	Opening up to a difficult emotion, thought, or memory of physical sensation
Perspective-taking	"Brain is not the same as mind, mind is not the same as you; brain is the computer, mind is the operating system, you are the one looking at the computer screen."
Sticky thoughts exercise	Patients are invited to write a painful thought or emotion on a paper that they attach to their clothes, then walk around the room greeting and reading the other participants' labels.
	Exercise repeated, but this time patients are asked to give a sweet and tender name to the emotion or thought as though naming a puppy.
	Debriefing
Observation distance (observer self)	"Leaves on a stream, I notice that I am having the thought"; other metaphors such as the tug of war with the monster
Homework	Patients commit to a values-based action to be executed before the next group.
Assessment	Re-rate values-behavior consistency on Bullseye exercise.
Evaluation of group by the participants	
Session 4	**Objectives**
Homework review	Debrief each patient's values-based actions
Intention-setting exercise	Thank yourself for what you've done already and what you are prepared to do next: intention for today's class (3 minutes)

Table 9–3.   Session-by-session agendas for an inpatient FACT
group *(continued)*

Session 4 *(continued)*	Objectives
About "self-compassion"	Learning to treat yourself with softness, an alternative to joining in with the inner critic; practicing awareness in the moment automatically leads you toward softness and allows you to keep going toward your life destination.
Compassion exercises	How would you treat a friend who was suffering?
	Wrap yourself in a blue blanket
	How to be "flaw-some"
About willingness	Voluntarily putting yourself in situations that matter to you, even though it puts you in harm's way emotionally
Willingness exercise	Obstacles course to values
Homework	Values-based action within the next 24–48 hours
Assessment	Re-rate Bullseye values-behavior consistency score
Evaluation of the session; future directions (e.g., outpatient ACT, mindfulness groups, individual therapy)	

Note.   FACT=Focused Acceptance and Commitment Therapy.

reassured by the small number of participants and agree more readily to participate. Because of the cognitive impairments often present in the acute phase of a psychiatric illness, patients may have difficulty understanding or retaining instructions concerning certain exercises. Working in a small group makes it easier to hold their attention and to work individually with each participant.

An overarching structure should be created for each group session. This reassures patients who have been uprooted from their usual daily routines and are still adjusting to life on the ward. Every session begins with an intention-setting exercise, which normally involves some type of silent self-reflection, followed by a patient-by-patient review of the between-group "homework" assignment that each participant agrees to (sessions 2–4). As noted in Table 9–3, the content of each session varies considerably as patients learn about the three core therapeutic processes of the ACT model, but the group always ends in the same way. At the end of each session, we ask patients to describe a values-based action they intend to take before the next group session. We then have them complete the Bullseye exercise (session 1) or go back to their completed Bullseye exercise and make a new rating on the "values-behavior consistency" target. Values-behavior consistency scores change surprisingly quickly in a positive direction, given the short duration of the group protocol. We also ask participants to rate the helpfulness of each session and to provide a confidence rating describing the likelihood they will follow through on their values-based homework assignment.

Impressive changes are often observed in patients who complete the FACT group. For some, it may be reflected in an increased openness toward participating in groups; for others, it stimulates a positive change in the therapeutic alliance; and for others, the experiential nature of the exercises helps them realize the negative consequences of using avoidance behaviors in life situations in which they would like to engage in values-based actions. Participation in a FACT group enables patients to redirect their focus from eliminating or controlling unpleasant internal experiences to putting important life priorities ahead of controlling unwanted feelings.

CLINICAL CONSIDERATIONS IN LEADING FACT GROUPS

The first inpatient FACT session may be quite difficult, from the therapist's viewpoint. This may be the first experience in a group therapy setting for some patients, who may have preconceived ideas about groups that make them wary and guarded. The subsequent three sessions run more smoothly because the ice has been broken and patients are reassured about not having to trot out their whole life story in such a public forum. In the third session, we invite patients to write about and share their unpleasant, sometimes shameful thoughts and experiences. Participants are frequently surprised to see how many of them share the same thoughts and emotions. The therapist encourages participants to come up with a sweet and tender name for their unpleasant private experience, asking them to name it as though it were a favorite kitten or puppy. Prior to this, in spite of clear instructions, participants will generally have somewhat diabolical names for their unwanted thoughts, feelings, or memories. The aim of this exercise is to promote acceptance of internal unpleasant experiences, demonstrate the universality of the human mind, encourage perspective-taking, and develop a stance of compassion toward feared and avoided experiences as well as toward oneself.

The cognitive impairment of patients in acute psychiatric distress, as well as medication-related sedation, often results in patients having difficulty grasping the abstract meaning of metaphors or participating in certain ACT experiential exercises. Sometimes, metaphors or experiential exercises may be interpreted in a concrete manner or taken literally by a patient. At the end of one raisin mindfulness exercise, some interesting recipes for raisins marinated in rum were offered by a participant. Patients who intellectualize can experience difficulty with metaphors such as the 180°-turnaround metaphor (see Table 9–3), which is designed to highlight the dangers of trying to make too many changes too fast. Such patients may propose elaborate explanations during debriefing as opposed to directly focusing on the physical experience of trying to rapidly change direction. Several questions and some prompting by group leaders may be required to get the patient to the desired response.

One may have to be more directive in an inpatient group than in an outpatient group, especially when it comes to roleplaying metaphors such as the "passengers on the bus." This metaphor illustrates the consequences and pitfalls of getting hooked on one's thoughts and emotions as well as the costs of avoidance in relation to pursuing one's values in life. It also highlights acceptance by having the driver allow the nasty passengers to ride on the bus without attempting to get them in order. The instructions for this exercise must be clear, explicit, and repeated frequently throughout the roleplay, which can last anywhere from 5 to 10 minutes. Group leaders must ensure the "passengers" are actively guided to develop the appropriate verbal distractions to get the bus driver to stop driving. Similarly, they may need to help "prime" the driver to make statements that reflect acceptance and a willingness to let the passengers "do their thing" while she keeps driving to her desired life destination. Participants sometimes take the instructions quite literally and may begin to physically interfere with the bus driver, bus drivers may forget their original destination, and some group members may be reluctant to play nasty passengers for fear of hurting their unit peers, whom they know by now quite well. Remind group members that this is a make-believe scenario, that they are only playing the content of the driver's mind, and that this will not hurt her. Conducting this physical metaphor exercise can sometimes seem choppy, tedious, and may appear to be futile, but it is remarkable how much participants learn from it. Participants often draw parallels with it during the obstacle course roleplay in the last session of the FACT group.

Sometimes, patients may agree to come to groups but will not actively participate or will refuse to talk or take part in the roleplay exercises. Accept their decision, because sometimes just being there is a step in the right direction for them. Sometimes this can be the very person who steps in and rescues a particularly arduous debriefing session of a roleplay or metaphor by hitting the nail on the head. Sometimes one may think an exercise is going horribly wrong and be tempted to step in and "fix it." One example occurred during a compassion exercise in which participants were first asked to describe how they would behave toward a friend in difficulty and then toward themselves. The aim of the exercise was to illustrate the discrepancy in one's behavior toward others (kind and comforting) versus oneself (harsh, judgmental, and punitive). One patient described how she would help a friend in difficulty in what seemed to be a very harsh and firm way. The group leader resisted the urge to intervene to ascertain if the patient had misunderstood the exercise, and in the second part, the patient described how she would relate to her own problems by pulling out her hair, screaming at herself, and banging her head against the wall while berating herself in a very derogatory manner. By comparison, her behavior toward her friend was relatively kind and gentle, and this stark contrast enabled the group leaders to see the extent of her harshness toward herself. Similarly, with mindfulness exercises, patients often continue to talk about pushing away their thoughts or trying to empty their mind of negative experiences. Although tactfully correcting these misconceptions is important, do not be too rigid about what is right and wrong and just be willing to recognize that in a short-stay inpatient unit, one is planting seeds that with further nourishment will one day germinate.

Sometimes, a patient's dysfunctional, unworkable behavior may be so ingrained that the patient has lost sight of its original function. One participant was adamant that the onset of his addictive behavior had been festive in origin and that using drugs and alcohol was not a strategy to avoid or escape from unpleasant feelings. He maintained that only in recent years, when his life stress level went way up, did using drugs and alcohol function as an avoidance behavior. When this was explored further in a curious and open manner, he discovered that a lot of his early addictive behaviors were in the service of sensation-seeking designed to help him avoid his intolerance of boredom and a feeling of emptiness.

ADJUNCTIVE ACT GROUPS FOR SELF-STIGMA AND MEDICATION ADHERENCE

Other ACT-oriented groups address the important clinical issues of self-stigma and nonadherence with treatment plans. These groups may run concurrently with the four-session FACT group. Again, some overlap and repetition between groups will occur, but this is useful because it enables patients to become more skilled at assessing the workability of their behaviors, being in the present moment, and practicing accepting, values-based, and compassionate responses toward themselves.

Stigma plays a major negative role in promoting self-defeating behaviors that may put the individual at risk for rehospitalization. As the old saying goes, people tend to live "down" to any derogatory label applied to them. In other clinical contexts, ACT has been shown to be a powerful treatment package for reducing stigma toward others as well as oneself. Hence, an important part of the ACT inpatient protocol is to aggressively undermine the stigmatizing attitudes and behavior of patients as well as the ward staff who care for them.

The stigma group consists of a single 90-minute session. The group's aim is enabling patients to take perspective on the way others (e.g., family, friends, work colleagues) view them because of their illness and on the manner in which they label themselves. Psychiatric inpatients often identify themselves as weak, inferior, and damaged. Overidentification with these provocative evaluations may result in feelings of shame and anxiety and exacerbate unhealthy, self-defeating avoidance behaviors (e.g., substance use, social withdrawal). In most cases, self-stigma is just an internalized version of the stigmatizing attitudes and behaviors of other players in the patient's social context. Although we cannot prevent others from engaging in stigmatizing behaviors, patients have some level of choice as to whether they choose to overidentify with these beliefs. Thus, the main focus of the stigma group is to help target and reduce *self-stigmatizing* behaviors. Functional analysis is repeatedly used to highlight environmental sources as well as the costs of self-stigma. Mindfulness exercises are used to promote awareness of stigma-based fear and shame—to highlight the alternative stance of self-acceptance and choosing to dis-identify oneself from any labels, diagnostic or otherwise, that have had a stigmatizing impact. One patient expressed a sense of relief after a perspective-taking exercise during which he realized he had several roles in life that had little or nothing to do with his struggles with bipolar symptoms. He had previously assumed everyone in every life context was responding to him based on the fact that he was "bipolar." During the perspective-taking exercise, he realized that what he had assumed to be other people's beliefs was actually his own inner critic chattering at him.

In the inpatient protocol, patients participate in a 90-minute ACT-oriented psychoeducation group on treatment adherence. This group teaches them to manage their own treatment using the measuring rods of workability and values-based living and to explore obstacles and behaviors that lead to nonadherence. Although the main emphasis of the group is on medication adherence, topics also include developing a healthy lifestyle through increased physical activity, making good dietary choices, and creating positive sources of social interaction.

The medication adherence group uses the ACT Matrix model (see Chapter 4). It helps patients notice the function of their behaviors and is a concrete way of showing how various behaviors may move them toward (values based) or away from (avoidance based) what is important to them in life. A matrix session may highlight the fact that taking prescribed medication allows patients to have more control over their lives and to move closer to their values. Another point of emphasis in the group is to explore the "legitimate" reasons patients have for stopping their medications. Patients may stop medication because of the fear or actual experience of unpleasant side effects, which they may or may not feel empowered to mention to their prescribing physician. The "reality" of taking a prescribed psychotropic medication is that the benefits of the medicine must be balanced against the risks. When patients feel emotionally unstable and unable to function, the benefits of taking a medication are so obvious that the risks, including the risk of side effects, dwindle in comparison. Once patients are partially or fully recovered, however, the balance between benefit and risk often will shift to the risk side. The ACT framework emphasizes that this is a natural human response. In other words, issues related to nonadherence are treated objectively by the group leaders, with curiosity and nonjudgment, rather than used as a basis for blaming and shaming patients.

TIPS FOR SUCCESS

An ACT inpatient program is centered around the philosophy that, although responding to and managing what can be severe symptoms of distress is important, the main goal of treatment is to improve patients' functional status and quality of life in their natural surroundings.

Biological interventions are delivered within a functional psychiatry framework, in which the goal is to target symptoms that interfere with real-life functioning.

Psychiatric diagnoses can be useful in professional contexts and discussions but are cautiously discussed at the patient–psychiatrist level due to the potential for patients to respond to such labels with passivity, self-blame, and pessimism.

Begin delivering the ACT "message" at the time of the initial admission interview with the attending psychiatrist and consistently thereafter during all sessions and meetings with members of the clinical care team.

A well-balanced inpatient program offers ACT interventions at the individual and group therapy and unit activity levels, requiring all members of the clinical care team, as well as unit staff, to be conversant in and comfortable with core ACT principles.

Short-term ACT groups are a particularly useful and powerful form of adjunctive therapy and are generally well liked by inpatient residents.

ACT-based groups that focus on self-stigmatizing attitudes and behaviors as well as medication adherence, placed in the context of
values-based chosen behaviors, can be highly impactful additions to
an inpatient program.

ACT Delivered in the Context of Unit Activities

Regardless of how many individual or group therapy sessions are delivered to any particular patient, the vast majority of the time spent by patients during an inpatient stay will be on the unit, mixing it up with other
inpatients and members of the unit staff. Indeed, members of the unit
nursing and support staff have by far the most contact with patients.
This means an effective inpatient ACT protocol must prepare unit staff
to function as ACT practitioners in their own right. This generally requires all unit staff receive training in, and exhibit buy-in to, the ACT
model. In Chapter 10, we examine the complexities of training unit staff
and offer a set of practical guidelines for doing so. For present purposes,
we simply highlight a few of the ways members of the unit staff can contribute to the creation of a hopeful, empowering ACT treatment milieu.

At the unit level, patients participate in daily, staff-guided mindful
movement sessions and controlled breathing exercises. Nursing staff can
run stand-alone sessions on communication skills, values, and committed action. All unit staff take turns leading a once-weekly "open forum"
psychoeducational class focusing on any issues that have arisen for patients on the ward. Again, the ACT Matrix approach is used, because it
is a practical and useful format for guiding these open forums. The following dialogue is taken from one such general unit meeting where the
focus was on learning to gauge the workability of behaviors. It illustrates
how the ACT Matrix can be used to reveal the "toward" or "away" functions of behavior and teach patients to notice distressing, unwanted experiences as simply events in the mind.

Patient 1: When I get anxious, I pray.
Staff member: How does praying work for you? What happens when
    you pray?
Patient 1: I don't think about the anxiety I have inside.
Staff member: When you stop praying, what happens then?
Patient 1: I feel anxious again.
Staff member: So, praying helps you in the short term but not in the
    long term. Where would you position praying on the matrix?
Patient 1: The top left-hand corner.
Patient 2: Isn't praying good? Some people are religious and are believ-
    ers, and prayer is important for them. There's nothing wrong with
    praying, is there?

Staff member: Of course there's nothing wrong with praying. It's the function of praying or the purpose it serves that's important. If you're religious and your relationship with God is important, and you pray to nourish your faith and bring you closer to your spiritual values, then prayer would go in the top right-hand corner. It's a positive behavior that helps you feel healthy inside. However, if you're praying to distract yourself so you don't have to feel your anxiety, then prayer serves the purpose of avoidance. In that case, it would go in the top left-hand corner. This isn't about whether praying is right or wrong, good or bad. It's about the purpose behind praying in the first place. Take, for example, staying in bed all day. If one is really physically exhausted or has a bad case of the flu and stays in bed during the day, where would you put that behavior?

Patient 2: In the top right-hand corner?

Staff member: Right! But if you're depressed, don't want to see anyone, and stay in bed all day even though you feel even more tired and depressed at the end of the day, where would you put that kind of staying in bed?

Patient 3: It could also go on the right top because it helps me rest up when I'm too depressed and too tired to do anything.

Patient 4: Yes, I have no energy and can't do anything when I'm depressed. Being in bed is the only place where I feel safe. When I sleep, I get some relief from my depression and worries.

Staff member: So, there's a feeling of being safe and having some relief from your mind when you're in bed as well as getting some rest. How does staying in bed work for you when you use it that way? Do you notice yourself feeling less tired and more chipper at the end of the day?

Patient 4: No, the tiredness doesn't go away; sometimes I feel even worse, and then I feel guilty and disgusted with myself for not doing all the things I should have done.

Patient 3: When I do it, it really irks my family.

Staff member: So, you notice that staying in bed does not restore your energy and you may even end up feeling more tired; it provides even more ammunition for your inner critic; and it annoys family members. In some ways, the solution of staying in bed has become a new problem. Where would you put staying in bed on the matrix?

Patient 4: In the top left-hand corner. It's an away move.

Staff member: Yes, notice the same behavior can be on both sides of the matrix. It's not staying in bed that's wrong, it's why you do it, what you're trying to achieve by doing it. So did staying in bed give you the result you hoped for or not?

Patient 5: That may be true for some of you, but I know there are times I feel so bad I just can't get out of bed, it's impossible. I know I'm not capable of doing it.

Staff member: Yes, sometimes in a bad depression the thought of getting out of bed is akin to the thought of climbing Mount Everest, and that can be a very painful experience. Just out of curiosity, where would you position the thought "I can't get out of bed, it's impossible; I know I'm not capable of doing it" on the matrix?

Patient 5: I guess it would be in the lower left part. It's an away-move type thought, right?

Summary

In this chapter, we demonstrated how ACT can be integrated into the daily routine of inpatient unit programs designed for short (5- to 7-day) inpatient stays. Thus far, the feedback from patients is favorable, and patient outcomes are much improved. More importantly, unit staff like the ACT model because of its humane, optimistic approach to patient care. ACT integrates well with and complements other therapeutic approaches often used on inpatient units, such as the "recovery" approach, which, like ACT, does not focus on symptom resolution but on the possibility for people with mental illness to lead meaningful lives in the presence of symptoms. Focusing efforts on strengthening the core processes underpinning psychological resilience opens up new avenues that can prevent both the psychiatrist and the patient from getting stuck in an avoidance-based agenda of symptom control and elimination.

Practicing ACT as an inpatient psychiatrist is highly gratifying and rewarding and gives meaning to the decision to pursue a career in psychiatry, particularly if one works in one of those all-too-familiar poorly resourced inpatient facilities where serious mental illness is rampant in the patient population and where a fatalistic attitude can insidiously install itself in treatment staff. It is essential to keep hope alive in staff and in patients; sometimes, temporarily, staff members become repositories of hope for their patients. At this point in our journey into the subtleties of inpatient-based ACT, it would be nice to find something deep, meaningful, and unforgettable to say, but for want of inspiration, Victor Hugo will have the last words: "There is nothing like a dream to create the future."

The Essentials

- A unit-wide ACT protocol can be a powerful adjunct to other forms of psychiatric management during an inpatient stay. ACT has been shown to improve the outcomes of inpatient treatment.
- The ACT protocol consists of individual treatment sessions conducted by various members of the treatment team, ACT delivered in a brief group therapy format, stand-alone groups addressing

self-stigma and medication adherence, and ACT Matrix interventions delivered by nursing staff as part of general ward meetings.

- An ACT process-based approach can be integrated into the initial admission interview by the attending psychiatrist.
- Use functional psychiatric diagnosis in a way that empowers patient engagement and minimizes the likelihood patients will react with passivity and pessimism and feel helpless and hopeless about their prospects for living a vital life.
- Medications can be used in a way that reinforces emotional avoidance or one that promotes patients' values and ability to function in life areas that matter.
- Four-session FACT groups are popular with patients and produce surprisingly strong results.
- Brief ACT groups can also focus on such topics as reducing self-stigma or adhering to medications.
- The ACT Matrix is a valuable tool for educating patients in the core processes of the ACT model and can easily be implemented by nursing staff with minimal training.
- All unit staff members are considered ACT providers, although roles and responsibilities will differ, and play a key role in delivering ACT-consistent patient education on a day-in, day-out basis.

Suggested Reading

Frögéli E, Djordjevic A, Rudman A, et al: A randomized controlled pilot trial of acceptance and commitment training (ACT) for preventing stress-related ill health among future nurses. Anxiety Stress Coping 29(2):202–218, 2016 25759942

Johns LC, Oliver JE, Khondoker M, et al: The feasibility and acceptability of a brief acceptance and commitment therapy (ACT) group intervention for people with psychosis: the 'ACT for life' study. J Behav Ther Exp Psychiatry 50:257–263, 2016 26480469

O'Donoghue E, Morris E, Oliver J, et al: ACT for Psychosis Recovery: A Practical Manual for Group Based Interventions Using Acceptance and Commitment Therapy. Oakland, CA, New Harbinger, 2018

Smallwood RF, Potter JS, Robin DA: Neurophysiological mechanisms in acceptance and commitment therapy in opioid-addicted patients with chronic pain. Psychiatry Res Neuroimaging 250:12–14, 2016 27107155

References

Bach P, Hayes SC: The use of acceptance and commitment therapy to prevent the rehospitalization of psychotic patients: a randomized controlled trial. J Consult Clin Psychol 70(5):1129–1139, 2002 12362963

Bach P, Hayes SC, Gallop R: Long-term effects of brief acceptance and commitment therapy for psychosis. Behav Modif 36(2):165–181, 2012

Ducasse D, René E, Béziat S, et al: Acceptance and commitment therapy for management of suicidal patients: a pilot study. Psychother Psychosom 83(6):374–376, 2014 25323551

Gaudiano BA, Herbert JD: Acute treatment of inpatients with psychotic symptoms using acceptance and commitment therapy: pilot results. Behav Res Ther 44(3):415–437, 2006 15893293

Gaudiano BA, Nowlan K, Brown LA, et al: An open trial of a new acceptance-based behavioral treatment for major depression with psychotic features. Behav Modif 37(3):324–355, 2013

Gaudiano BA, Davis CH, Epstein-Lubow G, et al: Acceptance and commitment therapy for inpatients with psychosis (the REACH Study): protocol for treatment development and pilot testing. Healthcare (Basel) 5(2):1–17, 2017 28475123

Jacob KS: Recovery model of mental illness: a complementary approach to psychiatric care. Indian J Psychol Med 37(2):117–119, 2015 25969592

Khoury B, Lecomte T, Gaudiano BA, et al: Mindfulness interventions for psychosis: a meta-analysis. Schizophr Res 150(1):176–184, 2013 23954146

Leamy M, Bird V, Le Boutillier C, et al: Conceptual framework for personal recovery in mental health: systematic review and narrative synthesis. Br J Psychiatry 199(6):445–452, 2011 22130746

Petersen C, Zettle R: Treating inpatients with comorbid depression and alcohol use disorder: a comparison of acceptance and commitment therapy versus treatment as usual. Psychol Rec 59(4):521–536, 2009

Prosser A, Helfer B, Leucht S: Biological v. psychosocial treatments: a myth about pharmacotherapy v. psychotherapy. Br J Psychiatry 208(4):309–311, 2016

Strosahl K, Robinson P, Gustavsson T: Brief Interventions for Radical Change. Oakland, CA, New Harbinger, 2012

Thekiso TB, Murphy P, Milnes J, et al: Acceptance and commitment therapy in the treatment of alcohol use disorder and comorbid affective disorder: a pilot matched control trial. Behav Ther 46(6):717–728, 2015 26520216

Tohen M, Hennen J, Zarate CM Jr, et al: Two-year syndromal and functional recovery in 219 cases of first-episode major affective disorder with psychotic features. Am J Psychiatry 157(2):220–228, 2000 10671390

Tyrberg MJ, Carlbring P, Lundgren T: Brief acceptance and commitment therapy for psychotic inpatients: a randomized controlled feasibility trial in Sweden. Nordic Psychology 69(2):110–125, 2017a

Tyrberg MJ, Carlbring P, Lundgren T: Implementation of acceptance and commitment therapy training in a psychiatric ward: feasibility, lessons learned and potential effectiveness. Journal of Psychiatric Intensive Care 13(2):73–82, 2017b

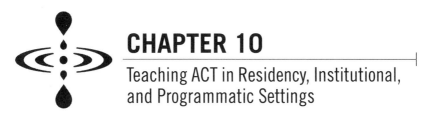

CHAPTER 10

Teaching ACT in Residency, Institutional, and Programmatic Settings

Vision, without action, is a daydream. Action, without vision, is a nightmare.

—Chinese saying

ACT is still in its relative infancy, having first appeared on the scene in 1999 with the introduction of the first comprehensive ACT text, now in its second edition (Hayes et al. 2011). Significant lag time always occurs between the introduction of a new clinical model and the uptake of the model within existing graduate medical education curricula. Thus, in many medical schools and psychiatric residency programs, systematic training in ACT is either not available at all or in the earliest stages of design. Even if several medical school or residency faculty members become interested in ACT, the tasks of building faculty knowledge and skill; developing training curricula for medical students, residents, and fellows in the basic theoretical principles of ACT; and ensuring clinical competency with ACT assessment, case conceptualization, and clinical intervention methods can be daunting.

Similarly, affiliated psychiatric health professionals, such as psychiatric nurses and nursing or medical assistants, may have received no training in the ACT approach during their clinical education. In these cases, the task becomes how best to add to their existing therapeutic repertoire so they can deliver ACT in the course of their normal job duties with a reasonably high level of fidelity to the model. In many institutional (inpatient psychiatric unit, partial/day hospital) or programmatic (day treatment, crisis respite care) settings, where the desire is to programmatically adopt the ACT approach, the intervention activities of all members of the multidisciplinary interprofessional staff must be consistent, regardless of who is interacting with the patient.

In this chapter, we address training issues and provide some possible solutions for each of these two very different domains. We start by examining how to integrate an ACT training component within a psychiatric residency context. We introduce a core competency training model that is highly consistent with the new milestones framework adopted by the Accreditation Committee for Graduate Medical Education (ACGME). The benefit of this core competencies approach is that ACT skills training can be integrated within the larger competency-based framework of the milestones approach, thus allowing ACT principles and techniques to be taught without creating unnecessary disruptions in existing residency program curricula.

Second, we examine some of the challenges involved in implementing an ACT treatment program for psychiatric inpatients or patients participating in a partial hospital or day-treatment program. This type of hospital-based initiative often not only involves the need to train unit staff in basic ACT principles but also requires the psychiatrist to create organizational buy-in for the ACT approach among hospital administrators and various hospital bureaucracies that might be entrenched in another or an "old way" of doing things. One of us (J.L.) has been involved in an ongoing process of creating an inpatient affective disorders unit in which ACT is the main treatment approach. We share the "learnings" from this initiative here, for those readers who might be interested in starting an ACT program within the inpatient context.

The Three Prongs of Residency-Based ACT Training

In this section, we examine three different educational components of ACT training that can be utilized either individually or in combination within a psychiatric residency program. Briefly, these three basic components are

1. Targeted source readings
2. Didactic education and behavioral rehearsal-based skill building
3. Practice-based core competencies training

Programs that implement only one of these components are likely to see less robust training effects than those that carefully integrate and balance all three components over the course of the residency experience. At the same time, the pragmatic reality facing most residency programs is that new residents are expected to acquire many different skills during their residency, and competing training needs often restrict the amount of ACT training that can be delivered in that time. Thus, our recommended approach involves "piggy-backing" ACT training onto other educational and training activities in which residents are already expected to participate. In some cases (e.g., functional psychopharmacology, contextual assessment), the ACT approach might be integrated with existing required educational curricula (e.g., general psychopharmacology, diagnostic psychiatric interviewing) to create a bigger "tool kit" for the young psychiatrist to use in practice. As we have stressed throughout the book, ACT is not in an "either/or" position with respect to more traditional forms of psychiatric practice; it is better thought of as a useful adjunctive approach that gives the psychiatrist additional leverage to enhance patient outcomes.

TARGET SOURCE READINGS

Until education and training in ACT becomes a regular component of medical school, it is safe ti assume that new psychiatric residents will have little, if any, exposure to the basic science underpinning ACT; the core principles of functional psychiatry or functional psychopharmacology; or the ACT clinical model proper. Thus, the educational process should start with residents being required to at least "speed-read" some basic source texts, which are outlined in Table 10–1.

Table 10–1. Core components of an ACT training program for psychiatric residents

Source text	ACT-relevant topic focus
Learning Acceptance and Commitment Therapy: The Essential Guide to the Process and Practice of Mindful Psychiatry (current book)	General overview of the basic science underpinning ACT, principles of functional psychiatry and behavioral psychopharmacology, and the core therapeutic mechanisms of the ACT model
Learning RFT: An Introduction to Relational Frame Theory and Its Clinical Application (Törneke 2010)	Introduces relational frame theory (RFT) in a "clinician friendly" way; allows for a basic understanding of the core, clinically relevant aspects of RFT
Brief Interventions for Radical Change: Principles and Practice of Focused Acceptance and Commitment Therapy (Strosahl et al. 2012)	Introduces ACT-consistent interviewing methods, case conceptualization models, and brief intervention strategies that fit the time demands of typical psychiatric practice
Learning ACT: An Acceptance and Commitment Therapy Skills Training Manual for Therapists, 2nd Edition (Luoma et al. 2017)	Self-guided training system for learning the core ACT processes that create psychological flexibility and methods for intervening with each of these processes

The resident's academic advisor and faculty preceptors should be willing and able to conduct impromptu "knowledge quizzes" about the "big ideas" surrounding the relational frame theory approach, the practice of functional psychiatry and functional psychopharmacology, and the core therapeutic mechanisms of ACT. This level of preparedness presumes faculty will also be familiar with these "big ideas."

DIDACTIC EDUCATION AND BEHAVIORAL REHEARSAL

It is becoming an increasingly accepted educational principle that medical residents learn much less when exposed to passive didactic training as compared with being required to engage in simultaneous or sequential learning activities designed to facilitate practice skills. This recognition has prompted widespread use of simulation labs in resident training across diverse disciplines and subdisciplines. As applied to psychiatric residents, this principle suggests that core didactic training in ACT is best achieved by having residents "learn a little" and "practice a lot." Rather than trying to introduce the entire ACT framework in a passive didactic lecture, a better approach is to break the ACT clinical approach down into manageable pieces that can be introduced one at a time, followed by dyadic or small-group roleplaying of core ACT skills.

The CARE framework (see Chapter 4) is an ideal way to "chunk" the ACT model, because one skill set in the CARE approach typically leads into the next. Thus, a simple framework for skill acquisition that is easy to understand and follow is available to psychiatric residents who are intent on learning ACT. Instructors should circulate among the practice groups during dyadic skill training and offer feedback and corrective modeling as needed. The quality of high-definition cameras on modern smartphones provides another positive source of learning: roleplays can be recorded in real time, with post-roleplay reviews being conducted in small groups or with the participation of the course instructor.

As mentioned, our recommended approach is to break ACT training down into "bite-sized" pieces. This allows for a more in-depth educational approach that leads to more refined, targeted skill building. Table 10–2 presents a four-session ACT didactic/skill training series that could be applied sequentially over the course of a residency year.

We recognize that the typical residency didactic schedule is very tight, and fitting four discrete learning sessions into a residency year may not be possible. The admittedly pragmatic guiding principle we try to follow is to have as many ACT didactic sessions on the schedule as possible and divide the content up accordingly. Also, having advanced residents attend the same series of ACT didactic training each year is not necessarily a bad thing. Individuals rarely master core ACT skills in just one training session, so repeated exposure to these same basic skills is a

Table 10–2. A four-session ACT training curriculum for psychiatric residents

Didactic session	Topics	Roleplaying exercises
Session 1: Context	Importance of context/functional analysis of presenting problems; change-oriented interviewing principles and strategies	*Mock patient interview:* Perform a full contextual and functional analytic assessment of the patient's presenting problems integrated within a typical differential diagnostic interview
Session 2: Avoidance	Recognizing and undermining patterns of avoidance; establishing impacts of avoidance with respect to patient values	*Mock patient interview:* Detect and bring patient into contact with examples of emotional and behavioral avoidance; initiate a "counter" conversation about the patient's values in life and the cost of following avoidance rules
Session 3: Reformulating and reframing rules	Reframing the patient's problem in a new light; using metaphors, physical exercises; creating values-based rule-following; changing the function of avoidance rules so they become approach rules	*Mock patient interview:* Practice redefining the patient's presenting problem from a values-based perspective and normalizing emotional pain as a reflection of what matters to the patient
Session 4: Experimenting	Guidelines for creating and conducting powerful behavior-change experiments; empowering and motivating patients to engage in self-directed behavior change	*Mock patient interview:* Help the patient identify "examples" of values-based approach behaviors; follow principles of strategic change and patient engagement; practice creating highly specific behavior-change plans with patient buy-in for follow through

positive educational strategy. In addition, residents who have already gone through the didactic/skill-building exercises in previous years can take on the mantle of "coach" for the new resident. Our experience has shown that being a coach or teacher often increases not only the student's skills but also the teacher's.

PRACTICE-BASED CORE COMPETENCY TRAINING

The new ACGME standards require psychiatric residents to demonstrate proficiency with at least two different systems of psychotherapy: supportive, psychodynamic, or cognitive-behavioral. The milestones model adopted by the ACGME assumes that psychotherapy training is both structured and ongoing across the course of residency training, allowing the learning process to be developmental. Such developmentally acquired skills continue to evolve long after the psychiatrist has left the residency environment.

Whereas some approaches to cognitive-behavioral therapy are more narrowly focused and will satisfy the requirements of one or two milestones, the contextual science underpinnings of ACT suggest it might be an appropriate vehicle for helping the typical psychiatric resident meet the standards for a larger span of milestones. For example, ACT includes developing skills associated with a functional analytic approach to psychiatric assessment and diagnosis and involves a rather unique approach to the practice of psychopharmacology. Then, the system of ACT contextual interviewing, case analysis, and clinical interventions is nested within the larger umbrella of functional psychiatry. ACT has also been studied and shown to be effective within a diverse array of racial and ethnic groups. Thus, we would argue that the time invested in training psychiatry residents in ACT, compared with other, more narrowly defined systems of psychotherapy, will have a greater impact on the development of general psychiatry skills.

Another salient feature of contextual behavioral science and the behavior analytic tradition underpins the ACT approach to training: the ability to conduct high-quality ACT is directly related to the use of specific, observable skills (i.e., psychiatrist behaviors) that can be assessed, improved upon, and mastered over time. We henceforth refer to these specific, observable skills as *core competencies*. These are the clinical skills that matter most in the application of the ACT model.

 Clinical Tool 23: ACT Core Competency Tool for Psychiatric Residents

---

Table 10–3 presents a framework for evaluating the core competencies that go into making up a competent ACT clinician. Thirty-two individual competencies are grouped into four basic practice domains (i.e.,

Table 10–3. ACT core competency tool for psychiatric residents

Rating: 1=poor; 2=developmental; 3=meets expectations; 4=exceeds expectations.

General interviewing competencies (milestone: PC 1, PC 4)	Rating
1. Communicates genuine belief that patient can engage in meaningful change at any point.	
2. Able to complete CARE interview sequence while conducting a casual conversation with patient.	
3. Able to integrate, summarize, and provide feedback on biomedical, psychological, and social aspects of patient complaints during clinical interview.	
4. Maintains brisk conversational pace and uses strategic questions to engage patient.	
5. Able to use interview strategies to locate and amplify sources of emotional pain for patient.	
6. Models stance of openness, nonjudgment, and curiosity during interview.	

Functional assessment competencies (milestones: PC 2, PC 4, PC 5, MK 1)	Rating
7. Implements streamlined contextual and functional assessment that is seamlessly integrated within psychiatric interview.	
8. Balances focus of assessment between symptoms, functional status, and quality of life.	
9. Able to isolate and analyze functional impairments that might be targeted by medications.	
10. Conducts evaluation of medication impacts by repeatedly measuring changes in functionally relevant patient behaviors targeted by medication.	
11. Conducts problem severity assessment early in each visit (1–10).	
12. Demonstrates ability to identify behavioral and emotional avoidance strategies.	
13. Able to uncover "cost" of avoidance by engaging patient in brief values clarification.	
14. Nonjudgmentally provides feedback about results of unworkable avoidance strategies.	

Table 10–3. ACT core competency tool for psychiatric residents *(continued)*

Case formulation competencies (milestones: PC 3, PC 5, MK 2)	Rating
15. Accurately conducts four-quadrant and/or flexibility profile analyses to profile patient's strengths and weaknesses.	
16. Accurately analyzes information from clinical interview within the CARE framework.	
17. Able to conceptualize and synthesize patient complaints within both functional contextual and biomedical frameworks.	
18. Accurately identifies treatable sources of functional impairment in patient's life context.	
19. Formulates appropriate functional targets for medication interventions.	

Clinical intervention and management competencies (milestones: PC 4, PC 5, MK 4)	Rating
20. Educates patient/significant others on complementary nature of somatic and behavioral interventions.	
21. Creates dialogue that both validates and changes patient's perspective on presenting problem.	
22. Selects, prescribes, and changes medication based upon observed impacts on functional targets.	
23. Demonstrates ability to activate core ACT therapeutic mechanisms.	
24. Helps patient "stay present" and function in an observer role.	
25. Helps patient practice acceptance of difficult internal and external experiences.	
26. Teaches patient to practice nonjudgment and nonreactivity.	
27. Teaches perspective-taking skills that allow patient to short-circuit unworkable self-stories.	
28. Helps patient make contact with deeply held values for living.	
29. Helps patient identify and experiment with new values-consistent approach behaviors.	
30. Moves flexibly among themes of workability, openness, and engagement.	
31. Follows principles of "small change" when designing interventions with patient.	
32. Collects confidence and helpfulness ratings at end of each session; adjusts goals as needed.	

Note. MK=medical knowledge; PC=patient care and procedural skills.

general interviewing, functional assessment, case formulation, clinical intervention and management). Each domain also relates specifically to certain ACGME milestones, allowing evaluations from ACT core competency training to be integrated with other sources of information pertaining to a resident's progress toward meeting those same milestones.

Any particular therapy session conducted by a psychiatric resident can be thought of as an exhibition of the resident's relative strengths and weaknesses with respect to individual core competencies or the larger domains within which they are nested. This feature of the ACT training system allows the trainer/supervisor to change the focus of supervision from one meeting to the next. A narrow focus will result in one or two specific skills being demonstrated and then applied by the resident. A broad focus might involve talking with the resident about the overall flow, or transition, between one subgroup of core competencies and another across the entirety of the session. Thus, a core competencies framework allows the trainer/supervisor to "zoom in" (micro therapy skills) or "zoom out" (macro therapy skills) during any particular supervision dialogue. Table 10–4 presents an example of a microskill-focused core competencies checklist—in this case, those required to meet competency standards specified in item 7 of the global competency scale ("Implements streamlined contextual and functional assessment that is seamlessly integrated within psychiatric interview" [see Table 10–3]). Many basic ACT clinical competencies can be approached in this manner: small therapist behaviors combine to create a larger core therapeutic process.

 Clinical Tool 24: Contextual Interviewing Microskills Evaluation

---

The core competencies approach also allows the trainer/supervisor to create a highly specific, customized plan of learning for each resident. Because ACT is a collection of many discrete therapist behaviors, individual differences in core competencies are to be expected. The goal is to be able to describe with some degree of precision the areas of strengths and weakness for each resident so an overall learning plan can be developed and revised as the profile of strengths and weaknesses changes with training and supervision. One resident may be adept at modeling curiosity, openness, acceptance, and mindfulness but struggle with case analysis and subsequently get lost when the time comes to deliver a targeted ACT intervention. A second resident may struggle with therapeutic relationship skills but have the natural ability to devise novel, creative ways to look at a patient's problem and what intervention would likely work. Both residents will struggle to deliver high-quality ACT interventions, but for different reasons. The first has established a solid working relationship with the patient but does not know how to capitalize on it.

Table 10–4.   Contextual interviewing microskills evaluation

Rating: 1=poor; 2=developmental; 3=meets expectations; 4=exceeds expectations.	
Love-work-play component	Rating
Establishes patient's living situation (who is in the home?)	
Establishes patient's relationship status (dating, married, single)	
Asks which family members are important in patient's life	
Asks who, if anyone, is a close friend (best friend, distant, online)	
Asks if any spiritual beliefs, practices, or philosophies impact patient's life	
Establishes source(s) of income (employment, student loans, Social Security)	
Discovers at least one pleasurable or fun activity for patient, present or past	
Health-protective behaviors component	Rating
Asks patient about sleep habits and sleep quality	
Asks patient about diet (home-cooked, fast food, fresh produce)	
Asks patient about exercise habits	
Health-risk behaviors component	Rating
Asks if patient ingests caffeine; if so, asks how much	
Asks if patient uses any tobacco products; if so, asks how much	
Asks if patient uses alcohol; if so, asks how much	
Asks if patient uses marijuana; if so, asks how much	
Asks if patient uses street drugs (opioids, cocaine, methamphetamine); if so, what kind and how much	
Problem analysis component	Rating
Asks when patient's current problem(s) started and current "triggers"	
Asks about things that make the problem worse and things that make it better	
Gathers brief history of problem: how has it developed over time; does it ebb and flow or is it always there; how severe is it right now relative to other times (better, about the same, or worse)	

Table 10–4. Contextual interviewing microskills
evaluation *(continued)*

Problem analysis component (*continued*)	Rating
Asks how problem is affecting important areas of living, how others in patient's life are reacting or are being affected	
Asks about patient's previous attempts to solve problem: What has worked? What hasn't worked?	
Asks what the patient's life would be like if the problem miraculously disappeared: What would the patient be doing differently in life? What would be important to patient?	

The second knows what to do but has not created a sufficiently strong relationship with the patient to get the patient to agree to try something different. By using the core competencies approach to "profile" each resident, the trainer/supervisor can avoid the pitfall of taking a "one size fits all" training approach. If training activities are matched to specific observed skill deficits on a resident-by-resident basis, the yield from what are often a very limited number of supervision hours can be significantly increased.

The emphasis in the core competencies approach on assessing observable behaviors helps the trainer/supervisor avoid another common pitfall: the tendency to talk about cases and hear verbal summaries of the resident's clinical activities without being able to confirm that these reports are accurate. Verbal summaries of patient–psychiatrist clinical dialogues, assessments, or intervention activities are basically socially constructed narratives designed to gain the supervisor's approval and thus are probably not accurate or complete analyses of what actually happened in the session. As long as the resident says the right things in the right order, no negative consequences will ensue. The highly general nature of these "explanations" does not do justice to the complexities of the in-session therapy environment, however. Most trainees do not "see" which clinical activities they engage do not work or diminish the patient's level of engagement. Indeed, therapists from all of the different mental health disciplines tend to overrate how well they are doing therapy and how well a patient is responding. This simple human truth makes ongoing clinical training and supervision a critical aspect of residency education.

Fortunately, the core competencies approach compels the trainer/supervisor to use whatever observational strategies are feasible in the clinical practice setting. Skill ratings really cannot be assigned on the basis of anything else. Direct observational assessments can only be made by using such strategies as conducting conjoint therapy sessions with the resident or directly observing him in practice, either by sitting in on the session as a "fly on the wall," viewing the session through a one-way mirror, or reviewing a video recording of the session. If none of these strategies is available, then engaging the resident in a simulated roleplay of a particular issue that has arisen during therapy is an option. Any training activity that requires residents to actively demonstrate core competencies is preferable to just talking about clinical cases. Of course, some clinical issues require verbal processing, such as when a resident's personal issues are functioning as barriers in the therapy process. Even then, after working through these issues, conducting a roleplay in which the resident demonstrates a new way of responding may be useful to unlock any therapeutic impasse.

Pre- (beginning of residency year) and post- (end of residency year) core competencies assessments are also a common practice designed to summarize a resident's general level of progress with learning psychotherapy approaches, including the ACT model. In this case, the results will be of great interest to the residency's clinical review committee, because each of the larger domains of ACT clinical competency is linked to specific milestones. In these more general evaluation exercises, the resident and the trainer/supervisor must be in sync in terms of how they see the resident's skill development process unfolding. To help create this shared viewpoint, they may find it useful to blindly and independently complete the core competencies rating system and then compare and contrast the results on an item-by-item and domain-by-domain basis. Ideally, both sets of ratings will be similar, with only a few minor deviations to discuss. However, if the ratings are very dissimilar across the board, this could be a sign of bad things to come, particularly if the resident consistently produces higher skill ratings than the trainer/supervisor. That being said, the advantage of using a behaviorally anchored core competencies system is that any disagreements will be focused on specific, observable, and assessable resident behaviors. Disagreements are less likely to be about vague, subjective matters that cannot really be resolved in a way that puts the disagreement to rest.

Another, far more positive scenario involves across-the-board discrepancies in core competency ratings in which residents underrate their skillfulness compared with ratings by the trainer/supervisor. This tends to occur in highly motivated, somewhat perfectionistic residents who use self-criticism as a primary source of motivation. Here, the trainer/supervisor might find a light touch of ACT to be useful for the resident to apply to herself. For example, residents might be encouraged to take a more self-compassionate stance toward their own personal flaws or imperfections. Whatever the outcome of the yearly core competencies evaluation process is, the last part of the evaluation sequence is for the trainer/supervisor and the resident to formulate a skill development plan for the next residency year. This helps anchor the training and supervision process and ensure everyone involved is working toward the same shared goals.

TIPS FOR SUCCESS

Teaching ACT in a psychiatric residency context is made easier by the fact that the ACT model incorporates and adds a functional component to such basic psychiatric skills as interviewing, case conceptualization, and pharmacological intervention.

The three main prongs of an ACT-based training program are:

- Targeted source readings
- Didactic instruction, practice simulations via roleplaying
- Practice-based core competency development

Core competencies are the specific behavioral skills a psychiatrist must acquire to deliver high-quality ACT assessment, case analysis, and treatment.

Core competencies can both be taught and evaluated at the "domain" level or at the level of specific clinical "microskills."

The core competencies approach requires the trainer/supervisor to focus on residents' specific, observable, ACT-consistent (or ACT-inconsistent) behaviors.

The best educational method for teaching ACT is direct observation of resident behaviors in psychiatric practice, such as

- Sitting in on live therapy sessions with residents
- Observing live therapy sessions through a one-way mirror
- Reviewing video recordings of sessions with residents

Bridging the Gap: Training Unit and Program-Level Staff in ACT

Within most inpatient, partial hospital, or crisis respite settings, training affiliated psychiatric providers and staff to work within a psychotherapeutic model is important because the treatment milieu influences the impact of psychotherapeutic interventions delivered by members of the clinical care team, such as psychiatrists, psychologists, and social workers. Tyrberg et al. (2017) noted the outcomes of an inpatient ACT intervention for psychosis might have been better if it had been supported by changes within the broader unit context that would have led to more

ACT-consistent responses by the unit staff. They stressed the importance of bridging the gap between ACT delivered by trained therapists and the daily clinical interactions between unit nurses and patients. Members of the unit staff, unlike psychiatrists and psychologists, are in constant contact with patients. Their often reflexive tendency to request increases in medication dosages or to implement more custodial measures when confronted with a patient experiencing heightened emotional distress can easily undermine the acceptance-based interventions that are the hallmark of ACT. Indeed, staff–patient interactions can easily reinforce a patient's avoidance tendencies.

For example, the following interview with a patient named Gloria was conducted by an attending psychiatrist who was accompanied by a medical assistant. Gloria was taking high doses of both a sedative atypical antipsychotic and a fast-acting benzodiazepine to help her deal with her anxiety attacks and control her impulsive avoidance behaviors, such as compulsive shopping, self-mutilation, and bingeing and purging. She had been diagnosed with both bipolar disorder and borderline personality disorder in early adolescence. Despite continuing to take these high doses of medicines, her condition has deteriorated over the past 2 years. At present, she is very attached to the idea that she needs medication to help her function at all, despite little objective evidence that this is the case. One of the aims of the current hospital stay is to use the ACT approach to enable her to relate differently to distressing internal experiences and to help her adopt more workable strategies for coping with her anxiety and impulsive, self-defeating behaviors. This segment of the interview focuses on the function of medication for her and how it is working.

> Gloria: I really want to go back on my medication. I know I can't manage without it; every time I decrease it or try to stop, I become more anxious, and things just spiral out of control.
>
> Psychiatrist: The main concern I have is how you're functioning when you're on the medication. Your experience, at least what you've told us so far, is that when you take your medication, you spend most of the time in bed, you withdraw from relating to your husband, and you feel overwhelmed when you have to take care of your kids.
>
> Gloria: Yeah, that's true. I have lots of anxiety even when I take the pills, but it will be even worse if I don't take the medicine.
>
> Psychiatrist: You've been taking these medications for some time, yet you're still struggling with anxiety, and you still seem to fall into using coping behaviors that don't seem to work very well in the long run. Medication isn't just about helping you feel less anxious; it's also about allowing you to do the things that lead to feeling a sense of satisfaction with your life. A medication that sedates you to the point where you spend all day in bed, even if it helps with anxiety to some extent, is not good for you in the long run. Would

you be willing to let us teach you some new ways to deal with anxiety and the urges you find so difficult to resist?

Medical assistant: You and I have talked about this on the unit. Your anxiety and bipolar behaviors are probably the result of your biology, of a chemical problem the medicine helps correct. You'll probably have these symptoms at some level for the rest of your life, and you'll have to take some kind of medicine to control those symptoms. We're just trying to find the right medicine for you.

Psychiatrist: Your husband says you have periods when you feel better and start to function around the house. Then, he says, you cut back on your medication. Do you notice any differences between those periods when you're able to cope with your anxiety and when your anxiety runs away with you? What do you do when you notice the anxiety is creeping up again? Does anything work besides taking medicine?

Gloria: Yes, I notice the difference when I cut back. I feel much more alert, energetic, and I actually begin to feel some hope that I could be a mother and a good partner for my husband. But I'm so afraid it won't last. Then I get very anxious that I'll get overwhelmed with anxiety again, and I can't calm myself down unless I take several Xanax.

Medical assistant: Another thing we've talked about is to keep taking your medications, even if you're feeling better, because your symptoms are bound to return if you stop using the medication. It sounds like when you stop taking your medicines, things fall apart really fast. That's why you should keep taking them.

This clinical dialogue illustrates how the responses of the medical assistant are inconsistent with the ACT approach and could easily undermine the overall management strategy the psychiatrist is trying to develop for this patient. Gloria might require medication assistance, but it is a question of for what purpose the medication is used and whether it improves her functional status. Most importantly, nothing the medical assistant is saying to Gloria is glaringly unusual. These kinds of messages get delivered repeatedly by various staff during a typical day on the unit and reflect a socially sanctioned view that the real goal of treatment is to get rid of the patient's distressing emotional and cognitive experiences. Without some type of progressive training in the principles of ACT, the patient very likely will hear apparently contradictory types of advice about what the goal of treatment is and what she must do to achieve that goal. The real problem to solve is how to convert the unit staff to an ACT-consistent framework for the daily management of the patient.

The challenges of training inpatient staff in a new psychotherapeutic model are eloquently summarized by Rosebert and Hall (2009), and this will resonate with any psychiatrist who has been involved in such work. A long, long list of potential obstacles must be addressed and solved:

countering staff resistances to functioning in a therapeutic role, counter-acting hospital administrators' narrow concept of the role of floor staff, dealing with unpredictable changes in staffing patterns and the overuse of temporary workers, balancing competing clinical and administrative requirements on staff, preventing staff from falling into a pattern of put-ting out "brush fires" and simply trying to guarantee patient safety, and bolstering what often amounts to weak management support.

Interestingly, Bower and Gilbody (2005) reported that treating the emotional needs of the patients was not among the tasks considered im-portant by the majority of the floor staff on an inpatient psychiatric unit. The therapeutic role of unit staff of all disciplinary backgrounds, and its importance in helping patients decrease alarming behaviors, is unrecog-nized and undervalued and therefore not formally included and pro-tected within unit work assignments. Hinshelwood and Skogstad (2000) speculated that unit staff unconsciously set up defense mechanisms to protect themselves from experiencing patients' anxiety and distress. Asking unit staff to engage in empathic, validating interactions with distressed patients threatens these defenses. Some may not consider it their role to have therapeutic interactions with patients and see this as just another unrealistic work requirement. Often, this point of view is reinforced by the attitudes and behaviors of hospital administrators, who may not regard psychotherapeutic interventions by unit staff as "real" interventions.

Staffing patterns and rapid, unpredictable changes in staff work as-signments are another common source of loss of program fidelity. Full-time employees often work irregular shifts with long hours and have several days off between shifts. This directly interferes with the unit's ability to ensure continuity in patient care. Unit staff also have to deal with crises on the unit and the unplanned admission of new patients, which can create rapid and unpredictable changes in who is actually able to function in a therapeutic capacity. In some contexts, staff may be wrenched from their therapeutic activities to fill staffing gaps in more understaffed medical and surgical wards or in other facility-based pro-grams. This can reinforce the idea that unit staff are just pawns on a chess board that can be sacrificed at the whim of the hospital administrator. Moving staff in this way undermines their efforts to ensure a consistent therapeutic approach is followed by all staff members on the unit.

In light of these challenges, one might be tempted to pose the ques-tion, "Why bother?" First of all, current best practices for inpatient psy-chiatric care recommend that therapeutic work, even if continued on an outpatient basis, be initiated immediately upon inpatient admission. Both patients and psychiatric professionals have demanded that more psychotherapeutic interventions be implemented during even brief in-patient stays (Mullen 2009; Walsh and Boyle 2009). An additional argu-ment is that the unit context is an ideal setting to begin treatments such as ACT that are based on a recovery model (Jacob 2015). The unit milieu is a highly controlled environment in which it is possible for an intense dose of psychological intervention to be delivered within a very short time period. Training unit or program staff is also a rewarding experience that serves the values of transmitting knowledge and increasing the quality of inpatient care. Finally, ACT interventions have been shown to have beneficial effects on staff well-being, perceived stress, and risk of professional burnout (Frögéli et al. 2016; Noone and Hastings 2009).

Based upon direct (and sometimes painful) experiences with training unit staff in the ACT approach, we describe some lessons we have learned that may help readers interested in developing an ACT-based inpatient, partial hospital, or crisis respite program. Many of our recommendations are consistent with the results of research studies of staff training, which are nicely summarized by Rosebert and Hall (2009).

FOCUS ON BUILDING ACTIVE LISTENING SKILLS

One of the most basic clinical skills we can teach unit staff is how to listen to, rather than judge, a patient. Unit staff often underestimate the value of actively listening and of encouraging the patient to express himself and observe and track his own experience. The urge or obligation to find a solution to the patient's problem often generates anxiety, may encourage avoidance of interacting with an obviously distressed patient, or may trigger excessive self-focused attention rather than a sincere desire to listen. The ability to listen, reflect, empathize, and validate is an important skill to develop in nursing staff.

FOCUS ON CLINICALLY RELEVANT SKILLS

The skills in which staff are trained must be seen as clinically relevant as well as specific, simple, and feasible to use within the established parameters of the unit or program. Most unit staff typically perform many duties at once and may be responsible for many patients. Thus, the time allowable for any one activity is likely to be limited. Even considering these very real constraints, unit- or program-level staff can be trained to deliver short, grounding mindfulness exercises such as those used in groups for psychosis (Johns et al. 2016). Within an ACT treatment milieu, staff members can be taught to use focused questions to help patients identify and name their emotions. They can learn to ask questions such as, "What do you do when the voices show up? Does that seem to help, or does it make it worse?" These simple, focused questions can help the patient see how she is relating to the symptom and may help foster a quick discussion about the possibility of trying a new strategy, such as acceptance. In the Tyrberg et al. (2017) study, unit staff rated the ACT workability questions as being particularly helpful in clarifying the issues with which patients were struggling.

ENCOURAGE SELF-DIRECTED LEARNING

Staff members interested in the ACT approach should be encouraged to seek out additional training opportunities, such as off-site conferences and workshops. In the ideal case, institutional support for such continuing education activities would be available for both covering the costs of training and allowing staff members to take education leave days. At a personal level, books can be purchased and made available to interested staff. Encouraging members of the clinical care team to find low-cost or free education and training resources, often internet based, can help build a higher level of basic staff knowledge about ACT.

DELIVER ONGOING TRAINING AND REINFORCEMENT

Staff training can be instigated at both a formal and informal level. At a formal level, 1- or 2-day on-site ACT workshops can be organized. In most institutions, such workshops are only likely to occur once per year, and what is learned may be discarded by staff soon after the training ends. Unfortunately, unit staff tend not to apply newly learned skills when they return to their unit after attending off-site trainings unless these new approaches become part of the culture and social norms of the unit. Contributing factors include a lack of confidence in themselves and a lack of interest in taking on the challenge of getting other staff members to apply newly learned concepts or skills. Sadly, one study showed that some staff see training workshops more as an opportunity to escape the unit for a day than as an opportunity to learn something new and exciting that would enhance their job performance and satisfaction (Tyrberg et al. 2017).

The drawbacks of single-dose staff trainings can be offset by adopting a strategy of delivering ongoing, more informal "mini-training" sessions that are integrated within existing unit routines. For example, the attending psychiatrist might use unit-level meetings to stimulate a case-based discussion of a recent patient issue that can be used demonstrate the use of ACT principles (Luoma and Vilardaga 2013). Remember that inpatient staff are a heterogeneous group with different educational backgrounds, professional skills, and differing levels of motivation. Furthermore, each unit staff is different in composition, "personality," and general receptivity to additional clinical training.

INVOLVE THE WHOLE STAFF

Another crucial consideration is the involvement of all members of a clinical care team and on-the-ground administrative staff in any transition to an ACT program, even though it is tempting to focus on the most enthusiastic and motivated staff. Concentrating too much positive attention on the early adopters may trigger resentment on the part of less motivated staff members and create a negative dynamic within the unit staff that, in effect, creates another barrier to implementation. Ironically, the more motivated staff members are also those most likely to leave the unit for other jobs because they are more likely to be seeking to further their careers. The lack of motivation in "nonadopters" may mask an underlying lack of self-confidence or fear of failure that can only be overcome by participating in ACT training. Recalcitrant staff should be included in all meetings and discussions about the design of the ACT program. Emphasize and reemphasize that the entire ACT transition is being done to improve patient care and to increase professional satisfaction among all members of the unit staff.

USE EXPERIENTIAL TRAINING METHODS

Experiential training can be done at a formal level through regular staff development and training sessions. One of the best ways to convert staff to an ACT state of mind is by helping them experience ACT concepts directly. One effective way of doing this is using experiential metaphors such as the "passengers on the bus" to help them relate differently to a patient who is "pushing their buttons." One staff member might play the difficult patient and, after discussing what might be pushing the patient to be difficult, other staff members play the patient's "passengers" (i.e., intrusive thoughts, impulses, emotional experiences, memories, distressing physical symptoms). The experiential nature of this exercise is an excellent way to increase staff understanding of the basic ACT model. These experiential exercises create a golden opportunity for staff to recognize that everyone has their own bus and passengers. The conversation often will shift to staff members talking about the passengers they tend to struggle with while doing their jobs. These interactions tend to produce a more compassionate, accepting, empathic attitude toward the experiences of patients on the unit. Through such sessions, staff can be encouraged to run stand-alone groups based on core ACT metaphors, particularly physical metaphors that are well suited for brief-group work, such as the "life path" (Strosahl et al. 2012). Encouraging staff members to run values-based groups is a good way to maintain an ACT focus, because the positive, encouraging emotional tone of such discussions generally makes it easier to talk about values with patients. Finally, allowing unit staff to participate as co-leaders in groups allows them to practice their ACT skills with the support of the psychiatrist, psychologist, or another professional member of the clinical care team.

MAKE ON-DEMAND SUPERVISION IMMEDIATELY ACCESSIBLE

Supervision often involves cultivating awareness among unit staff of their own thoughts and feelings in relation to both patient care and interactions with other staff members. Part of the attending psychiatrist's commitment is to be amenable to working with staff to help them increase their willingness to accept their own distress, acknowledge their fear of making mistakes, and allow patients to be in a state of emotional distress without feeling compelled to "fix it." Many of these moments of growth come up spontaneously during the workday, and thus the need to intervene with supervision is also immediate. The psychiatrist, or some qualified member of the clinical care team, should be available to provide curbside supervision to any affected unit staff member. Effective supervision involves helping affected staff learn to take perspective on their distressing personal experiences as well as their ongoing relationship to those experiences. Often, the combination of professional and personal life demands triggers high levels of distress. Thus, effective supervision often also increases the staff member's confidence in the ACT approach because it has worked in his personal life.

ENGAGE HOSPITAL- OR FACILITY-LEVEL MANAGEMENT

Enlisting the support of high-level administrators for implementation of an ACT-based program is an absolute must. Lack of management commitment seriously undermines training attempts and implies a lack of recognition of the staff's therapeutic activities. The psychotherapeutic work done by unit or program staff must be recognized as therapeutically beneficial and worth the time and effort involved. Ideally, administrators and program managers will agree to be present during staff training as a show of support for the important role staff play in making the ACT program work.

BE PATIENT AND PERSISTENT

Finally, converting a traditionally organized inpatient, day hospital, or crisis respite program into an ACT-based program is best thought of as an ongoing developmental process. Progress is not likely to be linear but rather a series of starts and stops. This requires the psychiatrist to keep her "eyes on the prize" and not get discouraged when the plan is going in the wrong direction. We must, and can, deal with different degrees of staff motivation, the hesitation of some staff members to adopt anything new, and the dampening effect of the sometimes overwhelming job demands made on the psychiatrist. Again, being able to take perspective on the unsteady process of organizational change allows the psychiatrist to be patient and accepting of the sometimes slow rate of change while at the same time persistently moving the unit or program in the desired direction. Perspective-taking prevents the psychiatrist from getting fused with her own thoughts and feelings and helps her concentrate more on the values-based plan for improving care on the inpatient unit and creating better long-term outcomes for patients.

TIPS FOR SUCCESS

Some powerful reasons for considering adopting ACT as a treatment framework at the unit- or facility-based program level include

- Such an approach leads to better clinical outcomes for patients.
- Outcomes are even better when all participating staff receive training and adhere to the treatment model.
- Training in ACT tends to result in higher levels of job satisfaction and reduced rates of professional burnout.

Common barriers to converting unit- or program-level staff to the ACT approach include

- Lack of recognition of the important role unit or program line staff play in promoting positive clinical outcomes
- Lack of administrative or management level support for activities that may not readily be reimbursable
- Unpredictable and chaotic staffing patterns and unexpected changes in staffing
- Resistance to adopting a more therapeutic role by unit- or program-level staff

Key steps to increasing the likely positive impact of staff training in ACT include

- Ensuring the new skills being taught are concrete, specific, and viewed as clinically relevant
- Offering various ongoing training experiences using different educational methods (e.g., didactic workshops, case discussions during staff meetings, on-demand supervision when staff are unsure how to implement ACT with a particular patient issue, experiential exercises that help staff connect ACT concepts

to their personal lives, and encouraging additional off-site training in ACT for interested staff)

Use the positive energy of early adopters while keeping skeptics and nay-sayers involved in the developmental process.

Be positive, patient, and persistent!

Summary

In this chapter, we examined several issues that are often addressed only well after a treatment such as ACT has gained notoriety as a potentially powerful adjunct to existing treatments or as a stand-alone treatment model in its own right: How do we train new students (residents) to be competent in delivering ACT as a result of their graduate-level education? How do we teach these new skills to psychiatric and mental health professionals who are already in the midst of their careers? In institutional and programmatic settings, which are normally staffed with a broad array of disciplines and different education levels, what is the best way to migrate a treatment model such as ACT into the existing treatment milieu? These questions do not have simple answers, because education and training paradigms, as well as institutional and programmatic practices, have their own "life." They do not typically change overnight of their own accord. It takes someone with vision, persistence, and a steady hand to stimulate change and keep it moving in the right direction despite it being an unsteady, and at times frustrating, process. We hope that the principles for instigating change, as well as the specific strategies for training and education discussed in this chapter, will give you a good start!

The Essentials

- The ACT model is a fairly broad theoretical framework that can significantly enhance the psychotherapeutic skill set imparted during medical school, general psychiatry residency, and fellowship training.
- Psychiatry residency training in ACT should involve a combination of three different educational methods:
  - Targeted source readings
  - Didactic training grounded in skill building
  - Core competencies training based in direct observational assessment

- Core competencies are select clinical skills that collectively contribute to a psychiatrist being a competent ACT clinician.
- Training in ACT clinical skills is best seen as a developmental process in which complex clinical activities are superimposed upon basic clinical activities.
- Teaching ACT to affiliated mental health professionals in agency and institutional settings requires active buy-in from administrative and medical leadership as well as patience and persistence from champions of the ACT approach.

References

Bower P, Gilbody S: Stepped care in psychological therapies: access, effectiveness and efficiency. Narrative literature review. Br J Psychiatry 186:11–17, 2005 15630118

Frögéli E, Djordjevic A, Rudman A, et al: A randomized controlled pilot trial of acceptance and commitment training (ACT) for preventing stress-related ill health among future nurses. Anxiety Stress Coping 29(2):202–218, 2016 25759942

Hayes S, Strosahl K, Wilson K: Acceptance and Commitment Therapy: The Process and Practice of Mindful Change. New York, Guilford, 2011

Hinshelwood RD, Skogstad W: The dynamics of healthcare institutions, in Observing Organisations: Anxiety, Defence and Culture in Health Care. Edited by Hinshelwood RD, Skogstad W. Hove, UK, Brunner Routledge, 2000

Jacob KS: Recovery model of mental illness: a complementary approach to psychiatric care. Indian J Psychol Med 37(2):117–119, 2015 25969592

Johns LC, Oliver JE, Khondoker M, et al: The feasibility and acceptability of a brief acceptance and commitment therapy (ACT) group intervention for people with psychosis: The 'ACT for Life' study. J Behav Ther Exp Psychiatry 50:257–263, 2016 26480469

Luoma JB, Vilardaga JP: Improving therapist psychological flexibility while training acceptance and commitment therapy: a pilot study. Cogn Behav Ther 42(1):1–8, 2013 23505991

Luoma JB, Hayes S, Walser R: Learning ACT: An Acceptance and Commitment Therapy Skills Training Manual for Therapists, 2nd Edition. Oakland, CA, New Harbinger, 2017

Mullen A: Mental health nurses establishing psychosocial interventions within acute inpatient settings. Int J Ment Health Nurs 18(2):83–90, 2009 19290971

Noone SJ, Hastings RP: Building psychological resilience in support staff caring for people with intellectual disabilities: pilot evaluation of an acceptance-based intervention. J Intellect Disabil 13(1):43–53, 2009 19332508

Rosebert C, Hall C: Training acute ward in-patient staff to use CBT techniques, in Cognitive Behavioural Therapy for Acute In-patient Mental Health Units: Working With Clients, Staff and the Milieu. Edited by Clarke I, Wilson H. New York, Routledge, 2009, pp 143–158

Strosahl K, Robinson P, Gustavsson T: Brief Interventions for Radical Change: Principles and Practice of Focused Acceptance and Commitment Therapy. Oakland, CA, New Harbinger, 2012

Törneke N: Learning RFT: An Introduction to Relational Frame Theory and Its Clinical Application. Oakland, CA, New Harbinger, 2010

Tyrberg MJ, Carlbring P, Lundgren T: Implementation of acceptance and commitment therapy training in a psychiatric ward: feasibility, lessons learned and potential effectiveness. Journal of Psychiatric Intensive Care 13(2):73–82, 2017

Walsh J, Boyle J: Improving acute psychiatric hospital services according to inpatient experiences. A user-led piece of research as a means to empowerment. Issues Ment Health Nurs 30(1):31–38, 2009 19148819

Index

Page numbers printed in **boldface** type refer to tables or figures.